Dieting For Dummies®

Where Calories Come From

Protein, carbohydrate, and fat make up the calorie contents of various foods. Although not considered a nutrient, alcohol also provides calories.

- ✔ 1 gram of **protein** contains 4 calories.
- ✔ 1 gram of **carbohydrate** contains 4 calories.
- ✔ 1 gram of **fat** contains 9 calories.
- ✔ 1 gram of **alcohol** contains 7 calories.

The remaining nutrients — water, minerals, and vitamins — do not provide calories, nor does fiber or cholesterol.

The Health Risks of Being Overweight

If you're having trouble staying motivated to eat healthfully and exercise, remember that being overweight increases your risk for developing one or more of these health problems:

- ✔ Diabetes
- ✔ Gallbladder disease
- ✔ Heart disease
- ✔ Hypertension (high blood pressure)
- ✔ Respiratory problems
- ✔ Some forms of cancer

Ten Rules for Healthy Living

There's more to good living than just counting calories. Remember these ten easy guidelines (and see Chapter 23 for more information):

- ✔ Eat a minimum of 3 servings of vegetables and 2 servings of fruit each day.
- ✔ Eat at least 3 servings of whole grains each day.
- ✔ Eat at least 4 servings of beans, lentils, or peas each week.
- ✔ Eat 3 meals and 2 to 3 small snacks a day.
- ✔ Eat breakfast.
- ✔ Limit soft drinks.
- ✔ Drink plenty of water.
- ✔ Limit caffeine to two servings or less a day.
- ✔ Limit salty foods.
- ✔ Limit the amount of saturated fat you eat.

...For Dummies: Bestselling Book Series for Beginners

FOR DUMMIES™
BESTSELLING BOOK SERIES FROM IDG

Dieting For Dummies®

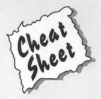

Cheat Sheet

Finding Your Healthy Weight Range

To quickly estimate your healthy weight range, first figure the weight for your height by using the appropriate formula:

Men: 106 pounds for 5 feet, plus 6 pounds per inch over 5 feet or minus 6 pounds per inch under 5 feet

Women: 100 pounds for 5 feet, plus 5 pounds per inch over 5 feet or minus 5 pounds per inch under 5 feet

You then calculate your range by subtracting and adding 10 percent of that weight. (See also Chapter 2 for the 1995 Dietary Guidelines for Americans weight chart.)

Knowing How Many Calories You Need to Burn to Lose Weight

Because there are 3,500 calories in a pound and 7 days in a week, you must cut your daily calorie intake by 500 to lose 1 pound a week (3,500 ÷ 7 = 500). To lose 1½ pounds, you need to cut 750 calories a day. A 2-pounds-a-week loss means eliminating 1,000 calories a day. A faster rate of weight loss is generally associated with weight regain and yo-yo dieting.

Eating less is one way to cut calories, but if you add exercise, you don't have to restrict your intake so severely to lose the weight you want to lose. And by adding muscle through strength-building exercises, you'll burn additional calories even when you're not exercising.

Calculating Your BMR

Your BMR, or basal metabolic rate, is what most people are referring to when they talk about metabolism. It is the number of calories that your body needs for basic involuntary body processes, like keeping your heart beating. A quick and easy way to approximate the number of calories your body needs for basal metabolism is to multiply your current weight in pounds by 10 if you're a woman or by 11 if you're a man. Additional calories are needed for digestion and activity. (See Chapter 4.)

...For Dummies: Bestselling Book Series for Beginners

Praise For Dieting For Dummies

"Jane Kirby knows her stuff. *Dieting For Dummies* is chockfull of solid facts about nutrition and weight. It tells you what your choices of foods and types of exercise can and can't do for weight control. The book fearlessly addresses fad supplements and diets and gives you the straight scoop."

— Shirley O. Corriher, Author of *CookWise*

"What a marvelous book for making changes in food habits. *Dieting For Dummies* demonstrates with simple facts why healthful and enjoyable eating go together. If you've looked all your life for the answer to losing weight and keeping it off, this book provides that answer with . . . practical tips and facts."

— Connie Diekman, M.Ed., R.D., FADA, ADA Spokesperson

"Jane Kirby has written a book that is as much for the brilliant as for Dummies. She provides good, solid advice as well as helpful hints in an easily understood form. Congratulations."

— Barbara Kafka, Author of *Soup: A Way of Life*

"Never has losing looked so good! Jane Kirby makes creating a healthy life — with great food, fun exercise, and a healthy attitude — within anyone's grasp."

— Robin Kline, R.D., President of the International Association of Culinary Professionals

"Despite the title of the book, going to Jane Kirby for your diet advice is the smartest thing you could do. As a registered dietitian and the former food editor of a fashion magazine, Jane has devoted her life to providing the kind of clear, reasonable information that will keep you healthy as well as slim."

— Joanne Lamb Hayes, Ph.D., Cookbook Author, Food Editor

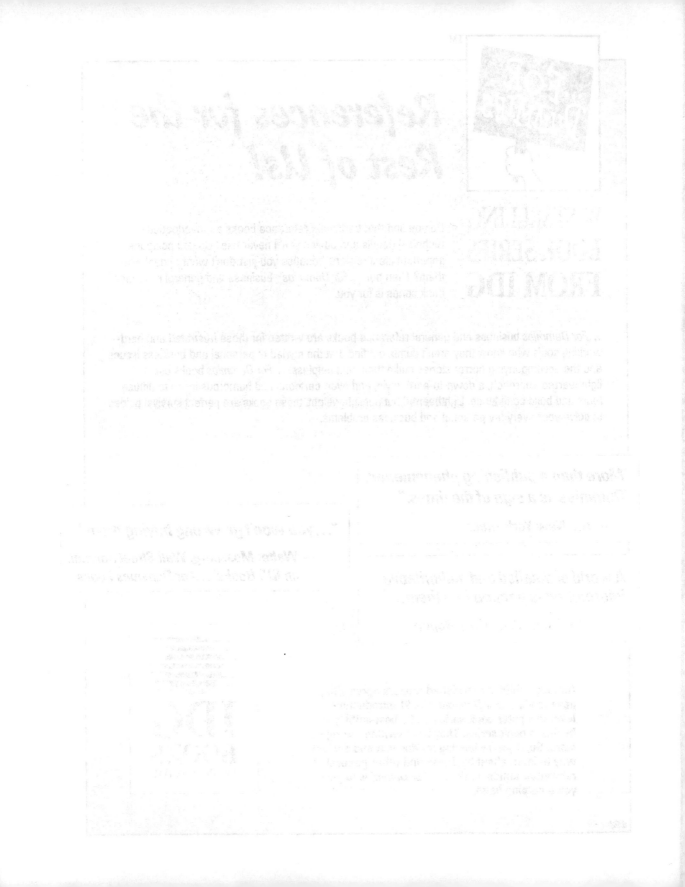

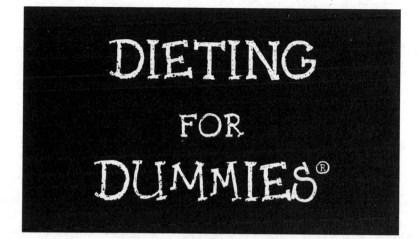

DIETING FOR DUMMIES®

by Jane Kirby, R.D., for the American Dietetic Association

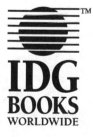

IDG Books Worldwide, Inc.
An International Data Group Company

Foster City, CA ♦ Chicago, IL ♦ Indianapolis, IN ♦ New York, NY

Dieting For Dummies®

Published by
IDG Books Worldwide, Inc.
An International Data Group Company
919 E. Hillsdale Blvd.
Suite 400
Foster City, CA 94404
www.idgbooks.com (IDG Books Worldwide Web site)
www.dummies.com (Dummies Press Web site)

Library of Congress Catalog Card No.: 98-88809

ISBN: 0-7645-5126-4

Printed in the United States of America

10 9 8 7 6 5 4 3 2 1

1B/RX/RR/ZY/IN

Distributed in the United States by IDG Books Worldwide, Inc.

Distributed by Macmillan Canada for Canada; by Transworld Publishers Limited in the United Kingdom; by IDG Norge Books for Norway; by IDG Sweden Books for Sweden; by Woodslane Pty. Ltd. for Australia; by Woodslane (NZ) Ltd. for New Zealand; by Addison Wesley Longman Singapore Pte Ltd. for Singapore, Malaysia, Thailand, and Indonesia; by Norma Comunicaciones S.A. for Colombia; by Intersoft for South Africa; by International Thomson Publishing for Germany, Austria and Switzerland; by Distribuidora Cuspide for Argentina; by Livraria Cultura for Brazil; by Ediciencia S.A. for Ecuador; by Ediciones ZETA S.C.R. Ltda. for Peru; by WS Computer Publishing Corporation, Inc., for the Philippines; by Contemporanea de Ediciones for Venezuela; by Express Computer Distributors for the Caribbean and West Indies; by Micronesia Media Distributor, Inc. for Micronesia; by Grupo Editorial Norma S.A. for Guatemala; by Chips Computadoras S.A. de C.V. for Mexico; by Editorial Norma de Panama S.A. for Panama; by Wouters Import for Belgium; by American Bookshops for Finland. Authorized Sales Agent: Anthony Rudkin Associates for the Middle East and North Africa.

For general information on IDG Books Worldwide's books in the U.S., please call our Consumer Customer Service department at 800-762-2974. For reseller information, including discounts and premium sales, please call our Reseller Customer Service department at 800-434-3422.

For information on where to purchase IDG Books Worldwide's books outside the U.S., please contact our International Sales department at 317-596-5530 or fax 317-596-5692.

For information on foreign language translations, please contact our Foreign & Subsidiary Rights department at 650-655-3021 or fax 650-655-3281.

For sales inquiries and special prices for bulk quantities, please contact our Sales department at 650-655-3200 or write to the address above.

For information on using IDG Books Worldwide's books in the classroom or for ordering examination copies, please contact our Educational Sales department at 800-434-2086 or fax 317-596-5499.

For press review copies, author interviews, or other publicity information, please contact our Public Relations department at 650-655-3000 or fax 650-655-3299.

For authorization to photocopy items for corporate, personal, or educational use, please contact Copyright Clearance Center, 222 Rosewood Drive, Danvers, MA 01923, or fax 978-750-4470.

is a trademark under exclusive license to IDG Books Worldwide, Inc., from International Data Group, Inc.

About the Authors

The American Dietetic Association is the largest group of food and health professionals in the world. As the advocate of the profession, the ADA serves the public by promoting optimal nutrition, health, and well-being.

For expert answers to your nutrition questions, call the ADA/National Center for Nutrition and Dietetics Hot Line at 900-225-5267. To listen to a recorded message or to obtain a referral to a registered dietitian (R.D.) in your area, call 800-366-1655. Visit the ADA's Web site at www.eatright.org.

Jane Kirby, a registered dietitian and a member of the American Dietetic Association, is editor and president of Kirby-O'Brien and Company, a nutrition and food communications firm in Charlotte, Vermont. She is the former editor of *Eating Well* magazine and the food and nutrition editor for *Glamour*. She served on the dietetics staff of the Massachusetts General Hospital in Boston, where she completed graduate work in nutrition. She holds a B.S. degree from Marymount College.

Jane has written nutrition and food articles for *American Health, Family Circle, Fitness, Food Arts, Glamour, Good Housekeeping, Harrowsmith Country Life, InStyle, Ladies Home Journal, McCalls, Woman's Day,* and *Working Mother* magazines and has been published in *The Journal of the American Dietetic Association* and *Nutrition Today.* She is also the author of *The 50 Best Salsas and Dips* (Broadway Books, 1998) and *Glamour's Guide to 30 Minute Meals and Effortless Entertaining* (Villard, 1987). She received the American Dietetic Associations's 1994 Media Excellence Award.

Introduction

• •

Does the world really need another book on dieting? More important, do you? Plenty of diet books out there make promises that this one doesn't. Lots tell you that losing weight and keeping it off is easy and effortless once you know their secrets. Well, we have a secret to tell you that the other books won't: Dieting gimmicks, such as eating only grapefruit or banning pasta, don't work. And that's precisely why you need this book. It's not about fad plans or take-it-off-quick schemes. It's about learning to balance healthful eating and exercise for a lifetime.

Here's another "secret" that the other books don't tell you but this one does: When you know the facts about how the exercise you do and the foods you eat regulate your weight, you can drop pounds and keep them off without ever eating another grapefruit — unless you like grapefruit, of course. We believe that knowledge is power: the power to *choose* to lose. That's what this book is all about.

You Can Trust Us

We know about losing weight. Here's what we bring to the table:

The American Dietetic Association is the largest organization of food and nutrition professionals in the world, with nearly 70,000 members. In other words, you can look to us for the most scientifically sound food and nutrition information available.

We realize that you're bombarded with confusing and often contradictory messages about food, nutrition, and dieting, in particular. You may be left confused and unable to translate the nutrition information you hear or read about into your everyday food choices.

Our members, with their extensive educational background, apply their knowledge of food, nutrition, culinary arts, physiology, biochemistry, anatomy, and psychology to help you translate nutrition recommendations into practical, clear, and straightforward advice.

This part also helps you determine why you eat the way you do. Personal preferences, emotions, hormones, and culture all influence your eating style. Once you understand what turns on your appetite, you're better prepared to get over overeating.

Also in this part, you can find advice for feeding an overweight child, as well as spotting and seeking help for an eating disorder.

Part III: A Plan for Healthful Living

Getting to and staying at a reasonable weight without sacrificing the enjoyment of great-tasting foods is what this section is all about. Healthful living is putting all the food and nutrition advice you read and hear into practice. You can find scientifically sound nutrition and weight-loss recommendations translated into practical and useful advice. You can also find how important exercise is to losing weight and creating a healthy environment for your new body.

Part IV: Shopping, Cooking, and Dining Out

Here's where the information about navigating the grocery store is located. Part IV also has affordable suggestions for stocking and outfitting your kitchen to make eating low-calorie easier. And when you're planning a meal out, read the recommendations given in this part before you go.

Part V: Enlisting Outside Help

When you can't go it alone, Part V has help for finding and working with health care professionals you can trust. Medications are a part of weight-loss treatment today, and because you need to be well informed before you take a weight-loss aid — be it prescription, an herbal remedy, or a standard over-the-counter issue — you need to read the information in this section. And because there's a sucker born every minute and a quack born every 30 seconds, you'd be smart to read the comprehensive section on weight-loss fads and scams before you get snookered.

Part VI: The Part of Tens

As do all the *...For Dummies* books, this one has a Part of Tens, too. Here, you can find lists of dieting myths, easy ways to cut calories, and tips for healthy living. Plus, we include more than ten of the world's best low-calorie recipes.

Appendixes

Appendix A is loaded with books, Web sites, and organizations that can help you in your search for more information about weight loss. All of them offer credible, useful, and trustworthy information. And if you like numbers and charts, look at the list of the nutrient values of many common foods that resides in Appendix B.

Icons Used in This Book

We've included icons in the margins of this book to help you find the information you're looking for more quickly. Here's a list of the icons and what they mean:

This icon points to a tip that can make the dieting process easier.

When you see this icon, you know that you're getting an important piece of information that's worth remembering.

This icon warns you of dieting myths and dangers. Be wary!

Because the dieting industry perpetuates many falsehoods, we've included this icon to point out information that you can count on — and some fun facts, too.

When we get a little technical and talk about scientific research, we use this icon. You can skip this stuff if it seems too far over your head, but it's good to know.

This icon demystifies the lingo that you so often hear when dieting is discussed. Learn what these terms mean and you'll sound like a pro in no time.

Where to Go from Here

People come in a wide range of heights, weights, and girths. One is not better than another. But staying within *your* healthiest weight range can help you achieve optimal health and well-being. Join us in this book, starting at whatever point you like, and you'll see through the fog of fads and myths. Read on and find out how to stop dieting and start living healthfully.

Part I
A Healthy Weight

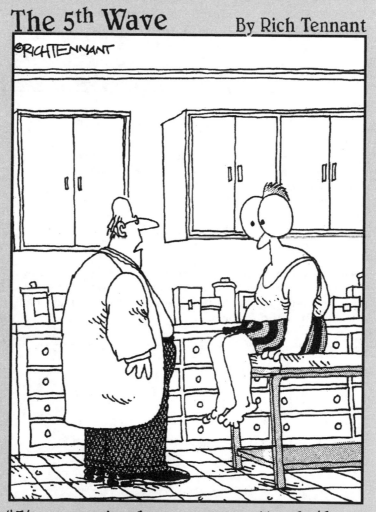

The 5th Wave

By Rich Tennant

"I'm surprised no one's noticed this before, but your weight gain appears to be a result of your eyes simply being bigger than your stomach."

In this part . . .

Before you even think about cutting calories, you need to understand how your weight affects your health. If you keep in mind that the point of losing weight is to make yourself feel better and improve your quality of life, then it's much easier to stay motivated. This part helps you see the weight-health connection and use it as a basis for your diet.

This part also helps you determine what weight will bring you optimal health. You may be surprised to find out that you can enjoy terrific health at a weight that's higher than what you consider "ideal."

Chapter 1

Exploring the Connection between Weight and Health

*I*f you've been trying to lose weight for much of your adult life, you're not alone. Excess weight is the number-one nutrition problem. The statistics are alarming: Of the ten leading causes of death in the United States, being overweight is a risk factor for half; and the number of Americans who are overweight is increasing. It's estimated that 55 percent (or 97 million) American adults and 15 to 20 percent of American children are overweight today!

This chapter can help you understand why being overweight is dangerous to your health and well-being. We hope that it helps you put the desire to lose weight in the proper perspective.

The Health Risks of Being Overweight

Obesity is not just a cosmetic problem; it's a health hazard. Being overweight puts a lot of stress on your body. Your lungs, heart, and skeleton need to work harder when you carry extra pounds of body fat. Try spending a few hours carrying around a 10-pound dumbbell. It's tiring, isn't it?

You may feel okay now and not worry about health problems. But your extra weight strains all your body systems, which increases your risk for developing one or more of these health problems:

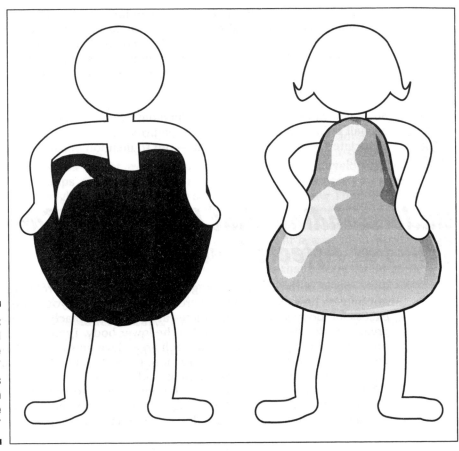

Figure 1-1:
Men tend
to be
"apples,"
whereas
women
tend to be
"pears."

For the most part, becoming an apple or a pear when you gain weight is an inherited tendency. Women are naturally predisposed to store fat in their lower bodies for use as energy during pregnancy and breast-feeding. However, your genes may play only a partial role. Smoking and drinking too many alcoholic beverages seem to increase fat accumulation in the stomach area in both men and women.

Making Health, Not Appearance, Your Weight-Management Priority

Sure, losing weight will result in a slimmer and trimmer-looking you. But your motivation for losing weight should be your health, not only your appearance. When you feel good, you'll look good, too.

You'll be pleasantly surprised at how much better you feel after you lose weight — physically as well as mentally. Walking up a flight of stairs or around the mall won't leave you breathless. Playing with your kids in the park will be a pleasure, not exhausting. You'll have more energy to do the things you want to do, and you'll have fun doing them!

As we've explained, maintaining a healthy weight is important for good health. But going on a diet and off, and on, and off, and on can be more harmful to your health than carrying a few extra pounds. This pattern, called *yo-yo dieting,* often results from trying to lose weight for appearance's sake, not health. It comes from quick weight-loss gimmicks and fad diets where you drop a few pounds and then gain them back, plus a few more. If you repeatedly lose and gain, changing your focus to maintaining a healthy weight may be the answer. Think long-term approach rather than fast results.

Long-term weight loss is a matter of attitude and conditioning. One of the reasons you bought this book is to find an answer to your weight problem. How many other diet books have you read? How many other books have you purchased? The diet book industry, which publishes nearly 40 titles annually, is built on the idea that diets are unsuccessful; otherwise, why would you need more than one book on the subject? Most diet books make promises that they can't deliver, because their concepts of dieting are based on the short-term. But successful weight losers and maintainers look at the long-term. This book encourages you to focus not on fads, but on weight-loss strategies that last.

Consider the differences in Table 1-1.

Table 1-1	Ways to Change Your Diet Attitude
Short-Term Diets	*Long-Term Life Goals*
Focus on the "don't"	Focus on the "do"
Swear off favorite foods	Concentrate on making healthier choices
Focus on denial	Focus on enjoying feeling better, healthier, and more energized
Set one answer "for life" goals	Establish flexible, short-term, attainable goals
Promise immediate results	Deliver success gradually
Allow no room for slips	Leave room for indulgences
Ban some foods	Encourage variety
Emphasize food	Emphasize healthy eating and exercise
Are extreme	Are gradual

Chapter 2
Assessing Your Own Weight

∙∙∙

In This Chapter

▶ Calculating your healthy weight range

▶ Comparing your weight to a weight chart

▶ Assessing how fat you are

▶ Determining your weight-related risk factors

∙∙∙

*W*hat exactly is a healthy weight? A healthy weight is a *range* that relates statistically to good health. Being overweight or obese is statistically related to weight-related health problems such as heart disease and hypertension.

Health care professionals use three key measurements to determine whether a person is at a healthy weight:

✔ **Body Mass Index (BMI):** A measure that correlates to how much fat is on your body

✔ **Waist size:** A measure that indicates the location of your body fat

✔ **Risk factors for developing weight-related health problems:** For example, your cholesterol level, blood pressure, and family history.

It's important to know that what *you* should weigh for optimal health may be quite different from what someone else should weigh, even if he or she is your same height, gender, and age. The information in this chapter can help you determine what weight is best for you — your *healthy weight,* not the lowest weight that you think you can reach.

Looking at the Number on Your Bathroom Scale

When you step onto your bathroom scale, the number shows you how much your total body weighs. This total includes fat, muscle, bone, and water.

Even though a healthy weight depends on more than the number on the scale, that number is a general starting point that you can use to assess your weight.

Once you know your weight, you can compare it to the healthy weight ranges of the "quick estimate" method or to the Dietary Guidelines for Americans weight chart. You can find both sets of numbers later in this section.

What if your weight falls above these ranges? For most people, that's less healthy. The further you are above the healthy weight range for your height, the greater your risk for weight-related health problems.

The "quick estimate" method

To quickly estimate your healthy weight, you can use this method. First, figure the weight for your height by using the appropriate formula:

Men   106 pounds for 5 feet, plus 6 pounds per inch over 5 feet or minus 6 pounds per inch under 5 feet

Women   100 pounds for 5 feet, plus 5 pounds per inch over 5 feet or minus 5 pounds per inch under 5 feet

You then calculate your range by subtracting and adding 10 percent. You'll be at the higher end of the range if you're a large-framed person or carry more muscle, and at the lower end of the range if you're small-framed with less muscle.

For example, if you're a 6-foot-tall man, your healthy weight range is 160 to 196 pounds:

- **Average-framed:** 106 pounds + 72 pounds (12 inches × 6 pounds per inch) = 178 pounds
- **Small-framed:** 178 pounds minus 10 percent (about 18 pounds) = 160 pounds
- **Large-framed:** 178 pounds plus 10 percent (about 18 pounds) = 196 pounds

The weight chart

For many years, the concept of an "ideal weight" was reinforced by specific height and weight tables with recommendations for two sets of desirable weights — one for ages 19 to 34 and another for ages 35 and older.

Today, we use the 1995 Dietary Guidelines for Americans weight table, which provides a generous weight range for determining a healthy weight. (See Figure 2-1.) Notice that a healthy weight is not a single spot on a graph; it's a range. However, don't view the range as a license to gain weight if you're at the lower end or in the middle. The upper limits in each category are for people who have greater amounts of muscle and bone, generally men and large-framed women.

Also, according to today's guidelines, a person's healthy weight range is the same regardless of age. Experts believe that the 10 to 15 pounds that many people put on as they age, although common, are not healthy.

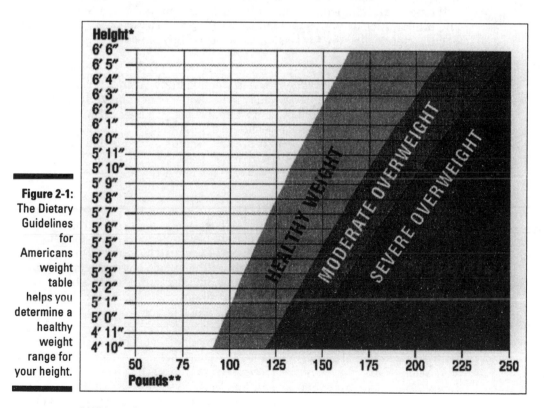

Figure 2-1: The Dietary Guidelines for Americans weight table helps you determine a healthy weight range for your height.

* Without shoes.
** Without clothes. The higher weights apply to people with more muscle and bone, such as many men.
Source: *Report of the Dietary Guidelines Advisory Committee on the Dietary Guidelines for Americans,* 1995, pages 23-24.

Figuring Out How Fat You Are

The "quick estimate" method and the ranges in the Dietary Guidelines for Americans chart (refer to Figure 2-1) can help you quickly compare your weight to the healthy weight range for your height. However, the location and amount of body fat you have are considered more important measures for determining whether you're at a healthy weight.

You have several ways to determine how much fat you have, which is often referred to as your *percent body fat.* Some methods, such as underwater weighing, are impractical but very accurate; some, such as skin-fold caliper and bioelectrical impedance measurements, are simple but often imprecise; and others, such as Body Mass Index (BMI) and waist size, are the methods of choice of health care professionals because they are considered easy and precise.

So why talk about the methods for determining body fat that are not the methods of choice? For one, you may read about them in magazine articles and books about weight loss. And most important, you may see them offered in health clubs, by commercial weight-loss programs, or even at a local university research facility. So here are the various methods and their limitations.

Underwater weighing

Underwater weighing is the most accurate method for determining your percent body fat, but it's the least practical because it's done with sophisticated equipment at university research facilities. This method is based on the premise that fat floats — think of how oil rises to the top in a bottle of salad dressing. Therefore, by submerging a body in a tub of water, you can determine how much of it is lean and how much is not.

How it's done: You sit in a large tank or tub full of water in a special chair with a weight belt around your waist. A trained technician then submerges you beneath the surface of the water as you force all the air out of your lungs. You must remain underwater for about 10 seconds so that the technician can record your weight. The technician repeats this procedure eight to ten times in order to determine an average.

The technician measures your body's volume by computing the difference between your body's weight measured in air and its weight underwater. The technician then calculates your body density by dividing your body mass by the volume of the water that it displaces, minus any air left in your lungs. After computing density, the technician uses another formula to determine your percent body fat.

Skin-fold thickness

Measuring skin-fold thickness (the amount of fat just under the skin) is a simpler method for determining percent body fat. When done by an experienced person, it is a very accurate predictor of total body fat.

However, this method can yield inaccurate results if not done by a skilled practitioner or if performed on an older person or on someone who is severely overweight. Given that the results can vary greatly depending on the practitioner, you should view the results skeptically.

How it's done: A person trained in skin-fold measuring, such as a doctor, dietitian, or health club staffer, measures your skin-fold thickness by using skin-fold calipers at the upper arm, upper back, lower back, stomach, and upper thigh. The technician takes two sets of measurements and obtains an average at each site. Then he or she converts the millimeters that the calipers measure and places those numbers in a formula to arrive at the percent body fat of your entire body.

Now you know where the expression "pinch an inch" comes from. It may not be scientifically precise, but if you can pinch a 1-inch-thick (or more) fold of skin on the back of your upper arm, you're probably overfat.

Bioelectrical impedance

Bioelectrical impedance is another relatively simple method for determining percent body fat, but it can produce inaccurate results if a person is dehydrated, overhydrated, severely overweight, or older with little muscle mass.

How it's done: A trained technician takes readings from a machine that delivers a harmless amount of electrical current through your body to estimate total body water, which reflects the amount of muscle or lean tissue you have. (Muscle contains water, and fat contains very little water.) The technician then determines the amount of body fat you have by taking the difference between your body weight and your lean tissue.

Body Mass Index

In addition to having their own limitations, underwater weighing, skin-fold thickness, and bioelectrical impedance measurements can be impractical for you as well as your health care practitioner for determining whether you're at a healthy weight.

Instead, doctors and dietitians recommend using Body Mass Index, or BMI, for determining whether you're at a healthy weight or overweight and therefore at a greater risk of developing weight-related health problems.

Assessing your weight based on your percent body fat

If you ever have the opportunity to get your specific percent body fat measured by underwater weighing, skin-fold caliper, or bioelectrical impedance, use these estimated guidelines to assess your weight.

	Percent Body Fat	
	Women	*Men*
Normal (optimal)	15 to 25 percent	10 to 20 percent
Overweight	25.1 to 29.9 percent	20.1 to 24.4 percent
Obese	Over 30 percent	Over 25 percent

BMI strongly correlates to the total fat on your body, and best of all, it's easy to determine and is applicable to all adults.

How it's done: Follow these steps to calculate your BMI:

1. **Convert your weight from pounds to kilograms.**

   Your weight (in pounds) ÷ 2.2 = your weight (in kilograms). For example, 132 pounds ÷ 2.2 kilograms = 60 kilograms.

2. **Convert your height from inches to meters.**

   Your height (in inches) ÷ 39.37 = your height (in meters). For example, 65 inches ÷ 39.37 meters = 1.65 meters.

3. **Calculate your Body Mass Index.**

   Your weight (in kilograms) ÷ [your height (in meters) × your height (in meters)] = BMI. For example, 60 kilograms ÷ (1.65 meters × 1.65 meters) = 22.03.

BMI is usually calculated in kilograms and meters, but if you feel more comfortable using pounds and feet, this formula will work for you:

$$\frac{\text{your weight (in pounds)} \times 704.5}{\text{your height (in inches)} \times \text{your height (in inches)}} = \text{your BMI}$$

Table 2-1 enables you to determine your BMI without doing any math. Here's how: Locate your height in inches in the left-hand column and follow the row across to your weight in pounds. Your BMI is at the top of the column at the intersection of your height and weight.

Table 2-1

BMI Chart

Weight in Pounds

Height in Inches	19	20	21	22	23	24	25	26	27	28	29	30	31	32	33	34	35	36	37	38	39	40
58	91	96	100	105	110	115	119	124	129	134	138	143	148	153	158	162	167	172	177	181	186	191
59	94	99	104	109	114	119	124	128	133	138	143	148	153	158	163	168	173	178	183	188	193	198
60	97	102	107	112	118	123	128	133	138	143	148	153	158	163	168	174	179	184	189	194	199	204
61	100	106	111	116	122	127	132	137	143	148	153	158	164	169	174	180	185	190	195	201	206	211
62	104	109	115	120	126	131	136	142	147	153	158	164	169	175	180	186	191	196	202	207	213	218
63	107	113	118	124	130	135	141	146	152	158	163	169	175	180	186	191	197	203	208	214	220	225
64	110	116	122	128	134	140	145	151	157	163	169	174	180	186	192	197	204	209	215	221	227	232
65	114	120	126	132	138	144	150	156	162	168	174	180	186	192	198	204	210	216	222	228	234	240
66	118	124	130	136	142	148	155	161	167	173	179	186	192	198	204	210	216	223	229	235	241	247
67	121	127	134	140	146	153	159	166	172	178	185	191	198	204	211	217	223	230	236	242	249	255
68	125	131	138	144	151	158	164	171	177	184	190	197	203	210	216	223	230	236	243	249	256	262
69	128	135	142	149	155	162	169	176	182	189	196	203	209	216	223	230	236	243	250	257	263	270
70	132	139	146	153	160	167	174	181	188	195	202	209	216	222	229	236	243	250	257	264	271	278
71	136	143	150	157	165	172	179	186	193	200	208	215	222	229	236	243	250	257	265	272	279	286
72	140	147	154	162	169	177	184	191	199	206	213	221	228	235	242	250	258	265	272	279	287	294
73	144	151	159	166	174	182	189	197	204	212	219	227	235	242	250	257	265	272	280	288	295	302
74	148	155	163	171	179	186	194	202	210	218	225	233	241	249	256	264	272	280	287	295	303	311
75	152	160	168	176	184	192	200	208	216	224	232	240	248	256	264	272	279	287	295	303	311	319
76	156	164	172	180	189	197	205	213	221	230	238	246	254	263	271	279	287	295	304	312	320	328

After calculating your BMI, you can determine whether you're at a healthy weight:

- ✔ **Healthy weight:** BMI of 19 to 24.9
- ✔ **Overweight:** BMI of 25 to 29.9
- ✔ **Obese:** BMI of 30 and above

Waist circumference

Even though health care practitioners use BMI as the measurement of choice, it is not a perfect measure of percent body fat when used alone. An athlete who is very muscular but who has a low percentage of body fat, for example, could have the same BMI as someone who is truly fat. Therefore, you also need to measure your waistline.

You can't use your waist size to measure an absolute percentage of body fat, but it does provide information regarding the *location* of your body fat. And knowing where your fat is located, along with your BMI, enables you to determine whether you are overweight and therefore need to lose weight. As explained in Chapter 1, fat that accumulates around your stomach area makes you more susceptible to a variety of health problems. People who accumulate fat around their waists (known as *apples*) are at greater risk for developing serious chronic illness than are people who collect fat on their hips and buttocks, known as *pears*.

How it's done: With a tape measure, measure your waist at the point below your rib cage but above your belly button. If your BMI is 25 to 34.9 and your waist size is more than 40 inches if you're a man or more than 35 inches if you're a woman, you're at an increased risk of developing serious weight-related health problems. Even if your BMI falls into the healthy weight range of 19 to 25, you're at a greater health risk if your waist size is larger than your hips or thighs.

Factoring in Your Personal Risk Factors

You may decide to lose weight based solely on the size of your waist, or by comparing your weight to the Dietary Guidelines for Americans weight chart, or by comparing your BMI to the BMI chart. But health care professionals use more than these measurements in analyzing your weight. They also look at your weight-related risk factors before determining whether the weight you're at is healthy.

The risk factors that health care professionals look for include the following:

- High blood pressure
- High blood cholesterol
- High blood sugar
- Evidence of arthritis in the knees or hips
- Respiratory problems
- Family medical history of weight-related health problems
- Risky behaviors: smoking, poor eating habits, and not exercising

If you're overweight without risk factors, many health care professionals suggest that you try to maintain your weight to prevent further gain instead of trying to lose weight. Or if your weight falls at the higher end of the healthy weight range and you have some weight-related risk factors, they may suggest that you lose 5 to 10 percent of your body weight to improve or lessen these risk factors.

Putting It All Together

Look back at where your weight falls on the Dietary Guidelines for Americans weight chart (at a healthy weight, moderately overweight, or severely overweight), your percent body fat (if you have access to this measurement), your BMI, and your waist size. Compare your numbers to the numbers in Table 2-2. Which column do you fit into?

Table 2-2	Healthy Weight or Overweight?		
		Healthy Weight	Overweight
BMI		19 to 24.9	Over 25
Percent body fat	Women	15 to 25	Over 25
	Men	10 to 20	Over 20
Waist size	Women	Varies	Over 35 inches (increased health risk when coupled with a BMI of over 25)
	Men	Varies	Over 40 inches (increased health risk when coupled with a BMI of over 25)

You probably don't need to lose weight if your weight is within the healthy range, if you've gained less than 10 pounds since you reached your adult height, and if you're otherwise healthy. However, you *can* benefit from losing weight if you're overweight and you

- ✔ Carry excess body fat around your stomach area
- ✔ Have weight-related risk factors
- ✔ Have a family history of weight-related health problems

Your doctor may even suggest that you lose a few pounds if you're within a healthy weight range but have health problems such as diabetes, high blood pressure, or arthritis.

The bottom line: Achieving and maintaining a healthy weight reduces your health risks. It also makes you feel better, increases your energy level, and boosts your confidence. In Part III, you can find out everything you need to know about eating and exercise to achieve and maintain your healthy weight.

Chapter 3

Are You Destined to Be Overweight?

*E*ating too much and not exercising enough are the fundamental reasons people gain weight. But genetics, metabolism, and environmental factors explain how large your appetite is and how efficiently your body uses the food you eat. Some of the reasons you gain weight are beyond your control, but that doesn't mean that you have to resign yourself to a life in the fat lane.

This chapter helps you figure out your own genetic predisposition and helps you manage those factors you *can* control. You can take inspiration from the fact that many people who suffered with being overweight for most of their lives have been able to lose weight and keep it off.

Will You Gain Weight?

Take this quiz to uncover your risk of gaining weight. Answer yes or no to the following statements, and then read on to find out more about the factors that are especially relevant to you.

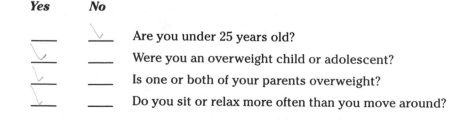

Yes	*No*	
	✓	Are you under 25 years old?
✓		Were you an overweight child or adolescent?
✓		Is one or both of your parents overweight?
✓		Do you sit or relax more often than you move around?

Yes	No	
___	___	Do you believe that eating fat-free or low-fat foods means that you can eat more of them?
___	___	Do you eat out often — especially at fast-food places?
___	___	Have you quit smoking in the last year?
___	___	Are you taking antidepressants or steroids?

If you're female:

___	___	Did you start menstruating earlier than age 11?
___	___	Have you never had a child, or do you have more than three children?
___	___	If you have had a child, did you gain the bulk of your pregnancy weight in the first trimester?
___	___	If you have had a child, did you gain more than 35 pounds during pregnancy?

A "yes" answer to any of these questions indicates that you may be at risk of weight gain. The following sections explain why.

Your age affects your weight

If you're an average American and you're under 25, it's likely that you're going to gain weight over the course of your lifetime. And if you're female, you'll gain weight for a longer period of time than a male will. According to studies published in the *Archives of Internal Medicine* 150, 1990, and in the *American Journal of Clinical Nutrition* 53, 1991, women gain an average of 16 pounds from age 25 to age 54, and then their weight starts to decline at about age 55. Men gain an average of 10 pounds starting at age 25 and stabilize at about age 45. They also begin to lose weight at about age 55. For both men and women, weight gain is highest in people aged 25 to 34 years.

Big children are often bigger adults

Children's health specialist William Dietz, Jr., M.D., Ph.D., has determined that three critical periods may exist for the development of obesity: the prenatal period, childhood between the ages of 5 and 7, and adolescence.

✔ Although more research is needed to fully understand the relationship between nutrition during gestation and birth weight to the onset of obesity later in life, several studies suggest a connection. For example, research shows that there is a greater prevalence of adult obesity in babies born to diabetic mothers who tend to gain an above-average weight during pregnancy and have large babies. Another study suggests that babies who are undernourished during the first two trimesters *in utero* have an increased risk of obesity as they age.

✔ In normal development during the first year of life, an infant's body weight — specifically the amount of fat (or adipose tissue) — is higher in proportion to the baby's height. Gradually, the weight-to-height ratio declines. Then, between the ages of 5 and 7, children naturally increase their fat stores. Nutritionists call this stage *adiposity rebound*. Some longitudinal studies suggest that children whose adiposity rebound occurs earlier (before the age of $5\frac{1}{2}$) are heavier and fatter adolescents and adults than children whose rebound is average (age 6 to $6\frac{1}{2}$) or late. Other studies, however, are needed to confirm these findings. The hypothesis is that children who rebound earlier grow fatter for a longer period of time.

✔ Other studies show that 80 percent of children who are obese during adolescence (ages 10 to 13) will remain obese as adults. Girls have a greater risk than boys for getting and staying overweight; in fact, several studies show that 30 percent of all obese adult women were obese in early adolescence.

See Chapter 10 for more information about helping children grow into healthy, non-obese adults.

Early dieters are big gainers

In a 1994 *Glamour* magazine survey of overweight women who started dieting when they were young, half the women reported that their adult weights are unhealthfully high. The younger the woman was when she started dieting, the higher her current weight is now. The study also found that those who dieted as children weigh more than women who first started dieting as teenagers or adults. But even those who dieted later in childhood did not escape — these women still described themselves at the high end of normal weight.

Nature or nurture?

Studies show that 80 percent of children born to two obese parents will become obese. Contrast that with the fact that only 14 percent of children born to normal-weight parents become obese. But studies on adopted children show that genetics account for only about 33 percent of a child's weight. Lifestyle factors, such as whether the family is active and their eating habits, are more important. Heredity only controls your metabolism — how fast or slowly you use calories.

The set point theory

Although the exact mechanism isn't clear, many health experts believe that each person is born with a genetically predetermined weight range that the body strives to maintain. Human bodies used this system to protect them from starvation when access to food wasn't as easy as a trip to the drive-through or a dash to the corner mini-mart. *Set point* is the weight a body naturally and easily maintains and is generally within a healthy weight range for most people. Unfortunately, this level is generally higher than most of us like, cosmetically speaking, and may explain why reaching a desired weight goal — especially those pesky 5 or 10 pounds — can be so difficult. Set points aren't set in stone; they may change from time to time, but then new set points tend to stay as fixed as the old one.

PRO SPEAK

In the genes

The research on genetics is promising. A gene called *ob,* which has been found in mice, offers a clue. It's responsible for the production of *leptin,* a hormone-like substance that helps the brain regulate appetite. Leptin, which is made in fat cells, travels to the brain, signaling to the brain that the cells have enough fat so that the appetite mechanism can be turned off. Researchers suspect that the brains of obese people have diminished capacities to recognize leptin in much the same way that diabetics have reduced sensitivities to insulin.

Another gene, known as *db,* also regulates leptin to reduce appetite, but it cranks up metabolism as well to control how fast or slowly calories are used. Scientists have found only *similar* genetic material in human DNA; unfortunately, they haven't yet found exactly the combination of genes or their structure that leads to obesity in humans — but they're working on it.

But the news isn't all bad. Set point also helps you return to your body's comfortable weight zone after you eat too much, such as during the winter holidays. Most people gain from 5 to 10 pounds between Thanksgiving and New Year's, but they naturally return to their pre-party weights by mid-February without having to starve themselves.

Don't move it; don't lose it

A study conducted by the Center for Disease Control found that 37 percent of obese people engage in no physical activity whatsoever. Whereas an athlete may burn up to 5,000 calories a day, a sedentary individual may begin to gain weight on as few as 1,800 calories. Regular exercise not only burns calories, but it also helps to build lean muscle, which in turn, burns more *calories* (see the discussion of body fat in Chapter 2).

Studies of children show that the more television they watch, the more they weigh. Experts credit this dubious honor to the fact that TV cuts down on physical movement, and the nonstop food cues that it delivers may prompt overeating. Adult TV watchers suffer a similar fate.

Faux food faux pas

Nutritionists call it the "Snack-Well syndrome" after the line of non-fat food products that people gobble up with abandon. It's believed that these kinds of products — which are fat-free but still contain substantial numbers of calories — are at least in part responsible for the increasing numbers of calories that Americans are eating — and in turn, America's expanding waistline. People have learned that fat-containing foods are fattening. But simply because a food has zero fat doesn't mean that it's a "free" food and that you can eat as much of it as you want. Yes, fat content is important, but when it comes to weight loss, total calories are even more important.

Some examples of how fat-free foods can be dangerous to a diet:

- A serving of Lite Cool Whip has the same number of calories as the regular kind: 25 per 2 tablespoons.

- A cup of nonfat vanilla yogurt has 223 calories, whereas the whole-milk version has a mere 24 calories more.

- Replacing a tablespoon of butter on a bagel with 2 tablespoons of jelly eliminates the fat but doesn't change the number of calories.

Fast food = fast fat

If you eat out frequently, especially in fast-food restaurants, you're probably eating more fat and calories than you want or need. Fast food has several problems. First, although low-calorie choices are available, most people don't order them. A typical fast-food meal averages 700 to 1,200 calories. Part of the blame rests on the fact that portion sizes are out of control. "Super-sizing" an order of fries or a soda may only cost a few cents more and seem like a bargain, but it comes at a big caloric price. A super-sized order of fries has a whopping 540 calories and 26 grams of fat (in comparison, a small order has 210 calories and 10 grams of fat) and a large 32-ounce cola has 310 calories, compared to 150 calories in a small.

Secondly, whether you eat in the restaurant or in your car, you're probably eating quickly — much too quickly. Researchers have consistently shown that one of the best ways to moderate how much you eat is to relax, eat slowly, and focus on your meal. People dining in restaurants at booths and benches that offer only about ten minutes of comfort — or worse yet, eat while driving — aren't focusing on enjoyable eating. They're wolfing down their meals so they can head off on their next errand or rush back to work. Particularly when it comes to fast-food chains, people tend to eat in response to outside cues such as advertising, bargain prices, convenience, and speed — very rarely for health or pleasure.

Up in (stead of) smoke

You may gain up to 10 pounds when you quit smoking, but most people return to their normal weights at the end of a year. The gain, according to research conducted at Kaiser Permanente in California and published in the *Journal of the American Dietetic Association* (1996; 11:1150-1155), seems to be due to eating extra calories in the first month after you quit, and peaks at about 6 months. Although it's not clear why quitting smoking leads to weight gain, it's likely that nicotine somehow increases metabolic rate, and quitting smoking lowers it.

A study published in the *American Journal of Public Health* (1996; Volume 86, Number 7) offers a solution. When researchers followed 9,000 women for 2 years, they found that light smokers (24 cigarettes or less per day) who quit and added 1 to 2 hours of vigorous physical activity each week averaged a $4^1/_2$-pound weight gain; formerly heavy smokers (25 cigarettes or more per day) averaged a gain of $8^1/_2$ pounds. Even more beneficial was exercising 2 or more hours per week. Light smokers had an average gain of just 3 pounds, and heavy smokers 6 pounds. By comparison, light smokers who quit but did not change their activity level gained 5 pounds on average, and heavy smokers nearly $9^1/_2$ pounds. Meanwhile, women who continued to smoke still gained, too: about 1 pound during the study.

Drug-induced gains

If you find that you're gaining weight on a long-term medication that your doctor has prescribed for you, discuss the possibility of switching to a different brand. Medications have different side effects, even if they're in the same class or family, so your doctor may be able to find one that works better for you.

For women only

If you're a woman, there are some inherent reasons why you gain weight more easily than a man.

Early puberty

According to research performed by Stanley Garn and his associates and reported in the *American Journal of Clinical Nutrition* (1986; 43:879-883), the earlier a girl reaches *menarche* (her first period), the heavier she's apt to be as an adult. Research indicates that if you had your first period at age 11 or younger, by age 30 you'll weigh between 9 and 11 pounds more than a woman who started after age 14. The study also found that more than 26 percent of early maturers were obese by age 30, compared to only 15 percent of girls who started their periods later in life.

Pregnancy

Many women hold on to 5 pounds or more following pregnancy, which they often never lose. That's especially true if you gain more than 35 pounds. However, this disheartening piece of news *doesn't* mean that pregnant women should severely limit their weight gain during pregnancy (the optimum maternal weight gain for a healthy 6$^{1}/_{2}$- to 8-pound baby is between 25 and 35 pounds). Rather, pregnant women should try to control the *rate* at which they gain weight.

If you gain most of your pregnancy weight early on (during the first 20 weeks, or about the first trimester) rather than during the last part of your pregnancy, you may have more trouble getting back to pre-pregnancy size. In the first trimester, the fetus needs very little energy, so any large weight gain — in excess of 5 to 7 pounds — goes to the mother's fat stores, not to the infant. During the first 3 months of pregnancy, you can expect a weight gain of 2 to 4 pounds. After that, the gain should be about 1 pound per week.

Many women lose about 10 pounds immediately following delivery and another 5 pounds in the first month or two. The rest of the weight usually continues to drop slowly over the next 6 to 12 months. How quickly you shed the weight depends upon several factors, including your calorie intake, your activity level, and whether or not you're breast-feeding. A strict weight-loss plan isn't recommended while you're nursing, because your body needs extra calories to produce milk. Losing 2 to 4 pounds a month won't affect your ability to nurse, but a loss of more than 4 or 5 pounds after the first month isn't recommended until you stop nursing.

Beating the Odds

Does weight loss seem harder than you thought? Don't despair. More than a third of the people followed by the National Registry of Weight Control (NRWC) reported that they had been obese since childhood. The NRWC is a database of nearly 2,000 individuals who have maintained a loss of at least 30 pounds for 5 years. Seventy-three percent of these indiviuals had at least one overweight parent. Yet even though the obesity cards were stacked against them, they were able to lose weight and keep it off. Almost all of them said that to lose or maintain their weight, they changed *both* their eating habits *and* their activity habits. Their words of weight wisdom:

- ✔ Choose meals that are lower in fat and calories, and watch portion sizes.
- ✔ Keep track of what you eat, and stay within your calorie limits.
- ✔ Learn to recognize and manage the cues that tell you to eat even when you're not hungry.
- ✔ Get physically active and stick with it.

Losing weight and keeping it off isn't necessarily easy. But the benefits of living at a healthy weight are worth it. Not only do you lower your risk for many diseases, including diabetes, high blood pressure, high cholesterol levels, heart disease, stroke, some forms of cancer, and arthritis, but you feel better, too — both mentally and physically.

Chapter 4
Calorie Basics

You eat calories. You count them. You shave them. You hate them. You have the calorie counts in most of your favorite foods memorized. You know that eating too many calories makes you gain weight, and that you lose weight when you eat fewer.

But there's lots more to calorie know-how than simply reading the numbers on food labels. Knowing *why* some foods have more calories than others and figuring out the number of calories your body needs to survive and thrive are the first steps in getting started on a healthy weight-loss plan. This chapter explains all about calories and tells you how to manage them.

What Are Calories, Anyway?

Although the technically correct name is *kilocalorie,* everyone, including dietitians, uses the shorter *calorie.*

Calories are simply a way to measure energy — the energy in food as well as the energy released in the body. Technically speaking, 1 calorie is the amount of energy necessary to raise the temperature of 1 gram of water by 1 degree Centigrade.

Part II
Developing a Healthy Relationship with Food

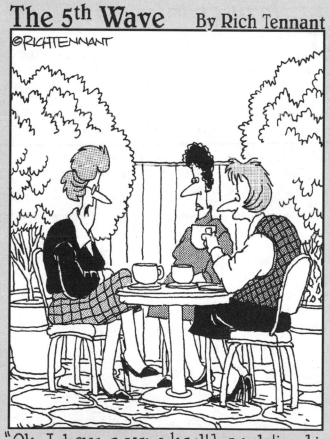

The 5th Wave   By Rich Tennant

"Oh, I have a very healthy relationship with food. It's the relationship I have with my scale that's not so good."

In this part . . .

One of the most difficult things about managing your weight is that you probably don't eat only because you're hungry. You may eat for a variety of reasons: anxiety, depression, stress, or even to celebrate. This part gives you tips for improving your relationship with the refrigerator, helping you control your eating by identifying when you're really hungry and when you're not.

Also in this part, you can find information about eating disorders — dieting gone too far — and about helping your children achieve and maintain a healthy weight.

Where Calories Come From

A calorie is not a nutrient, but certain nutrients provide calories. Protein, carbohydrate, and fat make up the calorie contents of various foods. Although not considered a nutrient, alcohol also provides calories.

- 1 gram of **protein** contains 4 calories.
- 1 gram of **carbohydrate** contains 4 calories.
- 1 gram of **fat** contains 9 calories.
- 1 gram of **alcohol** contains 7 calories.

The remaining nutrients — water, minerals, and vitamins — do not provide calories, nor does fiber or cholesterol.

Few foods and beverages are 100 percent of any one nutrient. Most foods and beverages are a *combination* of protein, fat, and carbohydrate (and sometimes alcohol), so a food's calorie count is the sum of the calories provided by each nutrient. Here's how it works:

A bowl of chicken noodle soup contains 3 grams of protein, 7 grams of carbohydrate, and 2 grams of fat for a total of 58 calories:

3 grams protein × 4 calories/gram	=	12 calories
7 grams carbohydrate × 4 calories/gram	=	28 calories
2 grams fat × 9 calories/gram	=	18 calories
Total	=	**58 calories**

Even though most foods are made up of two or more nutrients, foods are categorized by their predominant nutrient. For example, a bagel and a bowl of cereal are considered carbohydrate foods even though they also contain protein and, sometimes, fat. Even though a chicken breast is considered a protein food, not all of its calories come from protein. Chicken also contains fat, which contributes calories.

TECHNICAL STUFF

Calorie counts

Calories are rounded on food labels, so when you multiply the grams of protein, carbohydrate, or fat, you may come out with a different value than appears on the label. Foods that contain 50 calories or fewer are rounded to the nearest 5-calorie increment; foods with more than 50 calories are rounded to the nearest 10-calorie increment. And foods that have fewer than 5 calories can be listed as having 0 calories. Although you may think that this rounding seems misleading or inaccurate, keep in mind that a 10-calorie difference is actually negligible in the grand scheme of things.

How calories in foods are measured

Where do they get the calorie counts on food labels and in diet books?

The old-fashioned way: They burn it.

The scientists who measure calories in foods call this method *direct calorimetry.* They use an instrument called a *bomb calorimeter,* essentially a highly insulated box containing a special oxygen-rich chamber surrounded by water. A food sample is placed inside the chamber and is burned completely. The heat released raises the temperature of the water in the box. How high the water temperature rises determines how many calories are in the food. If the temperature of the water increases by 10 degrees Centigrade, for example, the food has 10 calories.

Not all calories are created equal. Foods that are considered *empty-calorie foods* really have nothing in them as far as nutrition goes, except for calories. Sugary foods like candy are prime examples. When you're restricting calories, you can make some room for empty-calorie foods, but don't build your diet on them. If you do, you'll miss out on valuable minerals, fiber, and vitamins.

The opposite of empty-calorie foods are *nutrient-dense* foods. Calorie for calorie, they pack a solid nutrition punch by providing a good amount of vitamins, minerals, and/or fiber in comparison to the number of calories they provide. In other words, you get a big nutrition bang for your caloric buck. An example of a nutrient-dense food is an orange. For a mere 60 calories, you get about 3 grams of fiber, 100 percent of your daily vitamin C requirement, and a good amount of folic acid.

How Many Calories Are You Eating?

Unfortunately, there's no magic formula for figuring out how many calories you eat on average — you simply have to track it. Buy a small notebook and write down *everything* you eat for 2 days during the week and 1 weekend day — including that handful of M&M's, the dressing you put on your salad, and the pat of butter you put on your potato. Don't forget to include beverages, too. People tend to eat differently on weekends than on weekdays, so including a Saturday or Sunday in your tracking is important.

Make sure, too, to accurately estimate the amount of each food you eat. Studies show most people grossly underestimate their portion sizes — and can't figure out why they don't lose weight on their "diets"! The problem, of course, is that most people just eat too much.

The best way to determine how much you're eating is to weigh and measure your food. Fill your plate with the typical amount of food you eat, and then use a measuring cup, spoon, or scale to determine your serving size. Most people find it easiest to write down what they ate immediately following each meal; otherwise, they tend to forget about the incidentals (like the glass of wine or soda, or the butter on the bread) and the amounts.

At the end of each day, go back and record the calories for each food you ate by using food labels or a book of calorie counts. You can usually find pocket-sized calorie count books in the grocery store checkout line — and more expanded versions in bookstores — that list hundreds of foods. Then simply tally the number of calories for each food based on the amount you ate, and total up for the day. After your 3-day recording period, add the total calorie counts together and divide by 3. This gives you the approximate number of calories (give or take a few) that you eat on average each day.

For more information about keeping a food journal, see Chapter 5.

Determining How Many Calories Your Body Needs

After you figure out how many calories you typically eat, the next step is to figure out how many calories you actually *need*. Not surprising, many people eat more calories than they truly need, resulting in excess weight.

Your calorie needs are unique to you and depend on a number of factors, including your age, sex, metabolism, activity level, and body size. To get a quick idea of your total calorie needs, multiply your current weight by 15 if you're moderately active or by 13 if you're not. The following sections talk about the factors that affect your calorie needs in more detail.

Your age

Calorie needs peak at about age 25 and then begin to decline by about 2 percent every 10 years. So if you're 25 years old and need 2,200 calories to maintain your weight, you'll need only 2,154 by the time you're 35; 2,110 at age 45; 2,068 at age 55; and so on. One of the reasons for the reduced need is that an aging body replaces muscle with fat, which (unfortunately) burns fewer calories than muscle does.

WARNING!

Don't try to cut calories dramatically

Don't cut your calorie level drastically in trying to lose weight; this strategy will backfire. Your body is programmed to defend your usual weight, so when calories are cut severely — to less than 800 to 1,000 a day — your meta- bolic rate adjusts to conserve the few calories you do give your body. Fortunately, when you overeat occasionally, your metabolism speeds up to burn the extra calories, too — ever striv- ing to maintain your normal weight.

Your sex

An adult man has less fat and about 10 to 20 percent more muscle than a woman of the same size and age. Because muscle burns more calories than fat does, a man's calorie needs are generally about 5 to 10 percent higher than a woman's.

The exception for women is during pregnancy and breast-feeding. During these times in your life, you definitely should *not* cut calories. In fact, you need to eat *more* calories — an extra 300 calories a day while pregnant and an extra 500 calories a day when breast-feeding. Consuming too few calories compromises a mother's health and the health of her baby.

If you're overweight when you become pregnant, talk with your doctor about an appropriate calorie level for you. Contrary to the old adage, pregnancy is not an excuse to eat for two (or three or more!), but you do need to be sure that you're taking in an adequate number of calories. The same goes for while you're breast-feeding.

Your metabolism

A living body needs a minimum number of calories to maintain vital functions like breathing and keeping its heart beating. This minimum number is called *Basal Metabolic Rate,* or *BMR.* It's what most people are referring to when they talk about metabolism.

You can compare your body to a car's engine: Some run efficiently, and others take lots of fuel to keep them moving. Researchers can predict BMR accurately by conducting a special test that measures how much oxygen the body uses within a set amount of time.

A quick and easy way to approximate your BMR without checking into a laboratory is to multiply your current weight by 10 if you're a woman or by 11 if you're a man. Your body needs about 10 to 11 calories (depending on your sex) for every pound you weigh to meet its basic needs. Therefore, a 150-pound woman needs about 1,500 calories a day; a 175-pound man needs about 1,925 calories. Additional calories are needed for digestion and activity.

You can find another, more accurate way to determine your BMR that factors in your age in Table 4-1.

Your genetic blueprint

The metabolic rate that you inherit from your family in part determines the number of calories your body needs to function — and you can't change this factor. That's why your friend who is at the same height, weight, and activity level as you are may be able to eat more calories than you and never gain weight.

Your body shape

Your body shape and size affect the number of calories you need. As explained earlier, muscle burns more calories than body fat does. So if you're rounder and have a greater proportion of muscle to fat, your metabolism is higher. Likewise, if you have more body fat and less muscle, your metabolism is lower and you have a greater tendency to store fat than does someone who is tall and thin.

If you're large, you burn more calories doing an activity than an average-sized person of the same sex and age does. The more you weigh, the more calories your body uses. That's one reason men, who are usually bigger and weigh more than women, need more calories.

Your activity level

When you're active, you burn calories. And if you burn (or expend) more calories than you eat, you lose weight. The kind of exercise you choose, and how long and how intensely you do it, determines exactly how many calories you burn. Some types of activity even help your body burn calories *after* you stop exercising — an added bonus!

Exercise, particularly resistance training, is also important to help minimize muscle loss that naturally occurs during weight loss. See Chapter 12 for more on how exercise helps you lose weight.

Putting it all together

Determining your body's total energy needs takes a bit of math — so grab a calculator and go figure! Follow these steps:

1. **Estimate your basic energy needs.**

   You can use one of two methods: Either multiply your current weight (in pounds) by 10 if you're a woman or 11 if you're a man. Or use the formula in Table 4-1, which factors in your age in addition to your sex.

   In the formula, *weight* represents your weight in kilograms, so translate your weight into kilograms by dividing the number of pounds you weigh by 2.2.

Table 4-1	How Many Calories Your Body Needs Per Day for Basic Energy Needs
Age	*Use This Equation to Calculate Your BMR*
Men	
18 to 30	[15.3 × weight (in kilograms)] + 679
30 to 60	[11.6 × weight (in kilograms)] + 879
Older than 60	[13.5 × weight (in kilograms)] + 487
Women	
18 to 30	[14.7 × weight (in kilograms)] + 496
30 to 60	[8.7 × weight (in kilograms)] + 829
Older than 60	[10.5 × weight (in kilograms)] + 596

Here's an example. Sue is a 45-year-old female who weighs 155 pounds. She calculates her BMR like this:

155 pounds ÷ 2.2 = 70.45 kilograms

70.45 kilograms × 8.7 = 612.92 calories

612.92 calories + 829 calories = 1,441.92 calories

So Sue's BMR — or the number of calories her body needs at complete rest to function — is roughly 1,442 calories.

If you figure Sue's BMR by using the shortcut method, her needs are about 1,550 (155 pounds × 10 = 1,550) — a bit higher than the full calculation, but still in the same ballpark.

2. **Determine your activity factor value.**

   How active are you? Find the description in Table 4-2 that best matches your lifestyle. If you have a desk job but fit in a dose of daily exercise (at least 30 minutes), consider yourself in the light or moderate category.

Table 4-2	How Active Are You?	
If, Throughout Most of Your Day, Your Activities Include . . .	**Your Activity Level Is . . .**	**Your Activity Factor Is . . .**
Sitting or standing; driving; painting; doing laboratory work; sewing, ironing, or cooking; playing cards or a musical instrument; sleeping or lying down; reading; typing	Very light	0.2
Doing garage, electrical, carpentry, or restaurant work; house-cleaning; caring for children; playing golf; sailing; light exercise such as walking for no more than 2 miles	Light	0.3
Heavy gardening or housework, cycling, playing tennis, skiing, or dancing; very little sitting	Moderate	0.4
Heavy manual labor such as construction work or digging; playing sports such as basketball, football, or soccer; climbing	Heavy	0.5

3. **Multiply your basic energy needs by the activity factor value that you determined:**

   _____ × _____ = _____

   BMR   Activity factor   Calories for activity

   Using Sue as an example, she multiplies her BMR of 1,442 by 0.3 because her activity level is light — running around after her kids, taking care of the house, and fitting in a 2-mile morning walk with her neighbors every other day. Sue needs 432.6 calories for her activity level.

   $$1{,}442 \times 0.3 = 432.6 \text{ calories}$$

4. **Determine the number of calories you need for digestion and absorption of nutrients.**

   Eating food actually burns calories. Digesting food and absorbing nutrients uses about 10 percent of your daily energy needs. Add together your BMR and activity calories, and then multiply the total by 10 percent.

$$(\underline{\hspace{2cm}} + \underline{\hspace{2cm}}) \times 10\% = \underline{\hspace{3cm}}$$

BMR calories   Activity calories   Calories for digestion/ absorption

The calculation for Sue's calorie needs for digestion and absorption looks like this:

1,442 calories + 432.6 calories = 1874.6 × 10% = 187.5 calories

5. **Total your calorie needs.**

Add together your BMR, activity, and digestion/absorption calorie needs to get your total calorie needs — that is, the number of calories you need to maintain your current weight.

$$\underline{\hspace{2cm}} + \underline{\hspace{2cm}} + \underline{\hspace{2cm}} = \underline{\hspace{2cm}}$$

BMR calories   Activity calories Digestion/ absorption calories   Total calories

To maintain her current weight of 155 pounds, Sue calculates her total calorie needs like this:

1,442 calories + 432.6 calories + 187.5 calories = 2,062 total calories

Setting a Reasonable Calorie Level for Weight Loss

To lose weight, you have to cut down on how much you eat — but not too much. If you try to cut too many calories, you may not lose any weight at all. When you cut calories severely, your metabolic rate slows to adjust to the lower calorie level. In addition, you probably won't be able to stick to your plan for very long because you'll be hungry all the time. This section can help you find the right balance of calories for you.

Too much food is not the only cause of obesity; lack of exercise is also part of the formula. So when you think about dieting, you need to redefine your definition to mean cutting calories *and* upping exercise. See Chapter 12 for more information about adding exercise to your daily routine.

How many calories you need to cut to lose weight

Because there are 3,500 calories in a pound and 7 days in a week, you can cut your daily calorie intake by 500 to lose 1 pound a week (3,500 ÷ 7 = 500). To lose $1^1/_2$ pounds, you need to cut 750 calories a day. A 2-pounds-a-week loss means eliminating 1,000 calories a day. A faster rate of weight loss is generally associated with weight regain and yo-yo dieting. Remember the tortoise and the hare: Slow and steady wins the race.

Look at how these guidelines affect Sue's weight-loss plans. She needs about 2,163 calories each day to maintain her current weight. To lose 1 pound per week, Sue needs to cut 500 calories a day, bringing her weight-loss calorie level to 1,663. To lose $1^1/_2$ pounds a week, her new calorie level would be 1,413 (2,163 − 750 = 1,413). Attempting to lose 2 pounds per week means that Sue's calorie allotment would drop to 1,163 calories. This amount, while still safe, may be too low for Sue's personal needs.

The 20 percent rule

Another way to determine your calorie needs for weight loss is called the 20 percent rule. This rule can be a healthier way to lose weight, especially if you're not eating many calories now and a reduction of 500 to 750 calories per day would put your calorie intake below 800 to 1,000 a day and therefore your metabolism into low gear.

First, you need to figure out the average number of calories you eat now. To do so, see the section, "How many calories are you eating?" earlier in this chapter.

After you determine the average number of calories you consume, simply subtract 20 percent. We'll use Maureen as an example. According to Maureen's food records, she eats about 1,800 calories a day and would like to lose 20 pounds. Here are her calculations:

1,800 calories × 0.20 = 360 calories

1,800 calories − 360 calories = 1,440 calories

If Maureen cuts her calorie consumption by about 360 calories to 1,440 calories, she can lose between $^1/_2$ and $^3/_4$ pound a week — a healthy rate of loss that won't leave her starving. In about 7 months, Maureen should reach her goal. Slow and steady, but she's more likely to keep it off than if she tried to lose it in half that time.

Chapter 5

Understanding Your Relationship with Food

*F*rom the time your mother or father hands you a cookie to quiet your crying, food becomes more than just a way to nourish your body. It's a way to nourish your soul as well. Regardless of your weight — and regardless of whether or not you realize it — you eat for different reasons: to celebrate, to calm, to feel comfort or joy, and, when times are darkest, perhaps to relieve loneliness and boredom. How you feel about yourself and your body is likely to be enmeshed in your relationship with food. Shame and guilt may also play a role in your range of emotions that affect how you deal with food.

In this chapter, we investigate the emotional reasons people have for eating even when they're not hungry. We help you understand why you eat when you do and give you some suggestions for replacing emotion-driven food habits with healthier behaviors.

Finding Out Whether You Are an Emotional Eater

The first step in discovering how emotions affect your eating is to understand your relationship with food. Answer the following questions as honestly as you can. Think about how frequently each question is true for you, and respond with words such as *sometimes, often, always,* and *never.* By analyzing your responses, you can better understand your triggers — and your strengths. Then refer to the sections that follow the questions to find out what your responses mean and understand how to deal with these issues.

✔ Do you eat even when you're not hungry? *Often*

✔ Do you crave certain foods and have trouble controlling the amounts of them that you eat? *Sometimes*

✔ Do you always clean your plate? *always*

✔ When faced with paperwork or a difficult task, do you find yourself in the kitchen or at the snack machine instead of doing the work? *Sometimes*

✔ Do you eat when you are stressed, angry, lonely, or tired? *Sometimes*

✔ Do you splurge on favorite foods when you're alone? *Sometimes*

✔ Do you feel guilty or unworthy when you eat foods you think you shouldn't — especially high-calorie foods, such as fried items or desserts? *often*

Eating when you're not hungry

If you eat when you're not hungry, you're not alone. Many people do. Unfortunately, physical hunger is often low on the list of reasons to eat. Many people eat because the clock says that it's time to, because people around them are eating, or because a food simply looks or smells good. The key is to learn to recognize these triggers and deal with the emotions behind them in ways not related to food. (Of course, if you're hungry, then you should eat.)

Craving favorite foods

If you can't resist your favorite foods, you're probably responding to a craving rather than hunger. What's the difference? A *craving* is based in emotions; *hunger* is rooted in biology. When you're hungry, any number of foods can satisfy you, but a craving is a highly specialized, very intense desire to eat a particular food or type of food. During a craving, the desire is sometimes so strong that you might go out of your way to get it. For example, when you crave potato chips, celery sticks just won't cut it.

According to a survey conducted by H. P. Weingarten, Ph.D., at McMaster's University in Ontario, Canada (published in the December 1991 issue of *Appetite*), 97 percent of women and 68 percent of men experience food cravings. Researchers believe that older people are generally less driven by cravings, particularly older men. Food cravings may also be dictated by the time of day — late afternoon or early evening is the prime time when cravings tend to occur. Hormones are thought to play a role as well. For example, during pregnancy and during certain times of a woman's menstrual cycle, food cravings are quite common. But dieters, especially those who frequently go on and off diets, tend to experience cravings most often. And their cravings tend to be strongest at the beginning of their diets.

Keeping a food journal

Most people don't make the connection between how they feel and how much they eat until they keep a food diary. A food diary is nothing more than a place to record the foods you eat, when you eat them, and how you're feeling when you eat. A small notebook that you can tuck into a pocket or purse will work. Just remember to do the following:

✔ **Record everything you eat.** That includes the swipe your finger made through the brownie batter. If you eat crackers, record how many. (Turn to Chapter 14 for suggestions on estimating portion sizes.)

✔ **Record your feelings.** What were you thinking or feeling when you ate? Were you angry, sad, or happy? Or just hungry?

✔ **Record information immediately after eating a food.** You don't want to forget anything or filter your emotions; your feelings may change later in the day. You're looking for clues to why you eat, not only to what you eat.

✔ **Record your physical activity.**

✔ **Analyze your diary at the end of the day and determine where improvements are needed.** Calculate the number of servings from each of the food groups in the pyramid (see Chapter 10). Determine the intensity of your emotions and how they affected your eating. Did you make your physical activity goal for the day?

✔ **Congratulate yourself for a day well done.** Or, if necessary, make plans to get back on the beam.

Dr. Marcia Levin Pelchar, a biological psychologist at the Monell Chemical Senses Center in Philadelphia, has conducted many research studies on cravings. In the July 1998 *Tufts University Health & Nutrition Letter,* she suggests that people who have been "dieting" for a long time probably don't experience cravings because diets that stand the test of time are usually sensible. These diets provide a wide variety of foods and don't require severe restriction or deprivation. Short-term, frequent dieters, on the other hand, tend to follow very restrictive, monotonous plans. The "banned" foods then become the focus of cravings — yearnings for those foods that one shouldn't eat.

How best to deal with food cravings? There's nothing that will stop a craving cold, and there's no "one size fits all" solution. Experiment with a few of the following tips to figure out which work best for you:

✔ **Substitute foods.** For example, try a glass of low-fat chocolate milk or a Fudgsicle instead of a chocolate candy bar.

✔ **Use portion control.** Buy smaller, single-size servings of favorite foods, such as ice cream, to satisfy the craving and quell the instinct to go overboard.

✔ **Give into the craving.** Don't eat around your craving in hopes that it will go away. You'll probably end up eating more food and calories than you would have if you simply gave in to your craving to begin with. Many people end up eating the craved food anyway after attempting to eat around it, because they still aren't satisfied.

Always cleaning your plate

Do you always feel compelled to clean your plate? Whether this mentality is due to well-meaning parents or a fear that you'll never eat a meal this good again, it's a particular problem for dieters. This kind of conditioning can be especially difficult for people who eat out often because restaurant portions can be gigantic and arbitrary. Restaurants plan their menus for economics and customer expectations, not health. (See Chapter 16 for more on eating out.) A solution is to order only from the kid's menu. And don't ask for "super-size" portions.

If finishing the bag of chips or the entire burger is your pattern, buy smaller sizes. Counter the fear-of-famine mentality by remembering that more is always available and that, yes, you *will* have a meal that good again.

Eating instead of working

Procrastination and boredom are very common reasons that people eat. It's a way to kill time and put off doing tasks that need to be done. Classic research on dieters and non-dieters performed at California State University (*Addictive Behaviors* 2, 1977) showed that when faced with monotonous tasks — in this case, writing the same letter over and over again — dieters and non-dieters alike ate more crackers. When they engaged in a stimulating mental activity such as a creative writing project, they ate fewer crackers. So if boring work or a big project is sending you to the fridge, try reaching for some ice water, raw veggies, or fruit before digging into the cookie jar. Or take a walk around the block or around the office to help clear your head.

Eating when you're stressed, angry, lonely, or tired

Eating to distract yourself from difficult emotions is not a constructive or healthy way to deal with your problems. The more deeply you feel the effects of your emotions, particularly the negative ones, the more you are apt to eat. For overweight people, this reaction may be especially problematic. A study conducted by Michael Lowe of Rutgers University and Edwin Fisher, Jr., of Washington University [*Journal of Behavioral Medicine* 6(2), 1983] compared the emotional reactivity and emotional eating of normal and overweight female college students. For 12 days, the women kept track of how they were feeling just before eating and recorded what and how much they ate. The results showed that the obese women were more emotionally reactive and more likely to engage in emotional eating than women of normal weight — but only at snack time, not at meals. The more emotional the women were feeling, the more they ate, and the heaviest women were the most emotional. However, the two groups did not differ in their reactions to positive, happy feelings, nor did they eat in response to good emotions.

If stress, anger, loneliness, or exhaustion is your trigger, work on non-food coping skills:

✔ Write out your feelings in a journal.

✔ Talk with a friend.

✔ Go for a walk, play with your pet, or ask someone for a hug.

✔ Release anger by pounding your fist into a pillow.

✔ Confront the person who is making you angry.

✔ Cry, if you need to.

✔ Practice breathing exercises, breathing in and out deeply, to help center yourself.

✔ Ask for time out or help on a project, if needed.

✔ Take a yoga or meditation class.

✔ Schedule time for yourself.

✔ Get a good night's sleep or take a nap.

Name that mood

People who belong to 12-step programs, such as Overeaters Anonymous or Alcoholics Anonymous, use techniques to keep from engaging in their addictive behaviors. One method is called HALT, which stands for Hungry, Angry, Lonely, and Tired. These physical and emotional feelings can masquerade as cravings for substances or behaviors. So if a 12-stepper feels the need to return to his or her self-destructive behavior, a quick inventory reveals what needs to be done. For example, you can relieve feelings of loneliness with a call to a friend or cure tiredness with a nap. The point is to recognize the triggers and deal with them rather than substitute unhealthy behaviors.

Psychologists know that giving your emotions a name makes them easier to deal with. Labeling makes feelings concrete, and therefore you can cope with them. If you engage in emotional eating, labeling what you're feeling when you eat may be the secret to eating less.

Eating healthfully around others but splurging alone

Overeating only when you are alone is usually the result of buying into the diet industry propaganda that you hear from television, well-meaning friends, and your own inner voice: "Don't eat too many calories," "You shouldn't eat that," "That cake is too fattening." Foods get labeled, and if you eat these "good" or "bad" foods, *you* become good or bad. These thoughts can make you restrict your eating so severely that when you are calm, alone, and not afraid of being judged, you splurge and enjoy all the foods that you otherwise think you shouldn't eat.

This kind of restrictive eating is a sure way to smother a natural sense of hunger (see Chapter 6 for more on appetite versus hunger) and keep the dieting treadmill rolling. Cognitive therapists know that when a negative thought ("I shouldn't eat that dessert" or "It's just going to end up on my thighs") leads to negative feelings ("I'm so fat; what a failure I am"), negative behavior (eating too much of the dessert and continuing to overeat) is sure to follow. Perception becomes reality.

You need to replace negative, irrational thoughts with positive, rational ones. One way is to get yourself out of all-or-nothing thinking. Pull back from the extremes and stay moderate. Get rid of "should" and "shouldn't." No food is all good or all bad, and neither are you. Quiet your own internal "food police" by listening to your sympathetic, caring, and loving voices. The conversation may sound something like this: "That cake sure looks good. I'd love to try it. My weight loss may slow down if I eat a big piece. So I'm going to have just a small slice. Yum, I sure will enjoy that. I will feel satisfied, and I won't have to forage for sweets later."

Feeling unworthy to eat or guilty about eating

Feeling unworthy to eat or guilty about eating also comes from the food police at work. And it's classic diet-think. Eating is not a moral issue, and neither is food. Eating and hunger are part of the human condition — you have to eat in order to live. You can squelch the food police by letting your nurturing voices be heard. Instead of thinking, "Do I deserve this?" ask yourself, "Am I hungry?" If your answer is yes, then eat.

Adjusting Your Attitude

It's a fact of life that society discriminates against overweight people. It starts in school, and anyone who has been larger than his or her classmates can tell tales of rejection and ridicule by thinner peers. That the prejudice is widespread in the business world, too, is well documented. And countless men and women can tell you that their weights and their dissatisfaction with their bodies keep them from getting close to other people or sometimes even enjoying sex with their spouses.

Being overweight takes a toll on your self-esteem and the way you relate to others. Self-esteem is key to your relationship with food, too. If you don't feel good about your body, you may not feel good about the food you put into it. And without a healthy relationship with food, your body image will plummet. It's a catch-22 situation.

This section is about body image: learning to feel good about who you are, regardless of your body size or shape.

Whose ideal are you?

According to research conducted by the Kellogg's corporation (published by the Opinion Research Corporation), women in the United States determine their ideal body size and shape from the way models in television ads and fashion magazines look, not from the way women look in real life. Women are obsessed about their weight, fueled by a society that sets an artificial standard for beauty based on the way models look. Women also believe that how they are described by men and by each other promotes the notion of an ideal woman, whom they will never be able to match.

The Kellogg's survey found that women tend to focus on the specific body parts they don't like, not on their bodies as a whole. They may like their hair color and think that they're tall enough, but only 14 percent of the women surveyed were happy with their weights. Almost a third of the women surveyed said that a woman's ideal weight is between 110 and 125 pounds, and half said that a weight between 126 and 145 is ideal. But in reality, there is no such thing as an "ideal" weight, because people are genetically programmed to be different shapes and sizes.

It's not surprising that so many women are confused about what they should look like. The role models look nothing like the average woman. In fact, if you think about it, it's the fashion models who don't conform to the standards of the average adult, not the other way around. Only 1 in 40,000 women has a supermodel-like body. 40,000! That's the population of a small city. That ratio means that out of the entire population of Ohio, only 135 women have model-perfect bodies!

Table 5-1 compares the average American woman to the media's and society's ideals, demonstrating that when it comes to selling clothes, life does not imitate art. In fact, it's getting further away from it. Marilyn Monroe, the pinup girl of the 1950s, wore a size 14 dress — the same size that many women in the United States wear today. This isn't to say that a size 14 is healthy for all women — that depends on your height and other factors. Someone who is 5 feet tall and a size 14 is probably not at a healthy weight, but someone who is 5'6" may be, even though she would still be considered on the "large" side by society's standards. The scary thing is that today's models, who are usually at least 5'8" or taller, typically wear only a size 6. And between 1955 and 1998, the measurements of a *Playboy* centerfold dropped by 35 percent.

Table 5-1	Female Role Models		
	Average Woman	*Mannequin*	*Model*
Dress size	12	6	6
Weight	138	—	120
Height	5'4"	5'10"	5'8" to 5'11"
Body measurements	37-29-40	34-25-34	34-25-34
Percent body fat	32	—	18

This phenomenon is not unique to women. Even male models and mannequins are smaller than the average American male. Table 5-2 illustrates the differences.

Table 5-2	Male Role Models		
	Average Man	*Mannequin*	*Model*
Pant size	34 to 36	30	30
Suit size	42 regular	40 regular	40 regular
Weight	170	—	145
Height	5'10"	6'	6'
Body measurements	42 chest	39 chest	39 chest
	34-36 waist	30 waist	30 waist
Percent body fat	23	—	15

The important point to take away from these charts is that you need to stop comparing yourself and your weight to unrealistic numbers. Even if you diet religiously, you probably won't end up with the body of a supermodel. Stop beating yourself up for not meeting standards that are so unrealistic and concentrate on the things you can do to make your body healthy. And learn to feel good about your progress, too.

One study of obese women — their average weight was about 218 pounds — conducted by Foster, et al., at the University of Pennsylvania did just that [see the *Journal of Consulting and Clinical Psychology* 65(1), 1997]. The women were asked to write down their goal weights and then the weight-loss amounts that they would consider "acceptable" and "disappointing." Most women set their goals 32 percent lower than their starting points (about 72 pounds). "Acceptable" was about a 25 percent loss (55 pounds), and the women considered a weight loss of only 17 percent of their starting weights (38 pounds) to be "disappointing."

After 6 months of dieting, exercising, and behavior modification and 6 months of maintenance, the average weight loss that these women were able to maintain was only 16 percent of their defined starting weights (or 36 pounds). They hadn't even reached their "disappointing" weight. Did they fail? No. These women can be called successful for several reasons: A weight loss of just 10 percent is enough to bring down high blood pressure, lower cholesterol and triglycerides, and improve overall health. And these women beat that goal by 6 percentage points.

More important, all the women were happy with their losses and were surprised to find that even though they hadn't reached the weight loss they initially called disappointing, they felt better physically and emotionally than they had expected.

The lesson is that accepting a weight loss that doesn't match the number you dreamed of is healthier than writing off the success as a failure and then giving in and gaining the loss back — plus a few more pounds. A healthier weight strategy is to maintain the loss for a few months and then reach for another 10 to 15 percent loss. Think of weight loss as moving down a flight of stairs — not a ramp — with landings to stop and evaluate your progress.

Unfortunately, most people don't give themselves credit for progress. They strive for perfection. Most people who consider themselves successful at maintaining weight loss lose about half the weight between their beginning weights and the "ideals" that they found on height-and-weight charts.

Is your body image accurate?

Society shouldn't dictate how people look. But in reality, it does. About 95 percent of females and 30 percent of males have issues about the way their bodies look. The thing is, it's the only body you have. So if you're not happy with your body, make the commitment to start taking better care of it. Exercise and stretch your body, fill it with the foods it needs to help keep you healthy and strong, and remember all the good things your body does for you. You may never look like a supermodel, but that's okay — virtually no one will. However, everyone can be healthy. When you start taking care of your body, you'll feel better about your body and about yourself. So get started today.

Here are some techniques to try if your body image needs improving:

- Remember that your perception of your body is a thought ("I hate my jelly belly"), but you feel it like an emotion ("I'm unlovable"). So if you can change the thought ("My stomach stayed round after the children were born"), you can change the emotion ("I'm happy that my body can give life").

- Use your body. It functions. Any woman who has breast-fed her child, for example, can explain the shift in thinking about her breasts as functioning entities rather than as sexual objects. Use your thighs to carry you through the woods, up a mountain, or down the street. Give them something to do rather than thinking of them as something to hide.

- Body images wax and wane. Some days, you may like your shape; other days, you may feel woefully inadequate. Think of times when you were not disappointed with your body. What were you doing? Do that activity more often.

- Do this simple exercise to find out whether your body image is accurate: Either alone in front of a mirror or with a kind and loving friend you trust, stand up straight and close your eyes. If you're a woman, stretch your arms out in front of you and indicate the width of your hips. If you're a man, do the same thing to indicate how thick you think your middle is. Now open your eyes and compare. Were you accurate? Many women with distorted body images think that their hips are much wider than they are. And many men may think that their bellies are larger than they are, too.

- Try not to play the mix-and-match, pick-and-compare body parts game with other people. You know, you'd like to have one woman's thighs, another's bust, or if you're a guy, one man's biceps and another's flat stomach. Remember that every body has great parts and not-so-great parts, and learn to appreciate your body for what it is. It's the only one you have!

- Give yourself credit for the physical attributes you do like, such as good teeth, great hair, sexy feet, a pretty belly button, or a lovely voice.

Chapter 6

Getting Over Overeating

In This Chapter
- ▶ Understanding the biology behind hunger
- ▶ Tuning in to your hunger signals
- ▶ Understanding the difference between cravings and hunger

How much you eat isn't a matter of willpower or lack of it. It's an inborn, powerful biological drive to assure human survival. Trying to override the system with diet and food restriction is counterproductive because it triggers the body's chemicals to turn on your appetite and increase hunger. Every time you undereat or deny your body's need for food, you actually crank into high gear a complex system of chemical reactions that tells you to eat. A vicious cycle? You bet. This chapter discusses some ways to get back in touch with your natural hunger cues — not the external or emotional cues that sometimes call you to eat whether or not you're actually hungry.

How Hunger Works

You may think that your hunger alarm is all in your stomach and that dieting is all in your head. But the truth is that hunger is regulated by a complex system of chemicals that communicate with all the systems of the body. Signals are sent back and forth from your brain to your body. What starts hunger depends on whether the signals come from sensory or mechanical origins.

The brain

Scientists have identified that a specific area in the brain, the hypothalamus, is in part responsible for processing eating behavior. The cells in the hypothalamus communicate with cells in other parts of the brain to coordinate the release and uptake of chemicals forming the feedback system that helps regulate how much and what you eat. The chemicals that the body releases help the brain cells communicate with cells in the other parts of the body.

What starts the chemical chain? Food can be the trigger that stimulates the brain to turn the desire to eat into the actual act of eating. How a food smells, what it looks like, how you remember it tasting — in short, its sensory appeal — excites chemicals within the brain. Another way the process starts is at a cellular level, when messages sent to the brain tell it that fuel is needed and that it's time to eat.

When the body needs nourishment, *neurotransmitters* (chemicals that transmit information to the neurons or brain cells) are released. Although more research is needed to help explain the exact mechanisms, one neurotransmitter called Neuropeptide Y (NPY) is thought to respond when the body needs carbohydrate. According to the theory, low levels of glycogen (carbohydrate in storage form in your body) and low blood sugar levels stimulate NPY's release from the hypothalamus. As NPY levels increase, so does your desire for sweet and starchy foods. While you sleep, your glycogen and blood sugar stores are used up, and they send a message to the brain to release NPY. It's no coincidence that our favorite morning foods are rich in carbohydrates — cereal, breads, bagels, and fruit. Skipping breakfast increases NPY levels so that by afternoon, you're set up for a carbohydrate binge. This craving for carbs is not the result of a lack of willpower; it's an innate biological urge at work. Stress and dieting are thought to trigger NPY production as well.

The serotonin-carbohydrate connection

Eating carbohydrates or other favorite foods turns off NPY by using a serotonin feedback system. Serotonin is another neurotransmitter, a brain chemical, that is associated with feelings of fullness and well-being. When serotonin increases, NPY decreases, telling your body that you have had enough food and that you can stop eating.

How carbohydrates may increase serotonin

Carbohydrates have been called "mood food" because many people find comfort and calmness from eating them. Carbohydrates may have a calming effect because eating them may increase the brain chemical called serotonin, a neurotransmitter that regulates sleep, mood, food intake, and pain tolerance. When levels are high, you're less irritable. But pasta isn't Prozac. The effects of eating carbohydrates are subtle.

The galanin-fat connection

Another neurotransmitter called galanin is released when fat stores need filling up. Research on galanin has been conducted only on animals, but the human appetite for fat is believed to act in a similar way. Laboratory animals that have been injected with galanin prefer high-fat foods to high-carbohydrate ones. And when the animals are given drugs that interfere with galanin production, their preference for fat decreases. How galanin works within individuals may help explain why some people store more fat than others do. In the evening, galanin levels tend to rise, which may be nature's way of making sure that people have enough calories to last them through the night without taking in more food.

Eating late at night has been associated with increased weight — not because the body processes calories differently after dark, but because hunger and fatigue late in the day can cause you to overeat.

CCK: The appetite control chemical

When you eat, food enters and fills your stomach and then travels to the intestinal tract. As the food is digested and the body's cells are fed, a chemical called cholecystokinin (CCK) is released. CCK sends signals to the brain to say "enough" by turning on feelings of satiety or fullness and turning off the appetite.

However, this chemical reaction doesn't work properly in some people. Researchers think that certain conditions, such as excessive dieting, anorexia (a form of self-starvation), and bulimia (a condition in which a person binges on huge amounts of food and then purges to get rid of what was overeaten) may affect many appetite-control body chemicals, including CCK. In bulimics, for example, researchers think that either the CCK mechanism doesn't work properly (so their brains never get the signal to stop eating) or the body's chemical systems become so desensitized that the person eats huge quantities of food quicker than the brain is able to signal satiety. The opposite effect may occur in anorexics — the CCK mechanism is so *over*sensitized that they feel full after only a few bites of food. When bulimics start eating normally, their CCK systems usually normalize. In a person with anorexia, the CCK hunger-satiety system also tends to normalize after he or she gains weight.

For more information about anorexia and bulimia, see Chapter 7.

Most people who have trouble with creeping weight gain eat not because they are hungry but because of appetite. What's the difference? Would you dig up a turnip and eat it dirty and raw? Or would you rather have a dish of Häagen Dazs? Hunger would force you to do the former; appetite is at work in the latter. But both have their origins in the brain, and both affect a series of chemical and hormonal reactions, which ultimately results in the physical act of eating. The key is to get back in touch with your natural hunger signals so that you eat when you're hungry, not just because you have an appetite.

How Dieting Makes You Hungry

Dieting experts and researchers Peter Herman and Janet Polivy have looked thoroughly at the biology and psychology of eating (see *Current Concepts in Nutrition* 16, 1988). They have found that dieters lose their ability to recognize subtle hunger clues, having suppressed them for so long that they feel hunger only when they are drop-dead ravenous. And when they eat, they overeat because they are no longer able to recognize subtle feelings of fullness. Their "biological indifference," as it has been called, is so ingrained that chronic dieters eat or don't eat based only on outside influences such as time of day, thoughts, and beliefs . . . not on what their bodies are actually telling them.

You can get back in touch with your hunger

Arbitrary portion sizes and years of parental instruction to "clean your plate" have conditioned people to ignore their innate ability to tell when they've had enough to eat. People eat down to the china pattern. They finish the whole portion simply because it's there, not because they really need to. Re-learning to recognize and respect your hunger and satisfaction signals takes time. These techniques can help:

- **Eat slowly.** Your brain needs up to 20 minutes to get the message that your body has had enough to eat.

- **Don't wait until you're famished to eat.** You're apt to overeat when you're absolutely flat-out starving. People who skip meals or eat skimpy meals often eat when they're ready to drop. Eating 3 meals and 2 or 3 small snacks is one way to make sure that you're never too hungry or too full. Remember, what counts is the total number of calories you consume each day, not how often you eat.

✔ **Pay attention to how you feel, and eat mindfully.** You need to eat slowly to recognize the sometimes-vague signals that you've had enough to eat. The goal is to internalize those feelings. Until you can hear and heed the conversations your brain and stomach are having, wear clothing with waistbands. Loose clothing may be more comfortable, but something snug around your middle can serve as a reminder to stop eating when it feels tight.

✔ **Buy only single servings of foods that you crave, or you may find it difficult to stop eating even when you're full.** Research at the University of Pennsylvania conducted by marketing professor Brian Warsink, Ph.D. [see the *Journal of Marketing* 60(3), 1996] looked at the way people use different-sized packages of cooking oil, spaghetti, M&M's, and other items. He found that many people use a product more freely when they aren't worried about running out, when price isn't important (larger packages are often cheaper than smaller ones), and when space is tight (larger packages take up lots of room). So if ice cream in the freezer tempts you, don't buy it in gallons. Single-sized servings, purchased one at a time, may be a wiser move.

Full but not satisfied? That may be your body's way of telling you that the meal you just ate was not well-balanced. Some researchers think that your body has a feedback system that tells your brain when it has enough carbohydrate, fat, and protein. When a meal is heavy in one nutrient and light in the others, you get little satisfaction from your meal.

Your body is sensitive to sensory fulfillment as well. Creamy textures and sweet flavors need to be balanced with crunchy and savory ones. That's one of the reasons one-food-only diets, such as the cabbage soup diet (see Chapter 20), are so frustrating: Besides being unbalanced nutritionally, they are unbalanced in flavor and texture.

Why you eat more premenstrually

If you just can't say no to premenstrual cravings, you have a good reason: Your body doesn't want you to. Interesting work at the University of British Columbia [see *The American Journal of Clinical Nutrition* 61(1), 1995] demonstrates what many women have suspected for some time: Women eat differently during the second half of their cycles — surprisingly, though, only if they have ovulated that month. Susan Barr, Ph.D., and her colleagues studied 42 women and compared their daily food intakes with their daily body temperatures. The women who had a rise in body temperature, signaling ovulation, had eaten more calories during the second half of their cycles. The women whose temperatures showed no change, and therefore had not ovulated, did not change their caloric intake.

When an egg is released and is not fertilized, the body secretes progesterone to start the menstrual flow. If no egg is released, the surge in progesterone does not occur. Progesterone has a thermogenic effect; in other words, it makes heat. To produce the heat, energy — in the form of calories — is burned. The women did not know when *or if* they were ovulating, proving that women subconsciously and automatically eat more to make up for the calorie deficit. The average increase was about 260 calories, but some women ate up to 500 extra calories a day. Women on birth control pills don't ovulate, so they don't experience progesterone's fuel burn.

What time is dinner?

Often, people eat not because they're hungry but because it's time to eat: another example of ignoring the body's messages. Eating based on time rather than hunger is one of the problems with the three-meals-a-day tradition. Sure, it's practical, but consider that on the three-squares plan, a body is expected to run for 5 hours between breakfast and lunch, 6 to 7 hours between lunch and dinner, and then 11 to 12 hours until breakfast (figuring that your breakfast is at 7, lunch is at noon, and dinner is between 6 and 7). If you're a breakfast skipper, you're hoping to go for about 16 hours without eating. But the human body needs to be fueled every 3 to 4 hours to prevent energy dips, metabolism slowdowns, crankiness, and cravings from interfering with life.

To help quell what may be legitimate hunger pangs, many people pick or graze on food throughout the day, not "counting" those mini-snacks as part of their food intake — a handful of popcorn here, a few pieces of candy there, half a piece of office birthday cake — you get the picture. The calories add up and keep people from being physically hungry because they've been eating all morning. But that doesn't stop most folks from sitting down to eat a full lunch when the clock strikes noon.

This doesn't mean that you should starve yourself all morning if you're hungry. Going past the point of hunger to ravenous can set the perfect scenario for overeating — eating beyond the point when hunger is satisfied. Re-train yourself to recognize feelings of hunger and respect them. Eat when you feel them, and stop when they stop. Don't eat when you're not hungry. This approach starts with eating breakfast, planning snacks, or eating only part of your lunch and saving the rest for a snack later on in the afternoon. Eat regular meals, but don't eat by the clock.

If you've been skipping meals or eating too infrequently, adjusting and recognizing your hunger signals will take some time. When you recognize one, wait 10 to 15 minutes. If you still feel hunger, eat. If you don't, you may have mistaken a hunger signal for another sensation.

Some people are so conditioned that they miss the normal signals of hunger. Look for these signals when you're tempted to eat:

- Difficulty concentrating
- Feeling faint
- Headache
- Irritability
- Lightheadedness
- Mild gurgling or gnawing in the stomach
- Stomach "talking"

Feeling stressed? Ask yourself: Am I biologically hungry? If you can no longer recognize your hunger signals, you'll have to rely on outside clues for a while. Ask yourself, has it been more than 5 hours since your last meal? Was it substantial enough? If you decide that you are truly hungry, eat. Make sure that the snack has carbohydrate, protein, and some fat for greater staying power. (See Chapter 24 for ideas for well-balanced, calorie-controlled snacks.)

If what you feel is not physical hunger, try to label the emotion and honor it. Then use one of these nurturing activities to deal with your emotional hunger:

- Arrange flowers
- Breathe in and out deeply
- Call a friend
- Count your blessings
- Dance
- Do a crossword puzzle
- Do yoga
- Feed the birds
- Get a massage
- Get a hug
- Give a hug
- Go to a museum
- Go window-shopping

- ✔ Laugh
- ✔ Listen to music
- ✔ Meditate
- ✔ Pet an animal
- ✔ Play childhood games, with or without children
- ✔ Read a book
- ✔ Rent a movie
- ✔ Ride a bike
- ✔ Sing
- ✔ Smell the flowers
- ✔ Take a bath
- ✔ Take a drive
- ✔ Take a nap
- ✔ Weed the garden
- ✔ Write your feelings in a journal

You call it dieting; your body calls it starving

When you go on a diet, your body doesn't know whether your goal is to squeeze into a small pair of jeans or to protect yourself from death from starvation. So it reacts in the only way it can: It hoards the calories that you give it. The psychological results of dieting and starvation are similar as well. People who are "always on diets" exhibit psychological behaviors similar to those of people who are starving in prison camps.

A landmark study done during World War II (see the *Journal of Clinical Psychology* 4, 1948) clearly shows how similar the effects of dieting and starving are. Normal-weight men who were conscientious objectors to the war were asked to restrict their eating for 6 months to lose about 25 percent of their body weight so that the effects of starvation could be studied. The men reduced their normal intake by about 25 percent; if they stopped losing weight, their intake was restricted even more. While they were being starved on their diets, they became increasingly focused on food; they collected recipes and replaced pinup pictures of women with pictures of food. They were irritable, upset, and argumentative. They became apathetic and lethargic. When they were allowed to regain their weight, they gorged themselves and didn't feel in control of their eating. They continued to be obsessed with food.

Chronic dieting

If you are a chronic dieter, you may be at risk of developing the same psychological characteristics of people who are starving: a tendency to eat excessively once you are "allowed" to eat, to become overly emotional, to have trouble concentrating, and to obsess about food and eating. How you answer the following question is a good indication of whether you're dieting too much: What would you do if the scale showed an extra 5 pounds?

If you're a dieter, you'd probably overeat. That's what researchers at the University of Toronto, Ontario, Canada found when they weighed dieters and non-dieters and told them that they weighed 5 pounds heavier or 5 pounds lighter than their actual weights (see the *Journal of Abnormal Psychology* 107, 1998). Dieters who believed that they were heavier experienced lowered self-worth and a worsening of mood that led them to relinquish their dietary restraint and overindulge in available food. Non-dieters and dieters who were told that they weighed 5 pounds less were not affected by the false weight feedback.

The bottom line

To get over overeating, you need to start listening to your body. As simple as it sounds, it's the only way to change your habits once and for all. If you're hungry, eat. When you're full, stop. Remembering these two simple rules puts you on the road to healthy eating for the rest of your life.

Chapter 7

Eating Disorders: When Dieting Goes Too Far

*E*ating disorders are a difficult problem to understand if you personally don't have one. They're difficult to treat and cure, too. And it's not only the person with the eating disorder who's affected; family and friends also feel the pain and anguish.

Eating disorders are a serious and growing problem in our society today. But just because you go on a diet doesn't mean that you'll get one. The vast majority of dieters don't turn their diet plans and activities into eating disorders. For those who do, however, the mental and physical consequences can be severe.

What causes eating disorders? Contrary to popular belief, eating disorders aren't just about being fat or thin, about food or weight. Instead, eating disorders are typically about self-esteem, depression, power, communication, or self-expression. Many factors can contribute, including society's emphasis on being thin and physically beautiful; prevalence of dieting in our culture; pressure by oneself or others that people should be perfect; and food and nutrition beliefs. Often, eating disorders begin when a person is dealing with a major problem or transition in life, such as alcoholism, death, divorce in the family, leaving home to go to school, or getting married. The person feels out of control and helpless and food provides them with unconditional comfort. Experts view eating disorders as a combination of physical, emotional, spiritual, and cultural factors gone awry. Eating disorders are very complex and take a long time to treat and cure.

How do you know if you're at risk for an eating disorder? The following questionnaire (which is reprinted with permission from Anorexia Nervosa and Related Eating Disorders, Inc., or ANRED) can help you decide whether you have an eating disorder or whether you are at increased risk of developing one. Circle the numbers of the items that describe you. The more items you circle, the more likely you are to have tendencies toward an eating disorder.

1. Even though people tell me I'm thin, I feel fat.

2. I get anxious if I can't exercise.

3. [Female] My menstrual periods are irregular or absent.

   [Male] My sex drive is not as strong as it used to be.

4. I worry about what I will eat.

5. If I gain weight, I get anxious and depressed.

6. I would rather eat by myself than with family or friends.

7. Other people talk about the way I eat.

8. I get anxious when people urge me to eat.

9. I don't talk much about my fear of being fat because no one understands how I feel.

10. I enjoy cooking for others, but I don't usually eat what I've cooked.

11. I have a secret stash of food.

12. When I eat, I'm afraid that I won't be able to stop.

13. I lie about what I eat.

14. I don't like to be bothered or interrupted while I'm eating.

15. If I were thinner, I would like myself better.

16. I like to read recipes, cookbooks, calorie charts, and books about dieting and exercise.

17. I have missed work or school because of my weight or eating habits.

18. I tend to be depressed and irritable.

19. I feel guilty when I eat.

20. I avoid some people because they bug me about the way I eat.

21. When I eat, I feel bloated and fat.

22. My eating habits and fear of food interfere with friendships or romantic relationships.

23. I binge eat.

24. I do strange things with my food (cut it into tiny pieces, eat it in special ways, eat it on special dishes with special utensils, make patterns on my plate with it, secretly throw it away, give it to the dog, hide it, spit it out before I swallow, etc.)

25. I get anxious when people watch me eat.

26. I am hardly ever satisfied with myself.

27. I vomit or take laxatives to control my weight.

28. I want to be thinner than my friends are.

29. I have said or thought, "I would rather die than be fat."

30. I have stolen food, laxatives, or diet pills from stores or from other people.

31. I have fasted to lose weight.

32. In romantic moments, I cannot let myself go because I am worried about my fat and flab.

33. I have noticed one or more of the following: cold hands and feet, dry skin, thinning hair, fragile nails, swollen glands in my neck, dental cavities, dizziness, weakness, fainting, rapid or irregular heartbeat.

The Many Faces of Eating Disorders

Eating disorders come in several forms. Anorexia nervosa, bulimia nervosa, and binge eating disorder are the most common and are described in detail later in this chapter. For information at a glance, Table 7-1 illustrates the specific similarities and differences among them.

Table 7-1 Anorexia Nervosa, Bulimia Nervosa, and Binge Eating Disorder: How They Differ and How They Are Similar

	Anorexia Nervosa	Bulimia Nervosa	Binge Eating Disorder
Estimated prevalence*	Up to 0.5-1.0%	Up to 1.0%	Up to 2.0%
Male versus female incidence	5-10% male versus 90-95% female	5-10% male versus 90-95% female	Unknown

(continued)

Table 7-1 *(continued)*

	Anorexia Nervosa	*Bulimia Nervosa*	*Binge Eating Disorder*
Typical age of onset	Early to middle adolescence	Late teens to early 20s	Any age, but usually not recognized until adulthood
Weight	Extremely thin and emaciated; < 85% of normal or ideal body weight	Near-ideal body weight, but often has weight fluctuations	Usually overweight or obese
Self-esteem	Low	Low	Low
Depression	Common	Common	Common
Substance abuse	Rare	Common	Rare
Rate of weight loss	Rapid	Repeatedly loses and gains weight or chronically diets without losing weight	Repeatedly loses and gains weight or chronically diets without losing weight
Past dieting	Yes	Yes	Yes

* Determining accurate statistics is difficult because physicians are not required to report eating disorders to a health agency, and because people who have eating disorders tend to deny that they have a problem and are very secretive about their behaviors.

Anorexia nervosa

A person may have anorexia nervosa when he or she diets to the point of weighing only 85 percent of ideal weight (or a BMI of 17.5 — see the chart in Chapter 2), fears gaining weight, is preoccupied with food, develops abnormal eating habits, stops menstruating, or, if male, experiences a decrease in sexual drive or interest in sex.

Anorexia nervosa is an eating disorder in which a person refuses to maintain his or her body weight at or above a minimally normal weight for his or her age and height. The person also has an intense fear of gaining weight or becoming fat, even though he or she is obviously underweight. Anorexia nervosa affects about 1 in 2,400 adolescents and tends to develop in early to mid-adolescence when body fat increases from 12 percent before puberty to about 20 to 25 percent after. This increase in body fat is not true weight gain in the adult sense, but a natural biological function of female development.

Ninety to 95 percent of anorexics are female and 75 percent of the young women who develop anorexia nervosa do not have a history of being overweight.

In addition to the physical changes that accompany anorexia nervosa, pronounced emotional changes such as irritability, depression, moodiness, and increasing isolation are also common. In fact, eating disorder experts have developed a profile of personality and family traits characteristic of a person with anorexia nervosa. Anorexics tend to be compliant, approval seeking, conflict avoiding, perfectionist, socially anxious, and obsessive/compulsive, with average or above-average intelligence. Their family environment may include a mother who is overprotective, critical, intrusive, and domineering and a father who is passive, withdrawn, and emotionally absent from the family. Although not every person who develops anorexia exhibits all or even some of these traits — nor may his or her family — they help paint a picture of the issues that many anorexia nervosa sufferers must struggle to overcome.

Do you (or someone you know) have any of the following symptoms? The more "yes" answers, the greater the likelihood that you (or he or she) may have anorexia nervosa.

- Skips meals, takes only tiny portions, and will not eat in front of other people
- Eats in ritualistic ways, such as cutting up food into extremely small bites or chewing every bite excessively, and creates strange food combinations
- Grocery shops and cooks for the entire household but will not eat
- Always makes excuses not to eat: "not hungry," "just ate with a friend," "feeling ill," and so on
- Becomes "disgusted" with former favorite foods such as red meat and desserts
- Will eat only a few "safe" foods; boasts about how healthy the meals he or she does consume are; drastically reduces or completely eliminates fat intake
- Says that he or she is too fat, even when this is not true, and has a distorted body image
- Becomes argumentative with people who try to help
- Has trouble concentrating
- Denies anger, making statements such as, "Everything is okay. I'm just tired and stressed."

✔ Withdraws into self, becoming socially isolated

✔ Often exercises excessively

Bulimia nervosa

Bulimia nervosa is characterized by recurrent episodes of binge eating followed by purging behaviors such as self-induced vomiting, misuse of laxatives or diuretics, fasting, or obsessive exercise, in an attempt to prevent weight gain from occurring as a result of the bingeing. Bulimia occurs in adolescents and young adult women but is relatively uncommon in men, and typically develops in the late teens or early twenties. Some authorities believe that as many as 10 percent of women are affected over their lifetimes. Clinically speaking, a person with bulimia nervosa binges at least twice a week, eats large amounts of food in a relatively short period of time, and then purges to rid his or her body of the unwanted calories. More than half of bulimics are severely depressed and often suffer from alcohol and drug abuse in addition to their eating problems. Unlike the anorexic, who is excessively thin, the bulimic is usually within a normal weight range, but his or her weight fluctuates.

Do you (or someone you know) have any of the following symptoms? The more "yes" answers, the greater the likelihood that you (or he or she) may have bulimia nervosa.

✔ Gorges, usually in secret, and may also buy special binge food; is uncomfortable eating around others

✔ Is usually at or around normal weight for height but has wide weight fluctuations

✔ Makes excuses to go to the bathroom after meals

✔ Buys large amounts of food that suddenly disappear

✔ Displays unusual swelling around the jaw and cheeks; knuckles may be scraped or calluses formed on back of hand from inducing vomiting

✔ Has dental enamel erosion or an excessive amount of dental caries due to vomiting

✔ Eats large amounts of food on the spur of the moment and feels out of control, unable to stop eating

✔ Doesn't seem to gain an excessive amount of weight given amount of food regularly consumed

✔ Often exercises excessively

- Frequently throws laxative or diuretic wrappers in the trash can, and may leave excessive numbers of empty boxes, cans, and food packages as well

- Runs water to cover the sound of vomiting, may use mouthwash and breath mints excessively, and may have a foul-smelling bathroom

- Can't explain the disappearance of food in the home or residence hall setting

- May engage in drug or alcohol use and/or in casual or even promiscuous sex

- Experiences mood swings; may experience depression, loneliness, shame, and feelings of emptiness (although may pretend to be cheerful)

Binge eating disorder

Binge eating disorder can happen at any age, but it's often not recognized until adulthood. It's similar to bulimia nervosa, but without purging activities. Victims of binge eating disorder eat large amounts of food at least twice a week, often in a relatively short time. They eat to escape from emotions, yet food makes them feel out of control. They often avoid social situations where food may be served but are preoccupied — even obsessed — with food, dieting, and their body weight. Most binge eaters are overweight or obese and may have obesity-related disorders such as high blood pressure, high blood cholesterol levels, or type 2 diabetes.

Do you (or someone you know) have any of the following symptoms? The more "yes" answers, the greater the likelihood that you (or he or she) have binge eating disorder.

- Frequently eats an abnormally large amount of food in a discrete period of time

- Eats rapidly

- Eats to the point of being uncomfortably full

- Often eats alone and in private to hide eating; in front of others, eats only small amounts

- Shows irritation and disgust with self after overeating

- Does not purge by vomiting, abusing laxatives, or vigorously exercising

- Is usually sedentary

Athletes with eating disorders

Although not quite as common as people with anorexia nervosa, bulimia nervosa, and binge eating disorder, athletes with eating disorders are surprisingly common among men and women who participate in sports and other activities that emphasize appearance and a lean body, such as ballet and other forms of dance, figure skating, gymnastics, running, swimming, horse racing and riding, and rowing. Wrestlers are especially vulnerable. In fact, some of the first studies on binge eating disorder were done on them. Before a match, it's common for wrestlers to binge to carbo-load and then purge so that they can qualify for a lower weight class.

Female athletes run a twofold risk of developing an eating disorder. They face all the usual conflict about their bodies, appetites, and needs for approval. But athletes also face the demands of sports that prize low body fat and unrealistic body shapes, sizes, and weights. For males, the pressures are different, which may account for their lower risk. Dieting is the primary risk factor for developing an eating disorder, and generally speaking, fewer men diet than women. Plus, many more of the male-dominated sports require strength and mass than traditionally female-dominated sports, so thinness is not as much of an issue.

Who Gets Eating Disorders?

Generally speaking, bright, energetic, attractive, conscientious, hard-working people of all races and economic classes get eating disorders. Ninety to 95 percent are female. They are most often between the ages of 12 and 25, although some cases have been reported in people much younger and much older.

People who are vulnerable to eating disorders also may have relationship problems, biological predispositions, and psychological disturbances that change their thinking. Many factors can trigger an eating disorder. The one thing that all those who suffer from eating disorders have in common is a history of dieting.

The Triggers of Eating Disorders

Eating disorders may be triggered for many different reasons. Dieting is one possible reason, some people argue, because the disorders share dieting as a common thread. They think that if dieting did not exist, there would be far fewer eating disorders and argue that people wouldn't get caught in the following cycle:

✔ Severe calorie restrictions make them ravenously hungry.

✔ They overeat in response to the unbearable hunger (bulimia nervosa and binge eating disorder).

✔ They panic about gaining weight, which brings them back to dieting and all the physical and psychological consequences that accompany food restriction. (See Chapter 5 for more on the mechanism of hunger.)

Of course, not all dieters develop eating disorders. And many of the reasons that people develop eating disorders may have little to do with food or dieting. This next section presents some of the major factors identified by ANRED.

Psychological factors

The label "perfectionist" describes many people with eating disorders. They demand success and excellence from themselves. Their achievements are many, but they may feel inadequate, defective, and worthless. Some people with eating disorders try to take control of themselves and their lives by managing their food and their weight, which gives them a sense of accomplishment. In addition, they see everything as either good or bad, black or white, fat or thin. And if thin is good, thinner is better. Some are searching for an identity. Dieting gives them the sense of self: "I am a successful dieter, therefore I matter. I diet, therefore I am."

Men get eating disorders, too

Only 5 to 10 percent of people with anorexia nervosa are male, and 5 to 10 percent of bulimics are male. Males tend to develop anorexia nervosa at older ages than females do. No statistics about the number of male binge eaters have been collected yet, but some researchers believe that males and females binge in equal numbers.

The factors that precipitate eating disorders in a male are similar to causes for females:

✔ History of being obese or overweight or dieting

✔ Involvement in sports that require thinness, such as running, track and field, horseback riding, wrestling (reduced weight means competing in a lower weight category), and body building (body fat and fluid reserves are depleted to increase definition)

✔ Involvement in professions that value thinness, such as modeling and acting

✔ Living in a culture or among people who value attractiveness and may judge men as critically as women

---

Biological factors

Genetics (at least in part) determine personality, and some personality types are more vulnerable to eating disorders than others. People who have low self-esteem and/or are socially anxious, value perfectionism, avoid conflict, and constantly seek approval from others are more likely to develop an eating disorder than are others who don't possess these traits.

Familial factors

The families of people with eating disorders often are overprotective and strict and have trouble resolving conflict. These families may value achievement and success and discount doubt and anxieties. Imperfections are criticized. These families may place a premium on physical appearance, making overt or teasing comments about someone's shape and size.

Social factors

Experts such as L. K. George Hsu, M.D., professor of psychiatry at Boston's Tufts University, believe that culture influences the onset of an eating disorder. We believe that body weight is determined by willful, conscious self-control. We are flooded by messages that being thin has its advantages. Like it or not, in our society, thinness is equated with attractiveness, and with that comes power, success, and popularity. Additionally, we have an abundance of food and an ever-increasing variety of cuisines and foods to choose from. It's an easy — and cheap — way to indulge, and advertisers often encourage it. We graze, never actually sitting down to a meal. Instead of eating socially with friends and families, hectic schedules drive us to eat alone. There are few "rules" for defining what makes an appropriate meal. Cereal for dinner? Sure. Cold pizza to start the day? Why not? And in the face of so many choices and opportunities for lack of "discipline," society considers loss of control over eating to be morally wrong. Fat people are labeled as failures — lonely, weak, and stupid. And so the conflict of appetite versus control begins.

The Medical Consequences of Eating Disorders

Make no mistake: Eating disorders — particularly anorexia nervosa — can be deadly. The following lists explain the many medical consequences of eating disorders.

Eating disorders may cause the following symptoms:

- In a person with anorexia nervosa, the heart muscle changes and its beat becomes irregular, potentially leading to cardiac arrest and death.

- Dehydration, kidney stones, and kidney failure may result in death.

- Liver damage (made worse if substance abuse is also a factor) may result in death.

- Menstruation often stops, even before extensive weight loss. This is called *amenorrhea* and can lead to infertility and bone loss or osteoporosis.

- Muscles waste away, resulting in weakness and loss of function.

- Slowed digestion caused by a lack of energy and diminished body function results in bowel irritation and constipation.

- Permanent loss of bone calcium leads to fractures and lifelong problems of osteoporosis.

- The person becomes intolerant to cold (especially in the hands and feet), and has sunken eyes, hair loss, bloating, and dry skin.

- The immune system weakens.

- Skin becomes dry and blotchy and has an unhealthy gray or yellow cast.

- Anemia and malnutrition may result.

- Fainting spells, sleep disruption, bad dreams, and mental fuzziness may result.

In addition to the complications in the preceding list, the following common medical complications associated with bulimia nervosa result from repeated cycles of bingeing and purging:

- Loss of muscle mass from excessive vomiting may occur.

- Vomiting and abuse of laxatives and diuretics flush sodium chloride and potassium from the body, resulting in an electrolyte imbalance. *Arrhythmia* (irregular heartbeat) can result, which can ultimately lead to heart failure and death.

✔ Stomach acids in vomit can erode tooth enamel, resulting in damage such as cavities and discoloration. The acids can go into the salivary glands in the month, causing swollen glands in the neck, stones in the salivary ducts, and "chipmunk cheeks."

✔ Self-induced vomiting can result in irritation and tears in the lining of the throat, esophagus, and stomach.

✔ Laxative abuse can create a dependence and result in an inability to have normal bowel movements.

✔ Abuse of medications to help induce vomiting, such as ipecac, can result in toxicity, heart failure, and death.

The medical consequences of binge eating disorder are most often associated with obesity and include the following:

✔ High blood pressure, elevated cholesterol levels, and elevated triglyceride levels, which may cause hardening of the arteries and heart disease

✔ Increased risk of bowel, breast, and reproductive cancers

✔ Increased risk of diabetes

✔ Increased risk of arthritic damage to the joints

Psychological Problems Associated with Eating Disorders

Tragically, a person with an eating disorder strives for control and self-esteem. But the disease produces the opposite effect. A person with an eating disorder may find that she or he must struggle with any of the following psychological problems in addition to the physical symptoms:

✔ Feels hopeless. May give up and sink into fatalism or denial. Depression can lead to suicide.

✔ Feels out of control and helpless to do anything about his or her problems.

✔ Suffers from anxiety and self-doubt.

✔ Feels guilt and shame.

✔ Is fearful of being discovered.

✔ Has obsessive thoughts and preoccupation with food and eating.

Treatment for Eating Disorders

Treatment works for at least 60 percent of people with eating disorders. They can return to and maintain healthy weights and eat normally. They can develop healthy relationships with people, raise families, and build careers.

But despite often intense treatment, about 20 percent do not recover fully. These people remain focused on food and their weight. They can't feel comfortable with friends or in romantic relationships. They work, but usually don't have meaningful careers.

The remaining 20 percent do not improve, even with treatment. Their lives continue to revolve around food and weight. Unfortunately, without proper treatment, up to 20 percent of people with serious eating disorders will die. But with therapy, the number of fatalities drops drastically to 2 to 3 percent.

The treatment for eating disorders is individual and specific to the person suffering. Because many factors contribute to the development of an eating disorder, a team approach makes for the best treatment. The professionals on the health care team include doctors, registered dietitians, psychologists or psychiatrists, and social workers. Counseling includes many stages, some in individual sessions and some in groups. But in general, the goals of treatment by the health care team include:

✔ Return and maintenance of normal or near-normal weight

✔ Ability to eat a varied diet of normal foods (not just low-calorie, nonfat, non-sugar items) and the elimination or major reduction of irrational food fears

✔ Restoration of relationships with family members and friends

✔ Learning of problem-solving and coping skills

Anorexia nervosa

More than 25 percent of patients with anorexia nervosa require inpatient hospitalization until they reach 85 percent of their ideal body weight. Outpatient programs are another good option for those who have not lost so much weight. Psychotherapy, family counseling, and medical nutrition therapy to help regain lost weight are part of the team approach needed to take on this disease. Drug therapy has not been effective in treating anorexia nervosa, although drugs may be used to treat depression and other psychological problems common to patients with this disease.

Bulimia nervosa

The treatment of bulimia nervosa is usually conducted on an outpatient basis. Psychotherapy is effective, especially in a group setting. Family counseling and medical nutrition therapy are also an important part of the treatment plan. Many psychiatrists prescribe antidepressants to treat bulimia nervosa because they may help reduce the frequency of purging episodes. Recently, Prozac won FDA approval specifically to treat bulimia.

Binge eating disorder

Treatment for binge eating disorder is similar to that used for treatment of bulimia nervosa, often including psychotherapy (especially cognitive behavioral therapy), family therapy, and medical nutrition therapy. Antidepressants may be effective in treatment as well.

What to Do If Someone You Know Has an Eating Disorder

If someone you know has an eating disorder, you can help. The problem is, the person who has the eating disorder may deny having a problem. That denial may leave you, the supporter, feeling powerless, confused, frightened, or even angry.

It helps to understand that people with anorexia refuse to believe that their eating patterns are abnormal. Binge eaters and those with bulimia are more likely to recognize that they have a problem, but they may still be skittish about seeking treatment. People with eating disorders may deny that they are too thin or that they purge or vomit, despite the mounds of evidence that you may be tempted to present to them. *Don't* push them — and *don't* show them documentation of your case.

Instead, first realize that eating disorders require professional treatment. Do some background research on treatment, referral centers, and support groups in your area (check with your local school system, university, medical center, or mental health center for recommendations and help). Ask your family doctor for an eating disorder referral. If you're a student, see the school nurse or school counseling center.

If you decide to talk to the person about the eating disorder, it's critical to do so in a nonthreatening, caring, and nonjudgmental way. Some important do's and don'ts:

- ✔ *Do* listen and be supportive.

- ✔ *Do* care and nurture.

- ✔ *Do* provide information.

- ✔ *Do* encourage professional help.

- ✔ *Don't* be judgmental.

- ✔ *Don't* dwell on eating, weight, or appearance.

- ✔ *Don't* insist that the person eat, not eat, or change attitudes about eating.

- ✔ *Don't* nag, criticize, or shame the person.

- ✔ *Don't* try to police or control the person.

- ✔ Most important, *don't* ignore the problem. Instead, help the person get the help that he or she needs.

Remember, too, that recovering from an eating disorder takes a long time. There's no such thing as overnight success. Just because symptoms are no longer visible doesn't mean that the disorder is cured. Changing behaviors and attitudes about food can take months or years. So hang in there — and be the support that your friend or loved one so desperately needs.

Where to Find Help

If you or someone you know is suffering from an eating disorder, look to these sources.

Information centers

American Dietetic Association
216 W. Jackson Blvd.
Chicago, IL 60606
www.eatright.org
Call 800-366-1655 for a referral to a registered dietitian in your area who specializes in disordered eating. For general questions, call 900-CALL-AN-RD (900-225-5267).

Anorexia Nervosa and Related Eating Disorders (ANRED)
P. O. Box 5102
Eugene, OR 97405
541-344-1144
An eating disorder information clearinghouse. You can download all the information via the Internet at www.anred.com.

Eating Disorders Awareness and Prevention, Inc. (EDAP)
603 Stewart Street, Suite 803
Seattle, WA 98101
206-382-3587
www.members.aol.com/edapinc

International Association of Eating Disorders Professionals
123 NW 13th Street, #206
Boca Raton, FL 33432
800-800-8126 or 561-338-6494
A referral center for treatment, as well as an association.

Massachusetts Eating Disorders Association (MEDA)
1162 Beacon Street
Brookline, MA 02146
617-738-6332
Open Monday through Friday, 10 a.m. to 4 p.m. EST. Gives referrals.

The National Association of Anorexia Nervosa and Associated Disorders (ANAD)
Box 7
Highland Park, IL 60035
847-831-3438
www.laureate.com
Offers free eating disorder information and prevention services, hotline counseling, support groups, and referrals to health care professionals.

Self-help groups

O-Anon for Family and Friends
General Service Office
P. O. Box 748
San Pedro, CA 90733
310-547-5226
Support services for families and friends of compulsive overeaters.

Overeaters Anonymous (OA)
P. O. Box 44020
Rio Rancho, NM 87174-4020
505-891-2664
An international self-help group for anorexics, bulimics, and compulsive overeaters. The office answers phone calls, distributes meeting lists, gives general information about the program, and sells literature.

Chapter 8

What to Do If Your Child Is Overweight

*I*f you live in the United States and have a child, there's a one in five chance that your child is overweight. Like the adult population, children are getting fatter. In fact, the number of overweight children has increased by more than 50 percent over the last 20 years, and the number of extremely overweight children has doubled. Because overweight children have a good chance of becoming overweight adults, they often enter adulthood at increased risk for a number of health problems, including diabetes, heart disease, high blood pressure, and stroke. In addition to health worries, fat children face painful social pressures from their peers.

If you're concerned about your child's weight, read this chapter and discuss your child's situation with your pediatrician. But think twice about starting your youngster on a weight-loss plan. Childhood weight issues are complex and varied. Don't impose adult diet or body standards on your growing child; serious emotional, psychological, and physical damage can result. Consult with your pediatrician first.

Why Children Are Overweight

Children become overweight due to either genetic tendencies, lack of physical activity, unhealthy eating habits, or a combination of these factors. In some rare cases, an endocrine disorder is to blame. Your pediatrician can perform an exam and blood test, if needed, to rule out this possibility.

Nurture or nature

Sometimes, the apple doesn't fall far from the tree. If a parent or sibling is very overweight, chances are that the child will be, too. The odds of a child becoming overweight increase dramatically if both parents are overweight. But why?

Researchers have been asking that question for some time. In a series of studies on twins, researchers found that the likelihood of becoming fat is estimated to be between 65 and 75 percent if you have a family history of obesity. (For comparison, the genetic risk for breast cancer is about 45 percent.) Researchers found that when identical twins were placed in separate adoptive homes, the twins' bodies looked more like each other's and those of their biological parents than the bodies of their adoptive parents — the homes in which they were raised. More recent work on twins shows that twins often share similar metabolic rates, eating styles, and food preferences, too, even when they are raised separately. The twin studies have been criticized by some experts for assuming that all environmental conditions are the same, which may or may not be true.

Genes alone don't sentence a child to a life of obesity. Many experts think that the way a child is raised is even more important. If nature is the genetic pool that humans swim in, then nurture is the location of that pool and the way it's maintained. Ethnic background, geographical location, and socioeconomic status may influence weight. In fact, contrary to the twin studies, many genetic experts argue that the inherited component of weight is much closer to 30 percent on average, compared to the 65 to 75 percent chance purported by the researchers who studied the twins. They argue that so many factors may be involved in determining weight that pinpointing the precise determinant is hard. They also point out that the role of genes varies from person to person — it may be 5 percent for one person, 95 percent for another.

Activity is key

It is crystal, in-your-face clear that a lack of physical activity leads to excess weight in both children and adults. Interesting is the correlation between the amount of time a child watches television and his or her weight. The more TV a child watches, the heavier he or she is. Experts think that there are two reasons for this phenomenon. First and foremost, while children watch TV, they are inactive and therefore burning few calories. Secondly, commercials often encourage consumption of high-calorie foods — and eating too many of them, of course, can result in weight gain. This also can be true for kids who spend a lot of time at the computer.

It's just baby fat, isn't it?

Your child's excess pounds are just baby fat, right? The answer may depend on *your* weight. A study of 854 children in Washington state found that obese children under 3 years old whose parents are not obese probably won't be obese as adults. But an obese child's risk of becoming an obese adult more than doubles if his or her parents are obese. And the longer a child remains overweight, the greater the likelihood that he or she will grow up to be an obese adult. Chapter 3 provides more detailed information about the critical time periods for childhood weight gain and how they relate to adult obesity.

Current eating trends and their impact on childhood weight problems

In childhood, as in adulthood, the more fat that people consume, the more calories they consume, too. And in turn, the more weight they tend to gain. That's because, bite for bite, a gram of fat delivers more than twice the number of calories that a gram of protein or carbohydrate does. Research performed at Brigham Young University [reported in the *Journal of the American Dietetic Association* 97(9), 1997] measured the amount of fat consumed by 262 children aged 9 and 10. Then the researchers compiled data on the children's weights, the parents' weights, and the level of the children's activity. The greater the amount of fat the youngsters ate, the more they weighed, even after genetics and activity level were factored in. The higher the amount of carbohydrates and fiber the children ate, the lower their weights. Fiber-rich carbohydrates are associated with lower body weights and a reduced risk of cancer and heart disease in adults as well.

Unfortunately, more children are eating their meals away from home (not including brown-bag lunches) and those meals are often higher in fat. Often, these meals are eaten at fast-food restaurants, where fiber-rich carbohydrates such as fruits, vegetables, and whole grains are hard to come by. Other common "food away from home" sources include stores, day-care centers, and school cafeterias.

Another trend is the shift from drinking milk to consuming more non-citrus juices, juice drinks, and other calorie-dense beverages. Not only has milk been squeezed out of children's menus, but the consumption of these other beverages that provide calories — and little but calories — has increased rapidly. The statistics are staggering; 3- to 5-year-olds in 1994 drank 15 percent less milk than 3- to 5-year-olds did in 1977. But they increased their juice consumption by 308 percent!

Some juice is fine, but drinking it all day long is not — no matter if it's a juice drink or 100 percent juice. Not only can constantly washing the teeth with juice lead to dental cavities, but consuming more than 12 ounces of it a day is associated with reduced height and increased obesity in 2- and 5-year-old children. (See *Pediatrics* 99, 1997.) Although counting a 4-ounce to 8-ounce glass of 100 percent fruit juice as one or two fruit servings per day is fine, in reality, juice accounts for 50 percent of all the fruit consumed by children. And juice isn't the best way to get all your fruit servings, because it doesn't provide fiber, which most children — and adults — don't get enough of in their diet. Table 8-1 shows how several popular juices compare nutritionally.

Table 8-1	Fruit Juice Nutrition Comparison			
	Orange Juice	*Grapefruit Juice (Unfortified)*	*Apple Juice*	*Grape Juice (Unfortified)*
Vitamin C	Excellent source	Excellent source	Not significant	Not significant
Potassium	Good source	Good source	Good source	Good source
Folic acid	Excellent source	Good source	Not significant	Not significant

Remember to count both juice and milk as servings from their appropriate food groups — they contain calories, but also some important vitamins and minerals. If you're looking to quench your child's thirst, go with water — it's refreshing, and calorie-free, to boot.

Determining Whether Your Child Is Overweight

Visually comparing your child's weight to those of his or her classmates and friends should give you a pretty good idea of whether your child is on the plump side. But if you like numbers, you can determine whether your child is overweight by using graphs or formulas. If your child is younger than 10 years old, follow these instructions:

Using Figure 8-1 if she is female or Figure 8-2 if he is male, plot your child's height and weight on the appropriate growth chart and determine which percentile he or she falls into.

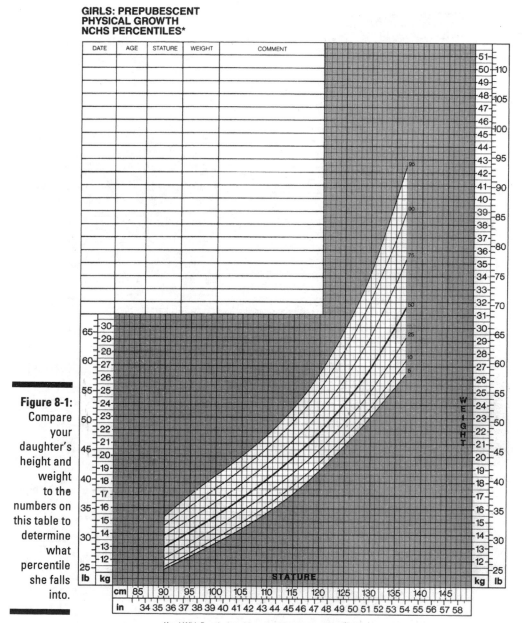

Figure 8-1: Compare your daughter's height and weight to the numbers on this table to determine what percentile she falls into.

Used With Permission of Ross Products Division, Abbott Laboratories Inc. Columbus, OH 43216

**BOYS: PREPUBESCENT
PHYSICAL GROWTH
NCHS PERCENTILES***

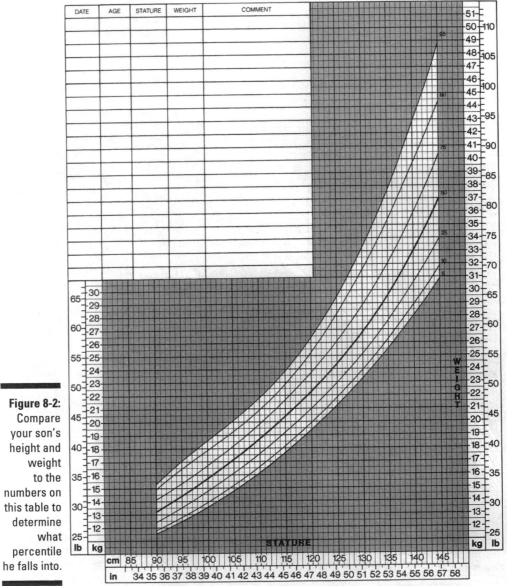

Figure 8-2:
Compare your son's height and weight to the numbers on this table to determine what percentile he falls into.

Used With Permission of Ross Products Division, Abbott Laboratories Inc. Columbus, OH 43216

As a general rule, a child who is at or above the 95th percentile is considered overweight.

For example, if a girl is 47 inches tall and weighs 60 pounds, she is above the 95th percentile and can be considered overweight. On the other hand, a girl who is 47 inches tall and weighs 53 pounds is in the 75th percentile and is not considered overweight.

For children older than 10, calculate their Body Mass Index (BMI) by using this formula:

$$\frac{\text{weight in pounds} \times 704.5}{\text{height in inches} \times \text{height in inches}} = \text{BMI}$$

For example, a 14-year-old boy who weighs 112 pounds and is 52 inches tall has BMI of 29:

$112 \times 704.5 = 78904$

$52 \times 52 = 2704$

$78904 \div 2704 = 29$

All juices are not created equal

Fruit flavor in a juice doesn't necessarily mean fruit nutrition. There are tons of juice-based beverages in supermarkets today and the nutritional value each provides varies. Some products you may think are loaded with juice don't contain much juice at all. A few tips on choosing juices:

✔ Be aware that all juice and juice products contain water and sugar. A drink labeled "100% fruit juice" contains naturally occurring sugars (fructose), whereas juice drinks, cocktails, ades, and beverages also have added sugars, such as high fructose corn syrup. However, our bodies don't use added sugar differently than the kind that nature puts in a fruit. Keep in mind, however, that the amount of added sugar will determine how many calories the juice drink contains.

✔ Read the label. Government regulations require that all juice-based beverages state the amount of juice they contain. If you opt for a product that's not 100 percent juice, you may be getting an item that contains mainly added sugar and water, with a bit of fruit flavoring thrown in for good measure. But know that 100 percent juice is not necessarily nutritionally superior. Because some juice beverages have added nutrients, they may provide more vitamin C, for example, than a product that is 100 percent real juice. However, a noteworthy difference between fruit juices and fruit drinks is that fruit juices often contain other important nutrients that fruit drinks aren't fortified with, such as folate in orange juice.

To determine whether a child is above the 95th percentile and therefore considered overweight, add 14 to the age of a boy and 13 to that of a girl. Therefore, for this boy:

$$14 + 14 = 28$$

His BMI (29) is greater than 28, so he can be considered overweight.

On the other hand, a 12-year-old girl who weighs 87 pounds and is 52 inches tall has a BMI of 23:

$$87 \times 704.5 = 61291.5$$

$$52 \times 52 = 2704$$

$$61291.5 \div 2704 = 23$$

12 years + 13 (for girls) = 27

Her BMI (23) is less than 27, so she is not overweight.

If Your Child Is Overweight

It's certainly hard for a child who is overweight — getting teased or called names, or being the last person picked for the kickball team. It's difficult for the parent, too. No parent wants to see his or her child left out of social events or hurt. If your child is overweight, you can help. But remember, the goal of weight control in children is just that: control, *not weight loss*. Instead of trying to help a child reduce his or her weight, let height catch up to weight by maintaining a slow rate of weight gain. The only exception is if the child's health is in danger because of the extra weight — and that's a decision to make with a physician.

Don't restrict food if your child is overweight. Restricting food sets up a binge mentality and metabolism similar to what a person experiences during starvation. Even after the restriction is lifted, the bingeing doesn't stop. Besides, no one has the right to withhold food from another person, even a child.

Food isn't the only thing that affects your child's weight — there are many psychological aspects to being overweight as a kid, too. If you want to help your child control weight, you can do many things to ensure that his or her self-esteem remains high, as the following sections explain.

Nurture a positive body image

Children learn by watching grown-ups. If you show your children good eating habits, they're more likely to follow your example. If you're constantly dieting and criticizing your body, they'll learn to disrespect theirs, too.

A study conducted by *Glamour* magazine on 4,000 young women (reported in the November 1994 issue) examined the effects that their mothers' dieting had on their eating habits. The study found that daughters of dieters were greatly affected by the subtle messages they received from their parents. The more often a mother dieted, the greater the likelihood that her daughter dieted, too, regardless of the child's age.

Let your children know that they are loved and perfect just the way they are. If they don't feel criticized by you for their size or shape, they will learn to accept and feel good about themselves. Let them share their thoughts about their size with you. Help them to learn that people come in all shapes and sizes and that their outsides have nothing to do with their insides. Chapter 7 offers much more information about why a positive body image and self-esteem is critical to the prevention of eating disorders, and why it plays such an important role in how people deal with food. Take a look.

Encourage physical activity

Sure, getting physical helps balance calories. But it also helps develop coordination and self-confidence. And habits that start now are more likely to follow your child into adulthood. Get the whole family involved in physical activity. Here are some ideas:

- Take walks together after dinner.
- Plan nature walks, hikes, and canoe trips for the whole family.
- Encourage your child to join school or community athletic programs — but only if he or she enjoys the activity. If it's not fun, the child won't do it, and it won't engender lifelong habits. Volunteer to coach or, at the very least, go to games and practice sessions.
- Take up sports that the whole family can do, such as inline skating, cross-country or downhill skiing, and backpacking.
- Get a rope and start jumping. Stage a family tournament.
- Teach children to ride bikes and swim at an early age. Dust off your bike, too; put on your suit and get into the pool with your kids.
- Turn off the TV. Better yet, unplug it. And limit computer and video game time.

Be sensitive about your child's size when selecting activities. Some activities will be difficult. His or her size may make movement difficult, uncoordinated, and embarrassing. And don't use physical activity as a form of punishment. One of the reasons many adults say they don't like to exercise is because as children they were made to work out as a form of discipline. Keep exercise fun.

Honor your child's body

As a parent, your job is simple — in theory, anyway. You must provide the what, when, and where food is eaten. Your child's job is to decide whether he or she will eat and how much. Whether your child is normal, underweight, or overweight doesn't matter. An overweight child should not be treated differently from other children.

A parent's responsibility is to:

- **Provide healthy food choices.** The Food Guide Pyramid (see Chapter 10) is a good place to start. When you plan a snack or meal, make sure that it includes protein, carbohydrate, and a little bit of fat. A carbohydrate-only meal or snack — such as noodles or an apple — satisfies quickly, but it doesn't have the staying power that protein and fat do. A hamburger patty or a handful of peanuts, which are mostly protein and fat, may have staying power but do not provide immediate satiety.

  Serve foods that are good sources of fiber, such as vegetables and whole grains, often. These foods have fewer calories than fiber-free foods that are high in fat and sugar, such as pastries and ice cream. Nutrition experts use this formula to determine kids' fiber needs: Take the child's age (up to 20 years old) and add 5. That's the number of grams of fiber needed daily. So a 6-year-old needs at least 11 grams of fiber per day and an 11-year-old needs 16 grams.

  It's also important to provide children with food regularly but not constantly. Children need to eat about every three hours; younger tykes may need to eat even more frequently. For adolescents who can eat more at one time, four hours between meals is fine. Don't allow children to panhandle all day with no beginning or end to the meal. Instead, schedule and serve snacks and meals at predictable times. Make snacks substantial enough to be filling, but not so large that they ruin an appetite for an upcoming meal.

- **Manage the environment as much as you can.** What food you serve and when you serve it are important. *Where* is the third leg of a parent's responsibility. Following are some tips for establishing a good meal-time environment:

  - Limit eating to one or two rooms in the house — preferably the kitchen and dining room.

- Insist that children sit while eating.

- Eat your meals together as a family as much as possible. Keep the TV off and books and toys out of sight to encourage conversation.

- Sit and eat with your child. You create a healthy social environment and serve as a role model, too.

✔ **Be a good example.** Eat the same foods that you expect your child to eat. If you want him or her to drink low-fat milk, you should have some, too — not a soda. Eat slowly and allow your child to set his or her own pace. That shows respects for his or her individual eating rhythm.

✔ **Never use food as a reward or punishment.** This approach will backfire. Studies on children and their parents show that when food (such as dessert) is given as a reward for eating another food (such as a vegetable) or food is withheld as a punishment for not eating vegetables, children decrease their desire to eat the vegetables.

✔ **Remember that it's a child's responsibility to decide whether to eat — not yours.** A child may not be hungry at one meal but may make up for it and eat heartily at the next. Trust his or her body to decide. Studies that measure children's intake show a tremendous variability over the course of a day. However, when researchers calculated the calories consumed over several days, the results showed very little difference in total calories from one day to another.

✔ **Let a child decide when to stop eating.** People are born with an innate sense of knowing when to eat and when to stop. Unfortunately, outside influences have taught most adults to ignore these signals. The best approach you can use to help children control their weight — now and in adulthood — is to encourage them to trust, honor, and listen to their own internal hunger and fullness signals. Offering advice (such as "I think you've had enough") or regulating the amount of food that a child is allowed to eat teaches distrust and fear of hunger, and may leave a child powerless and unable to take responsibility for his or her own body.

Frequently Asked Questions

If you have questions about your child's diet, you're not alone. Most parents, at one time or another, are concerned that they may not be doing the right thing when it comes to feeding their kids. You may have asked yourself these same questions.

What should I do when my child's classmates taunt him about his size?

It's undoubtedly hard for a child — and his parents — when he feels left out or is teased by peers. Other children can be cruel when a person is "different" and not realize how terrible they can make an overweight child feel. Take the time to talk regularly to your child about his feelings. Assure him that the inside of a person — not the outside — counts and that you love him no matter what his weight. Overweight children need support, acceptance, and encouragement from loved ones.

What do I do when my child refuses to eat vegetables?

Just like adults, children should aim for five servings of fruits or vegetables a day. They're good sources of fiber, they're packed with vitamins and minerals, they're low in fat, and they're important for good health and development. Even if your child isn't crazy about vegetables, you can get her to eat them — and happily — by using these tips:

- ✔ **Offer cut raw veggies as snacks.** Many kids prefer uncooked vegetables to cooked ones, and especially like to dip them. Try bean dip, hummus, salsa, or plain, low-fat yogurt flavored with seasonings as an accompaniment.

- ✔ **Know that bright colors and crisp textures are kid winners.** Steam or microwave veggies in a small amount of water to keep from overcooking them. You want them to be firm to the bite.

- ✔ **Sneak them in!** Add peas to mac and cheese; add shredded carrots or other vegetables to spaghetti sauce, lasagna, chili, tuna fish salad, or even peanut butter.

- ✔ **Bake them in.** Try low-fat zucchini and carrot muffins — your kids won't know what hit them!

- ✔ **Stir in finely chopped veggies.** Add them to meatloaf, ground turkey, ground beef, rice, or mashed potatoes.

- ✔ **Start a garden.** Most kids will eat vegetables that they grow themselves — and are proud to share the bounty with the rest of the family.

Out of sight, out of mind

The sight and smell of food can be a powerful appetite turn-on — a bogeyman of temptation for overweight children who may be especially sensitive to food cues. You don't have to ban all high-calorie foods from the house, but do limit temptation and put away the cookie jar, or don't fill it. Have bowls of fruit ready instead. The point is not to take the fun out of food, just to offer healthier, less calorie-dense options more often than nutrient-poor ones.

How do I keep my child from trading her healthful lunch for a candy bar?

Parents have been asking this question for years. A candy bar is a big temptation to most kids, and once they're out of your sight, they're out of your control, for the most part. However, you *can* help them eat healthfully even when you're not around to monitor their eating by packing items that they enjoy eating. Children often enjoy eating a little bit of a lot of things — it adds surprise and fun to their meals. Plan easy-to-eat foods like baby carrots, cherry tomatoes, cucumber slices, and pepper strips along with low-fat dip. Use a cookie cutter to turn an ordinary sandwich into an extraordinary shape. Score the rind of an orange or tangerine so that it's easier to peel, or offer fruit salad. Low-fat pudding or a few low-fat cookies are fine, too.

Most important, if you get children to help plan and prepare their own lunches, they're more likely to keep them than trade them — after all, they made them!

What are some low-calorie and healthful snacks that children can eat in the car?

Unless you must be in the car during a regularly scheduled meal or snack time, don't feel that you need to provide food. Filling idle time in the car with eating gives food too much entertainment value. You don't want to condition your children to equate riding in the car with eating, which trains them to ignore their appetites and eat for the wrong reasons. Food should be served so that children eat and only eat. When they focus their attention exclusively on the meal, without distractions, they're far more likely to recognize their innate but subtle appetite clues of hunger and satiety.

However, when schedules don't allow for dining-room meals, your youngsters will welcome snacks. Staying hydrated is most important, especially if the heat or air conditioner is running nonstop. Water is the best choice. Whole-wheat crackers, not-too-sweet cookies (such as ginger, vanilla, or graham crackers), and fruit are the healthiest snacks to carry.

What's wrong with skipping breakfast?

Many parents allow their children to skip breakfast. Parents may reason that the children aren't hungry that early in the morning, and by skipping breakfast they avoid a bunch of calories. However, eating breakfast is important because it shifts the body out of starvation mode and into action. When a body thinks that it's starving, it hoards energy by slowing down the burning of calories. Concentration becomes difficult. A child often becomes cranky and isn't able to run, play, or jump with much enthusiasm. A school-aged child won't do well in morning lessons.

The healthiest breakfasts are a combination of whole grains, some form of low-fat or fat-free milk, yogurt or cheese (for calcium and protein), and a little fat. Like any meal, avoid eating sweet breakfast foods without balancing them with fiber, protein, or fat because the sugar load can backfire in an energy crash. Be practical: Breakfast can be as simple as a granola bar or half a tuna sandwich and milk, or as homespun as a warming bowl of hot cereal sweetened with raisins. The important thing is to be sure that your child eats something every morning.

How much fast food is too much?

One or two meals of burgers, fries, and shakes aren't going to ruin a week's worth of healthy eating. But keep in mind that fast foods lack variety and generally contain too much fat and salt and very little fiber. The environment isn't conducive to relaxed eating. And the prepackaged serving sizes don't encourage eating and stopping based on internal clues.

One way to add variety is to offer lots of vegetable-rich, crunchy, fresh foods at breakfast, lunch, and snack time. Another way is to expand the kinds of restaurants you visit. Try Mexican food one night, pizza another, and a seafood dinner occasionally, and add in Asian cuisine. Not only do these various cuisines allow your children to open their taste buds to new foods and experiences and add adventure to their meals, but they also add variety — which means that they'll get a wide array of vitamins and minerals in addition to enjoying their food.

Part III
A Plan for Healthful Living

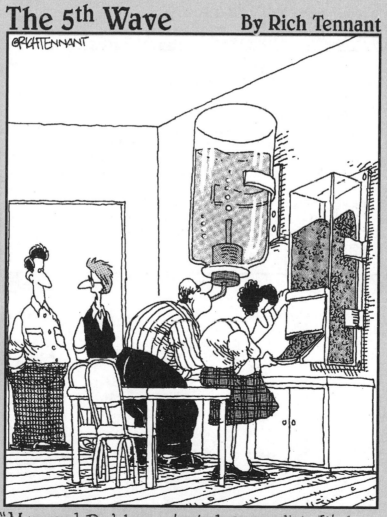

The 5th Wave   By Rich Tennant

"Mom and Dad have started a new diet. It's been proven quite effective when used on hamsters."

In this part . . .

After you understand how your weight affects your health, how your body processes calories, and how other factors besides hunger can affect your eating habits, you're ready to put a dieting plan in place. This part tells you how to set up a healthful eating plan, work physical activity into your lifestyle, and maintain your healthy weight for a lifetime. It also talks about those trendy fat substitutes and artificial sweeteners and how they fit into your diet, separating the truth from the "too good to be true."

Chapter 9

Eating for Your Health: The Dietary Guidelines for Americans

In This Chapter

▶ Making the Dietary Guidelines work for you

▶ Getting enough fiber

▶ Understanding how drinking alcohol may affect your health

*W*hile dieting, it's easy to forget that there are a lot of important reasons to eat. Instead of spending time calculating your calorie intake and expenditure with Scrooge-like precision, take the Tiny Tim approach and focus on all the good things that foods give you — like fiber, vitamins, minerals, and, of course, pleasure! Don't just concentrate on how many calories or how much fat is in a food (what you probably consider its "negatives"). In this chapter, you can find out how stepping back and looking at the big picture is the best thing that you can do for your weight, as well as your general well-being.

Many kinds of dietary recommendations come from government-funded organizations and health associations. Some recommendations are detailed and specify quantities of nutrients that you should consume daily, such as the Daily Values that you see on food labels and dietary supplement labels. Others, such as the Food Guide Pyramid and the Dietary Guidelines for Americans, are more general in nature — but they're hardly vague.

Both the Food Guide Pyramid and the Dietary Guidelines for Americans form the basis of good nutrition and health. Chapter 10 focuses on the Food Guide Pyramid and explains the different food groups and the number of servings that you need from each food group to stay healthy. This chapter examines the Dietary Guidelines for Americans and describes how to make food choices that help you get enough, but not too much, of the nutrients that your body needs for good health.

Here are the seven 1995 Dietary Guidelines for Americans, published by the U.S. Department of Agriculture, U.S. Department of Health and Human Services:

- ✓ Eat a variety of foods.

- ✓ Balance the food you eat with physical activity — maintain or improve your weight.

- ✓ Choose a diet with plenty of grain products, vegetables, and fruits.

- ✓ Choose a diet low in fat, saturated fat, and cholesterol.

- ✓ Choose a diet moderate in sugars.

- ✓ Choose a diet moderate in salt and sodium.

- ✓ If you drink alcoholic beverages, do so in moderation.

It's important to remember that guidelines are just that — suggested steps that you can take to ensure good health. Remember, too, that these recommendations are for eating patterns over several days, not for single meals or foods. For example, if you decide to eat a piece of birthday cake at your daughter's party, that's fine; you haven't ruined your diet or your eating habits. What counts is that over the course of time, your eating habits are generally low in fat, high in fiber, include plenty of fruits, vegetables, and whole grains, and are at an appropriate calorie level for you.

The Dietary Guidelines apply to all healthy Americans ages 2 and over. They provide sound nutrition advice and are updated every 5 years to incorporate the most up-to-date nutrition knowledge. The following sections take a look at each of the guidelines in detail.

Eat a Variety of Foods

For health, it's important to vary the foods you eat, because you can't get all the nutrients in the amounts you need from any one food. For example, peaches supply vitamin A but not vitamin B_{12}. Yogurt provides vitamin B_{12} but not vitamin C.

Lack of variety is one reason that single-food reduction diets, like the grapefruit diet, are not a good idea. Besides being B-O-R-I-N-G, they're nutritionally unbalanced.

Generally, eating a wide variety of foods is not a problem for most people. Serving sizes, however, are a different story. Many peoples' perceptions of what constitutes a serving are out of whack — usually much larger than recommended. We talk about serving sizes in more detail in Chapter 10.

Balance the Food You Eat with Physical Activity — Maintain or Improve Your Weight

Physical activity is just as important to good health as a well-balanced diet. Many Americans gain weight as they get older, increasing their risk of high blood pressure, heart disease, stroke, diabetes, certain cancers, and other illnesses. To maintain your body weight, you must balance the calories in the foods (and beverages) that you eat with the calories that your body uses. To lose body weight, you need to use up more calories than you eat.

Being active is an important way to use energy, or calories. But many Americans spend their leisure time being inactive — watching television or playing on their computers. To burn calories, get up and get moving! For more information about fun ways to get active, see Chapter 12.

Choose a Diet with Plenty of Grain Products, Vegetables, and Fruits

Whole-grain breads and cereals, pasta, rice, vegetables, and fruits are key parts of a varied diet because they provide vitamins, minerals, complex carbohydrates (starch and dietary fiber), and other substances that are important to good health. They're also low in fat — as long as you eat them without butter or creamy sauces. Few people eat enough of these foods, though, whether or not they're trying to lose weight.

Packing a fiber punch

Dietary fiber, which is found only in plant foods, is one of the most important components supplied by whole grains, fruits, and vegetables. Eating enough fiber helps the bowels function properly; can alleviate symptoms of chronic constipation, diverticular disease, and hemorrhoids; and may lower your risk for heart disease and some cancers. Because different foods contain different types of fiber, make sure to choose a variety of fiber-rich sources every day. And because other components of fiber-containing foods may be partly responsible for the health benefits of a high-fiber diet, make sure to get your fiber from foods as opposed to supplements.

People who eat high-fiber diets generally weigh less than those who don't. This may be true, in part, because fiber-rich foods are filling and people who eat enough of them feel full, so they aren't hungry for "extras" like cake, candies, and other low- or no-fiber treats.

There are two kinds of dietary fiber:

- **Soluble fiber** has been proven to help decrease blood cholesterol levels, thereby reducing the risk of heart disease. Soluble fiber slows the absorption of glucose, which may help to control blood sugar levels in people with diabetes. Soluble fiber is found in foods like oats and oat bran, barley, brown rice, beans, and many vegetables and fruits (like apples, oranges, and carrots).

- **Insoluble fiber**, also known as *roughage,* is mainly responsible for keeping things moving along your digestive tract. Good sources of insoluble fiber include whole-grain breads and cereals, wheat and corn bran, many vegetables (like green beans and potatoes), and the skins of fruits and vegetables.

Most grains, fruits, and vegetables are two-thirds insoluble and one-third soluble. Fruit tends to be 50-50, and the fiber in oatmeal, barley, and legumes is about 65 percent soluble. Some manufacturers provide the amount of soluble or insoluble fiber on Nutrition Facts panels, but it's not required. Typically, you just see the total amount of dietary fiber provided. A quick tip: A food is considered to be a "good" source of fiber if it provides at least 2.5 grams per serving.

Oddly enough, there's never been a Recommended Dietary Allowance (RDA) for fiber because it isn't considered a nutrient in the way that vitamins and minerals are. Unlike vitamins, minerals, and other nutrients, fiber can't be digested. Fiber's relationship to good health and long life is so compelling, however, that the National Academy of Science, the organization that writes the RDAs, has fiber on the agenda for a future evaluation panel. There is, however, a Daily Value (DV) established for fiber, which is listed on food labels (see Chapter 14).

Health professionals recognize how important fiber is to your health. You need about 20 to 35 grams of fiber each day (a mix of soluble and insoluble) — which is a lot, considering the amount that most Americans currently eat. On average, people consume only about 11 grams of fiber — less than half the minimum amount recommended. If you don't eat enough fiber, find ways to get more into your diet. Just be sure to add it gradually to give your body time to adjust. And drink plenty of fluids, too, to help the fiber move easily through your digestive tract.

Filling up with fiber

TIP

Looking for quick and easy ways to add fiber to your diet? Try some of these delicious tips:

✔ For a side dish, have ¹/₂ cup of lentils (5 grams), cooked dried beans (7 grams), or a cooked whole grain, such as wheat berries (2 grams) or cracked wheat (3 grams). Mix it with ¹/₂ cup of vegetables, such as peas (3 grams), green beans (2 grams), or spinach (1 gram).

✔ Make an opened-faced sandwich with a sliced tomato (1 gram) and a slice of whole-grain toast (2 grams). Top it with 1 ounce of low-fat mozzarella.

✔ Select your cereals wisely. You have tons of high-fiber cereals to choose from now — some offering up to 10 grams per serving! Look for cereals that provide at least 2 grams of fiber per serving.

✔ Reach for fiber-rich fruits and think of them as ingredients, not just as snacks — especially a pear (4 grams), an apple (3 grams), a couple of figs (3 grams), 1 cup of strawberries (3 grams), or a banana (2 grams). Add them to salads, cereal, and yogurt or use them as a topping for pancakes and waffles.

✔ Make short-grain brown rice a staple (4 grams of fiber per cup). It has a rich, nutty flavor and tastes much better than the long-grain variety. If you can't find it at your local supermarket, check health food stores or Asian supermarkets.

✔ Sneak vegetables in wherever you can — pizza, soups, stir-fries, rice, sandwiches, and pasta dishes. The sky's the limit!

✔ A surprising source of soluble fiber is reduced-fat foods. The guar gum that many reduced-fat foods contain in place of fats is soluble fiber. *Caution:* This doesn't give you license to replace fresh produce and whole-grain products with faux fats, but they do contribute a marginal amount of healthful fiber. For example, one piece of Entenmann's fat-free chocolate loaf cake contains 1 gram of fiber, as does one fat-free oatmeal cookie (a full-fat one contains only ¹/₂ gram). Surprisingly, even 2 tablespoons of fat-free ranch dressing has ¹/₂ gram of fiber.

More reasons to eat more plant foods

In addition to fiber, plant foods contain many other compounds that help promote good health:

✔ Phytochemicals — which include hundreds of naturally occurring, beneficial substances — are abundant in plant foods. Although the role of phytochemicals in promoting health isn't certain, researchers think that they may help protect against certain cancers and heart disease.

✔ Plant foods are among the best sources of *folate,* a B vitamin that, among its many functions, reduces the risk of a serious type of birth defect.

✔ Minerals such as potassium, calcium, and magnesium, found in a wide variety of vegetables and fruits, may help reduce the risk of high blood pressure.

✔ Antioxidant nutrients, like vitamin C, beta-carotene (which forms vitamin A), and vitamin E, may also reduce the risk of cancer and certain other chronic diseases.

Choose a Diet Low in Fat, Saturated Fat, and Cholesterol

Yes, you do need *some* fat for good health. Fat supplies essential fatty acids and helps your body absorb the fat-soluble vitamins A, D, E, and K. But eating too much saturated fat and dietary cholesterol is linked to increased risk of heart disease. And because fat has more calories than protein or carbohydrate, cutting down on fat is also the easiest way to cut calories. All kinds of fat, regardless of how saturated or unsaturated they are, have 9 calories per gram and should comprise no more than 30 percent of your total calories. Dietary cholesterol does not provide calories, but it too should be limited — to less than 300 milligrams per day.

When wheat bread isn't really what you think

You've decided to really focus on making sure that you get enough fiber in your diet. So you pick up a loaf of wheat bread instead of your usual white variety. But be careful — just because a bread is brown in color or calls itself wheat bread, it doesn't mean that it's *whole* wheat bread.

All bread — white or wheat — is made with wheat flour. But in some breads, the flour is refined. These brown breads get their darker color from caramel coloring, not from the type of flour used. By law, any bread labeled *whole wheat* must be made from 100 percent whole-wheat flour, although the amount used can vary depending on the brand. The type of flour that's first in the ingredient list is the one present in the greatest amount.

To find high-fiber breads, read Nutrition Facts panels and ingredient lists. For maximum fiber impact, choose breads that list whole-wheat or whole-grain flour as their main ingredient.

The number of calories that you consume determines the amount of fat that you can have in your diet. No more than 30 percent of your daily calories should come from fat.

Calorie Level	Daily Fat Gram Allowance
2,000	Less than 65 grams
1,800	Less than 60 grams
1,600	Less than 53 grams
1,400	Less than 46 grams
1,200	Less than 40 grams

To quickly determine your fat gram allowance, drop the last digit of your calorie intake and divide by 3. For example:

1,500 calorie diet = 150 ÷ 3 = less than 50 grams of fat

Choose a diet low in saturated fat

Fats are made up of both saturated and unsaturated fatty acids and are categorized by the predominate kind of fatty acid they contain. Research shows that a diet high in saturated fatty acids causes blood cholesterol levels to rise even more than eating large amounts of dietary cholesterol does. The fats from meat, milk products, and tropical oils are the main sources of saturated fats in most American diets. Lesser amounts of saturated fat come from vegetable oils.

Less fat + more calories + less exercise = more weight

In 1977, Americans were getting 40 percent of their calories from fat. Ten years later, fat intake dropped to 34 percent. By 1994, that number was down to 33 percent. (Thirty percent is the recommended maximum.) Looks like America is on the low-fat track, right? Wrong. Although changes in the way consumption data was gathered may be to blame, another reason may be that between 1977 and 1994, the total number of calories that Americans ate rose 7 percent. So although the percentage of calories from fat looks like it decreased from 1977 to 1994, the drop may have been due to an increase in total calories consumed. And considering that 30 percent of men and 45 percent of women say that they rarely or never exercise, it's easy to understand why 55 percent of Americans are considered to be overweight or obese today, compared to only 20 percent in 1977.

As a guideline, remember that any fat that is solid or semi-solid at room temperature (think of butter and the fat on beef and other meats) is predominately saturated fat. Your diet should provide less than 10 percent of calories from saturated fat.

On the Nutrition Facts panel, 20 grams of saturated fat (less than 10 percent of calorie intake) is the Daily Value for a 2,000-calorie level. That translates into a 13-gram maximum of saturated fat in a 1,200-calorie diet.

When you eat fat, choose unsaturated

Unsaturated fat is classified as either *monounsaturated* or *polyunsaturated*. Monounsaturated fats are found predominantly in canola oil, olive oil, peanuts, and avocados; you get polyunsaturated fats from most other vegetable oils, nuts, and high-fat fish. Eating foods that contain either type of unsaturated fat in place of foods containing saturated fats can help reduce your blood cholesterol level. However, monounsaturated fats reduce only the harmful low-density lipoproteins (LDLs) and leave the protective high-density lipoproteins (HDLs) in place. Research shows that polyunsaturated fats reduce both LDLs and HDLs.

Trans fatty acids are a type of fatty acid formed during *hydrogenation,* which makes a fat stable and solid at room temperature. For example, stick margarine is made by hydrogenating vegetable oil. A fatty acid becomes more saturated during hydrogenation. So the softer the margarine, the less saturated it is.

Most varieties of fish contain omega-3, a type of polyunsaturated fatty acid that is associated with a decreased risk of heart disease in certain people.

Choose a diet low in cholesterol

Your body (specifically, the liver) can make all the cholesterol it needs. This type of cholesterol is referred to as *blood cholesterol*. But cholesterol also comes from foods that you eat; it's known as *dietary cholesterol*. You can get dietary cholesterol *only* from animal sources, such as egg yolks, meat (especially organ meats like liver), poultry, fish, and higher-fat dairy products. Plant foods do not contain cholesterol.

Often, foods that are high in cholesterol are also high in saturated fats. Although it was once believed that dietary cholesterol was mainly responsible for raising blood cholesterol levels, researchers now know that saturated fat is the main culprit that causes your body's cholesterol factory to work overtime. For more information about saturated fat, refer to the "Choose a diet low in saturated fat" section, earlier in this chapter. The Nutrition Facts panel lists the Daily Value for cholesterol as 300 milligrams, no matter what your calorie intake is.

Figuring out the fats

Confused about which foods contain significant amounts of saturated, polyunsaturated, or mono-unsaturated fat? Here's a quick look at which foods contain which types of fat:

Saturated	Polyunsaturated	Monounsaturated
Butter, lard	Corn oil	Canola oil
Dairy products (except nonfat)	Fish oils	Olive oil
Meat and poultry	Cottonseed oil	Peanut oil
Palm oil, palm kernel oil,	Safflower oil	Other nut oils
coconut oil	Sesame oil	
	Soybean oil	
	Sunflower oil	

Fat-busting tips

✔ Use fats and oils sparingly.

✔ Eat plenty of grain products, vegetables, and fruits.

✔ Choose lean or extra-lean meats, fish, and poultry, and trim off any visible fat. For beef, look for the word *round* or *loin* in the name, which indicates that it's a lower-fat cut — like sirloin, ground round, or top round.

✔ Use small amounts of low-fat salad dressing, whipped butter or margarine, and low-fat or fat-free mayonnaise.

✔ Use herbs, spices, lemon juice, and fat-free or low-fat salad dressings for seasoning.

✔ Consume few high-fat processed meats, such as sausage and cold cuts.

✔ Up your intake of beans (such as kidney, pinto, and Great Northern) and bean products. Not only are most of these foods nearly fat-free, but they're also a good source of protein and fiber.

✔ Choose fat-free or low-fat (1%) milk, fat-free or low-fat yogurt, and reduced-fat or low-fat cheeses.

Choose a Diet Moderate in Sugars

Sugars, which are simple carbohydrates, are found naturally in many foods, including milk, fruits, some vegetables, breads, cereals, and grains. And sugars are sometimes used as preservatives and thickeners; they're also added to foods during preparation, during processing, and at the table.

In the process of digestion, the body breaks down carbohydrates (with the exception of fiber) into sugars. Interestingly, no matter whether the sugar is added or naturally found in a food, your body can't tell the difference because, from a chemical standpoint, all sugar is the same. For example, whether you eat canned fruit packed in natural juices or canned fruit packed in heavy syrup, your body digests it in exactly the same way. The difference is that fruit packed in its own juices is much lower in calories than fruit packed in syrup because juice contains less sugar than syrup does.

Contrary to popular belief, sugar does not cause hyperactivity or diabetes. But it can cause dental cavities and supply unnecessary calories. Sugary foods are usually low in nutrients, too, so eat foods with added sugar sparingly if you want to lose weight.

Sugar shows up on food labels in many forms. If one of the terms in the following list appears as the first or second ingredient on a food label, or several are used in a single product, it's an indication that the food is probably high in sugar. It also means that the food has sugar added to it because the sugars that are naturally present in foods are not listed in the ingredients. The USDA Dietary Guidelines offer the following examples:

- ✔ Brown sugar
- ✔ Corn sweetener or corn syrup
- ✔ Fructose
- ✔ Fruit juice concentrate
- ✔ Glucose (dextrose)
- ✔ High-fructose corn syrup
- ✔ Honey
- ✔ Invert sugar
- ✔ Lactose
- ✔ Maltose
- ✔ Molasses
- ✔ Raw sugar
- ✔ [Table] sugar (sucrose)
- ✔ Syrup

Sugar substitutes

Sugar substitutes such as sorbitol, saccharin, and aspartame are ingredients in many foods. Most sugar substitutes do not provide significant calories and therefore may be useful in the diets of people who are concerned about calorie intake. Foods containing sugar substitutes, however, may not always be lower in calories than similar products containing sugars, so check labels. Unless you reduce the total number of calories you eat, the use of sugar substitutes will not help you lose weight. For more information on sugar substitutes, see Chapter 11.

Keep in mind that many reduced-fat and fat-free products are high in sugar, which also keeps their calorie contents high; so check labels before you decide to splurge. Finally, unlike the ingredient list, the Nutrition Facts panel on most food products includes sugars (which include both naturally occurring and added sugars), so it's easy to see at a glance how much sugar a food provides.

Choose a Diet Moderate in Salt and Sodium

Many foods naturally contain sodium, albeit usually in tiny amounts. Although some people add salt to their food at the table, most dietary sodium in the U.S. diet comes from foods to which salt has been added during preparation or processing. Many foods that are high in sodium don't taste salty, so beware.

Salt is chemically known as sodium chloride. Although sodium accounts for only part of table salt, most people use the words *salt* and *sodium* interchangeably.

Sodium plays an important role in the body, helping to regulate fluids and blood pressure. But if you consume too much salt, you may need more calcium because the excess salt may cause your body to excrete calcium in your urine.

The Nutrition Facts Label lists a Daily Value of 2,400 milligrams per day for sodium. Just 1 teaspoon of salt contains 2,300 milligrams of sodium — almost your entire day's allowance!

Sodium and weight gain

Eating too much sodium may make the number on the scale jump, but that's probably water weight, not fat. In time, your body will adjust and rid itself of the extra sodium.

Sodium and high blood pressure

Many studies have shown that eating a lot of sodium is associated with high blood pressure. Sodium does not cause high blood pressure any more than sugar causes diabetes, but research indicates that people at risk for high blood pressure — because it runs in their families — may reduce their chances of developing this condition by consuming less sodium. Other ways to help decrease high blood pressure include losing excess weight if you're overweight, eating enough fruits and vegetables for adequate potassium, getting sufficient calcium through low-fat and fat-free dairy products, and keeping alcohol consumption moderate to low.

Consuming sodium in moderation

✔ Limit the amount of salt you add to foods during cooking and at the table. Measure the amount you use so that you don't overdo. A sprinkle here and a sprinkle there can add up quickly. Remember: Taste before you shake.

✔ Season with spices, herbs, fruit juices, and vinegars rather than salt to heighten the flavor of your food.

✔ Gradually cut back on the amount of sodium that you consume. It takes about two weeks for your palate to get accustomed to the reduced amount — but your taste for salty foods will change.

✔ Use fresh and plain frozen vegetables. Not only are they lower in sodium than vegetables in sauce, but they're generally lower in calories, too.

✔ When selecting canned foods, select those labeled without salt, low-sodium, or reduced-sodium. Or with regular canned beans or vegetables, rinse before preparing.

✔ Many frozen dinners, packaged mixes, canned soups, and salad dressings also contain considerable amounts of sodium. Again, choose low- or reduced-sodium versions when possible.

✔ Use condiments such as soy and other sauces, pickles, olives, ketchup, and mustard in moderation. They are high in sodium.

✔ Fresh fruits and vegetables are a lower-sodium (and lower-calorie) alternative to salted snack foods — and they still provide the "crunch" factor.

✔ If you eat out frequently, be sodium-conscious. Request that foods be prepared without added salt; ask for sauces and dressings on the side; and pay attention to the terms that signal a high sodium content: *smoked, pickled, au jus, soy sauce,* or *in broth.*

If You Drink Alcoholic Beverages, Do So in Moderation

Beer, wine, and spirits may enhance your enjoyment of meals, but they supply calories and few or no nutrients. Dieters who eliminate alcoholic beverages save about 150 calories per 12-ounce bottle or can of beer or 8-ounce mixed drink, and 100 calories per 5-ounce glass of wine. In addition, the alcohol in these beverages has physiological effects and is harmful when consumed in excess. If you're an adult and you choose to drink alcoholic beverages, consume them only in *moderation,* defined as no more than one drink per day for women and no more than two drinks per day for men. (One drink equals 12 ounces of regular beer, 5 ounces of wine, or 1.5 ounces of 80-proof distilled spirits.)

If you're on this list (which was compiled by the USDA and can be found in their Dietary Guidelines), you shouldn't drink, even in moderation. The health risks for you outweigh any benefits:

✔ **Children and adolescents.**

✔ **Individuals of any age who cannot restrict their drinking to moderate levels.** This is a special concern for recovering alcoholics and people whose family members have alcohol problems.

✔ **Women who are trying to conceive or who are pregnant.** Major birth defects, including fetal alcohol syndrome, have been attributed to heavy drinking by the mother while pregnant. While there is no conclusive evidence that an occasional drink is harmful to the fetus or to the pregnant woman, a safe level of alcohol intake during pregnancy has not been established.

✔ **Individuals who plan to drive or take part in activities that require attention or skill.** Most people retain some alcohol in the blood up to 2 to 3 hours after a single drink.

✔ **Individuals using prescription and over-the-counter medications.** Alcohol may alter the effectiveness or toxicity of medicines. Also, some medications may increase blood alcohol levels or increase the adverse effect of alcohol on the brain.

More isn't better

A little alcohol may be good, but more isn't better. Moderate drinking, especially of wine, is associated with a lower risk for coronary heart disease in some individuals. Yet a higher alcohol intake raises the risk for high blood pressure, stroke, heart disease, certain cancers, accidents, violence, suicides, birth defects, and overall mortality (deaths). Drinking too much alcohol may also cause cirrhosis of the liver, inflammation of the pancreas, and damage to the brain and heart.

Chapter 10

Putting Healthful Eating Guidelines into Practice

*T*his is the chapter you've been waiting for. It pulls together all the information you've amassed on healthy eating and makes the Dietary Guidelines (see Chapter 9) easy to put into practice.

The Food Guide Pyramid is the main tool that we recommend using to help plan your diet. But it's not the only pyramid out there — the Asian Pyramid, Latin American Pyramid, Movement Pyramid, and Mediterranean Diet Pyramid are just a few of the others. You name it; someone's got a pyramid for it. The Food Guide Pyramid, however, is the original.

The Food Guide Pyramid

The Food Guide Pyramid (shown in Figure 10-1) is considered the "mother" of all pyramids. It's flexible, practical, and visual, so no matter what your eating preferences are, you can make it fit your lifestyle. Remember the Basic Four Food Groups concept? Think of the pyramid as its modern offspring, albeit with a few changes. There are now five groups instead of four (fruits and vegetables are separated), plus the tip of the pyramid, where fats, oils, and sugars reside. You can read more about each group later on in this chapter. In addition to the variety message, the Food Guide Pyramid emphasizes balance and moderation in your overall diet.

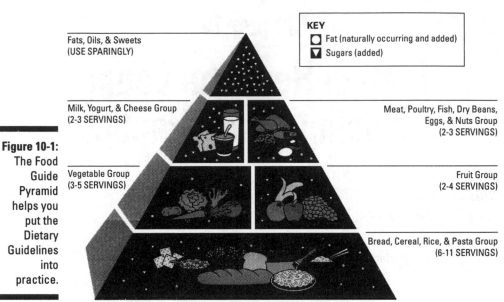

Figure 10-1:
The Food
Guide
Pyramid
helps you
put the
Dietary
Guidelines
into
practice.

Source: U.S. Department of Agriculture/U.S. Department of Health and Human Services

The Food Guide Pyramid contains the building blocks for a healthy diet. If you follow the recommended servings listed for each food group in the pyramid each day and eat lower-fat, -sugar, and -sodium choices within each group, you're sure to get enough protein, vitamins, minerals, and dietary fiber without getting excessive amounts of calories, fat, saturated fat, cholesterol, sodium, added sugars, or alcohol.

Notice that a range of servings is given for each block, or food group, of the pyramid. If you choose the lower number of servings from each group, you'll consume about 1,600 calories. If you eat the maximum number of servings, your calorie level will be more in the range of 2,800 calories.

The serving sizes are designed to help people maintain their weights depending on how active they are. The lower number is intended to provide adequate nutrition for sedentary women, and the upper limit is for active teenage boys. Individuals who want to lose weight need to stick to the lower number of servings and sometimes go lower still. (Figure 10-4, later in this chapter, gives you a look at the Weight-Loss Pyramid.)

Fats and added sugars are concentrated in foods located at the tip of the pyramid. But they're also in foods found in the other food groups. When you choose foods for a healthy diet, take the amount of fat and added sugars in those foods into consideration.

Remember:

> ✔ Choose lower-fat foods from each of the food groups.
>
> ✔ Go easy on fats and sugars added to foods in cooking and at the table.
>
> ✔ Choose fewer foods that are high in sugars — candy, soft drinks, and sweet desserts.

Using the pyramid can help you identify where the bulk of your calories are coming from. Unfortunately, many people create a top-heavy pyramid by eating too much fat and sugar and not enough grains, fruits, and vegetables, as shown in the Actual Consumption Pyramid in Figure 10-2.

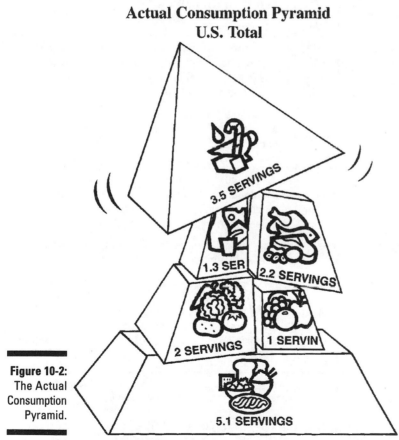

Actual Consumption Pyramid U.S. Total

3.5 SERVINGS

1.3 SER

2.2 SERVINGS

2 SERVINGS

1 SERVIN

5.1 SERVINGS

Figure 10-2:
The Actual
Consumption
Pyramid.

Source: National Cattlemen's Beef Association

Understanding What Makes a Serving

Of course, few people eat foods that fit neatly into one of the pyramid blocks. Pizza, for example, can be counted as dairy, grain, and, depending on the topping, either meat or vegetables or both. A cheeseburger piled high with lettuce and tomato and a bit of mayonnaise counts as a serving from each of the food groups.

Table 10-1 lists the sizes of many foods that constitute one serving. Check out the discussions of the individual food groups for an extended and detailed list of serving sizes.

Table 10-1	What Counts as a Serving
Food Group	*One Serving Is . . .*
Bread, Cereal, Rice, and Pasta	1 slice of bread; half a hamburger bun or English muffin; 1 small roll, biscuit, or muffin; 5 to 6 small or 3 to 4 large crackers; $\frac{1}{2}$ cup cooked cereal, rice, or pasta; 1 ounce ready-to-eat cereal.
Fruit	One whole fruit, such as a medium apple, banana, or orange; half a grapefruit; a melon wedge; $\frac{3}{4}$ cup fruit juice; $\frac{1}{2}$ cup berries; $\frac{1}{2}$ cup chopped fresh, cooked, or canned fruit; $\frac{1}{4}$ cup dried fruit.
Vegetable	$\frac{1}{2}$ cup cooked vegetables; $\frac{1}{2}$ cup chopped raw vegetables; 1 cup leafy raw vegetables, such as lettuce or spinach; $\frac{1}{2}$ cup cooked beans, peas, or other legumes*; $\frac{3}{4}$ cup vegetable juice.
Milk, Yogurt, and Cheese	1 cup milk, 8 ounces yogurt, $1\frac{1}{2}$ ounces natural cheese, 2 ounces processed cheese.
Meat, Poultry, Fish, Dry Beans, Eggs, and Nuts	Amounts should total 2 to 3 servings (for a total of 5 to 7 ounces) of cooked lean meat, poultry without skin, or fish per day. Count 1 egg; $\frac{1}{2}$ cup cooked beans, peas, or other legumes*; or 2 tablespoons peanut butter as 1 ounce of meat.
Fats, Oils, and Sweets	Use sparingly.

* Note that you can count dry beans, peas, and other legumes as either a serving of vegetables or a serving of meat, but the same bowl of beans can't count as a serving from both groups.

You've heard it before: It's not only *what* you eat, but also *how much* that's important. As people eat more foods from restaurants and convenience stores, it's difficult to remember how large a serving should be. Portions of takeout food are much larger than the standard portion sizes defined in the

Food Guide Pyramid. Even cookbooks are instructing people to serve larger portions. For example, the 1964 edition of *The Joy of Cooking* recommends cutting a 13-x-9-inch pan of brownies into 30 bars; the 1997 version is cut into 16 bars.

Table 10-2 illustrates a few discrepancies between what most people consider an "average" serving and the size that the USDA's pyramid recommends [see Young and Nestle in the *Journal of the American Dietetic Association* 98(4), 1998].

Table 10-2	How Large Is Medium?	
Food	*USDA (In Ounces)*	*Perceived as Average (In Ounces)*
Bagel	2.0	4.0
Cookies	0.5	1.0
Muffin	1.5	5.5
Potato	3.9	6.5

Looking at the Food Groups

All your favorite (and not-so-favorite) foods have a place on the Food Guide Pyramid. Foods are grouped together because their nutrient content is similar. And each of the five food groups, which we describe in detail in the following sections, supplies your body with some of the nutrients that you need for good health. Remember, some of the foods in the various groups may be higher in fat or added sugars than others, so if you're watching calories, focus on the lower-fat options that contain less added sugar.

The ground floor: Grains (6 to 11 servings)

Grains form the foundation of healthy eating; they are low in fat and provide essential vitamins, minerals, and fiber. This group is the source of complex carbohydrates in your diet. But eating too many calories here without getting beneficial nutrients is also common. Croissants, donuts, cookies, muffins, cake, and other higher-fat and -sugar items all belong to this group, but they provide more calories than nutrients and should be kept to a minimum.

Make sure that at least three of your grain servings each day are whole grains — whole-wheat bread or cereal, for example. Use the ingredient labels to find the products with whole grains: You want whole wheat or other whole grain to be the first ingredient. Sugar, oil, and fats should be last on the list, if they appear at all.

Serving sizes for grains include the following:

- ✔ 1 slice of bread
- ✔ Half a hamburger or hot dog bun
- ✔ Half an English muffin or bagel
- ✔ 1 small roll, biscuit, or muffin (about 1 ounce each)
- ✔ 1 ounce ready-to-eat cereal
- ✔ 5 to 6 small crackers (saltine size)
- ✔ 2 to 3 large crackers (graham cracker square size)
- ✔ 4-inch pita bread (white or wheat)
- ✔ 3 medium hard breadsticks, about 4³/₄ inches long
- ✔ 9 animal crackers
- ✔ ¹/₂ cup cooked cereal, pasta, or rice
- ✔ One 7-inch flour or corn tortilla
- ✔ 2 corn taco shells
- ✔ Nine 3-ring pretzels or 2 pretzel rods
- ✔ ¹/₅ of a 10-inch angel food cake
- ✔ ¹/₁₆ of a two-layer cake
- ✔ 3 rice or popcorn cakes
- ✔ 2 cups air-popped popcorn
- ✔ 12 tortilla chips

Second tier: Fruits and vegetables

Fruits and vegetables form the next layer of the pyramid. Both provide important vitamins, minerals, and fiber. Without high-fat toppings such as butter and whipped cream, they're also naturally low in fat (with few exceptions).

Fruits (2 to 4 servings)

Breakfast is a good place to begin building up fruit servings. You may already start your day with a glass of juice. Add a mid-morning snack of fruit and have some for dessert at lunch or dinner, and you've made your goal of three to four servings a day.

Make at least one serving each day a citrus fruit. Orange and grapefruit juice are standard options, but don't forget about the many varieties of oranges (navel, temple, Valencia, blood, and mandarin) and grapefruits (Ruby Red, white, and pink) that are available, as well as tangerines, tangelos, kumquats, and ugli fruit, which are also considered citrus fruits.

When choosing fruit, reach for fresh or, if canned, packed without added sugar. Experiment with new fruits that you haven't tried before — figs, guava, starfruit, or prickly pears, for example. Try less-common varieties of favorite fruits, such as Winesap or Rome apples; Casaba, Persian, or Santa Claus melons; or Comice or Seckel pears. Blend fresh or frozen fruits together with a dollop of low-fat yogurt, a splash of orange juice, and a ripe banana for a scrumptious fruit smoothie. Toss citrus segments, grape halves, or strawberries with mixed greens with a low-fat poppy seed dressing for a pretty and nutritious salad. Or sprinkle fresh or dried fruits on cereal, on frozen or regular yogurt, into muffin batter, or into rice and stuffing dishes.

With so many fruitfully delicious options to choose from, you'll never have to eat the same fruit twice in a week. Use these guidelines to determine serving sizes for fruits:

- ✔ One whole fruit (a medium apple, banana, peach, or orange; or a small pear)
- ✔ $1/2$ grapefruit
- ✔ Melon wedge ($1/4$ medium cantaloupe or $1/8$ medium honeydew)
- ✔ $3/4$ cup juice
- ✔ $1/2$ cup mandarin or clementine orange sections
- ✔ $1/2$ cup cut-up fresh fruit
- ✔ $1/2$ cup cooked or canned fruit
- ✔ $1/2$ cup frozen fruit
- ✔ $1/4$ cup dried fruit
- ✔ 5 large strawberries or 7 medium strawberries
- ✔ $1/2$ cup raspberries, blueberries, or blackberries
- ✔ 11 large cherries
- ✔ 12 grapes
- ✔ $1^1/2$ medium plums
- ✔ 2 medium apricots or clementines
- ✔ $1/8$ medium avocado (but beware of its high fat content!)
- ✔ 7 melon balls (or $1/2$ cup melon)
- ✔ $1/2$ cup fruit salad (made without mayonnaise)
- ✔ $1/2$ medium mango
- ✔ $1/4$ medium papaya

- 1 large kiwi fruit
- 4 canned apricot halves, drained
- 14 canned cherries, drained
- 1 1/2 canned peach halves, drained
- 2 canned pear halves, drained
- 2 1/2 canned pineapple slices, drained
- 3 canned plums, drained
- 9 dried apricot halves
- 5 prunes

Vegetables (3 to 5 servings)

If it weren't for French-fried potatoes and tomato sauce on pizza and pasta, many people wouldn't get any vegetables at all. Too bad, because vegetables are mostly water, so they're a great way for dieters to expand their meals. Vegetables are a great source of vitamin C, folate, beta-carotene, minerals, and fiber — and practically no fat.

Use these guidelines to determine serving sizes for vegetables:

- 1/2 cup vegetables, cooked or chopped raw
- 1 cup leafy raw vegetables, such as lettuce or spinach
- 1 medium tomato or 5 cherry tomatoes
- Seven to eight 2 1/2-inch carrot or celery sticks
- 3 broccoli florets
- 1/3 medium cucumber
- 10 medium green onions
- 13 medium radishes
- 9 snow or sugar peas
- 6 slices summer squash (yellow or zucchini)
- 1 cup mixed green salad
- 1/2 cup cole slaw or potato salad
- 1/2 cup leafy cooked greens, such as kale, Swiss chard, or spinach
- 2 spears broccoli
- 1 medium whole green or red pepper, or 8 rings
- 1 artichoke
- 6 asparagus spears

✔ 2 whole beets, about 2 inches in diameter

✔ 4 medium Brussels sprouts

✔ 1 medium ear of corn

✔ 7 medium mushrooms

✔ 8 okra pods

✔ 1 medium whole onion or 6 pearl onions

✔ 1 medium whole turnip

✔ 10 french fries

✔ 1 medium baked potato

✔ 3/4 cup sweet potato

✔ 1/2 cup tomato or spaghetti sauce

✔ 1/4 cup tomato paste

✔ 1/2 cup cooked dry beans (if not counted as a meat alternate)

✔ 3/4 cup vegetable juice

✔ 1 cup bean soup

✔ 1 cup vegetable soup

Some vegetables are "starchy" and calorie-dense; others are mostly water. If you're watching your weight, limit your starchy vegetables to one or two servings per day, and make the remainder of your veggie servings nonstarchy. Table 10-3 lists examples of starchy and nonstarchy vegetables.

Table 10-3	Vegetable Variations
Nonstarchy Vegetables	*Starchy Vegetables*
Asparagus	Beets
Broccoli	Cassava (yuca)
Brussels sprouts	Corn
Cabbage	Lima Beans
Cauliflower	Peas
Celery	Potatoes
Chicory	Pumpkin
Cucumbers	Rutabaga
Eggplanta	Sweet Potatoes
Escarole	Taro

(continued)

Table 10-3 *(continued)*

Nonstarchy Vegetables	*Starchy Vegetables*
Green beans	Turnips
Greens (such as collard, kale, mustard, and turnip)	Winter squash
Lettuce	Yams
Mushrooms	
Okra	
Peppers	
Radishes	
Sprouts	
Summer squash	
Tomatoes	

Looking for ways to up your veggie intake? Try these delicious ideas:

- ✔ Pile a sandwich high with lettuce, tomato, and vegetables.

- ✔ Start every meal with a salad made with a mix of dark green varieties of lettuce and colorful vegetables, drizzled with just a bit of low-calorie dressing.

- ✔ When you need a snack, reach for cherry tomatoes, celery, or sweet pepper strips. Many supermarkets carry small packages of celery or carrot sticks in their produce sections. They make good lunch box (or briefcase) snacks for kids of all ages.

- ✔ Toss pasta with steamed broccoli, carrots, and other veggies and top with a smidgen of Parmesan cheese for pasta primavera. Or add finely chopped veggies — such as carrots, onions, cooked eggplant, squash, or chopped spinach — to pasta sauce.

- ✔ Toss a can of veggie or tomato juice into your briefcase for a quick pick-me-up (and a serving of vegetables to boot!).

- ✔ Top a baked potato with thick vegetable salsa or stir-fried vegetables.

Third tier: Animal foods and products

Moving up the pyramid, you find foods that come mostly from animals — the Dairy group and the Meat, Poultry, Fish, Dry Beans, Eggs, and Nuts group. Foods from this level contribute important nutrients such as protein, calcium, iron, and zinc.

Cruciferous vegetables

Cruciferous vegetables — bok choy, broccoli, Brussels sprouts, cabbage, cauliflower, kale, collards, kohlrabi, mustard greens, radishes, rutabaga, turnip, and watercress — are the cancer-fighters from the garden. They're called *cruciferous* because their flowers or buds form a cross. Besides helping to protect against colon and rectal cancer, they're also good sources of calcium, iron, and folate.

Meat and meat alternates (2 to 3 servings equivalent to a total of 5 to 7 ounces

Two to 3 ounces of meat, poultry, or fish (about the size of a deck of cards) is an adequate amount of protein for a meal. Choose the select grades of beef, veal, and lamb to make sure that you get the least-marbled meats. Also, opt for lean cuts of meat such as those from the round, loin, or leg (beef sirloin, ground round, or top round; pork tenderloin or loin chop; or leg of lamb). Select lean and extra-lean ground beef. Unless you're eating fat-free cold cuts, be extra cautious in the deli; many have more fat than lean meat per slice. Most fish are naturally lean.

Trim all visible fat from meats before cooking and remove the skin from poultry before eating. And use lower-fat cooking methods, such as roasting, broiling, and grilling instead of frying, sautéing, or pan-frying.

Legumes, such as dried beans and peas, are a good substitute for meat in this group. And as a bonus, they're fat-free. Eggs, nuts, and seeds are also packed with protein and make suitable substitutes for meat. Just beware that nuts and seeds are quite high in fat — and therefore calories.

Check out these options to meet your protein needs:

Meats (each counts as 1 serving):

- ✔ 2 to 3 ounces cooked lean beef, pork, veal, or lamb without bone
- ✔ 2 to 3 ounces cooked poultry without skin or bone
- ✔ 2 to 3 ounces cooked fish without bone
- ✔ 2 to 3 ounces drained, canned fish

Meat alternates (each counts as 1 ounce, about ¹/₃ serving):

- ✔ 1 egg (yolk and white) or 2 egg whites
- ✔ ¹/₂ cup cooked dry beans (if not counted as a vegetable)
- ✔ 2 tablespoons peanut butter

✔ ¹/₄ cup seeds, such as sunflower or pumpkin seeds

✔ ¹/₃ cup nuts, such as walnuts, pecans, or peanuts

✔ ¹/₂ cup baked beans

✔ ¹/₂ cup tofu

Meat and fish products (each counts as 1 ounce, about ¹/₃ serving):

✔ 1 ounce lean ham or Canadian bacon

✔ 1¹/₂ frankfurters (10 per pound)

✔ 1 frankfurter (8 per pound)

✔ ¹/₄ cup drained canned salmon or tuna

✔ ¹/₃ cup drained canned clams or crabmeat

✔ 4 Pacific oysters or 11 Atlantic oysters

✔ 6 medium shrimp

✔ ¹/₄ cup drained canned lobster or shrimp

Dairy products (2 to 3 servings)

The Milk, Yogurt, and Cheese group shares the third tier of the pyramid with the Meat, Poultry, Fish, Dry Beans, Eggs, and Nuts group. Like foods in the meat group, dairy foods are a good source of protein. They're also some of the best sources of calcium and contribute vitamins A and D to your diet as well. A word of caution: Dairy foods can be very high in fat, so reach for fat-free, low-fat, part-skim, or reduced-fat cheeses, ice cream, frozen yogurt, ice milk, and fluid milk products when you're watching your weight.

Dairy delicious ways to get calcium and protein in your diet include the following:

✔ 1 cup milk or buttermilk

✔ 1 cup yogurt

✔ 1¹/₂ ounces natural cheese

✔ 2 ounces processed cheese

✔ 2 cups cottage cheese (it's lower in calcium than most other cheeses)

✔ ¹/₂ cup ricotta cheese

✔ ¹/₂ cup dry nonfat milk

✔ ¹/₂ cup evaporated milk

✔ 1 cup frozen yogurt or 1¹/₂ cups ice milk

Alcohol in your diet

Although alcohol isn't technically part of the pyramid, keep in mind that like items from the pyramid's tip, you get calories but no nutrients in each and every glass. Limit your consumption to no more than two drinks per day if you're male and one drink per day if you're female. A serving of alcohol is defined as

- 12 ounces of beer
- 1½ ounces of hard or distilled spirits (80 proof)
- 5 ounces of wine

Don't mistake cheese for the only ideal protein alternative to meat. Sure, it delivers some protein, but it also comes with lots of fat. If you choose not to eat meat from the meat group, go for water-packed tuna, bean and bean spreads such as hummus (made with a minimal amount of tahini paste), and soy products such as tempeh and tofu. Or choose reduced-fat cheeses or lower-fat varieties, such as feta, baby Swiss, and part-skim mozzarella.

The tiny tier: Fats, oils, and sweets

Just because this group is on the top of the pyramid doesn't mean that it's the best group. Instead, this placement means that, like a penthouse, few people can spend much time there. Scan the following list and you'll see plenty of foods that you probably eat frequently. Most of these foods contribute practically no nutrients other than sugar, fat, and calories. You don't have to *eliminate* them from your diet, even if your goal is to lose weight, but you *do* have to eat them sparingly. Besides, you get plenty of fat when you eat foods from the other groups.

Fats:

- Bacon and salt pork
- Butter
- Cream (dairy or nondairy)
- Cream cheese
- Lard
- Margarine
- Mayonnaise

> ✔ Salad dressing
>
> ✔ Shortening
>
> ✔ Sour cream
>
> ✔ Vegetable oil

Sugars:

> ✔ Candy
>
> ✔ Corn syrup
>
> ✔ Frosting (icing)
>
> ✔ Fruit drinks (unfortified)
>
> ✔ Gelatin desserts
>
> ✔ Honey
>
> ✔ Jam or jelly
>
> ✔ Maple syrup
>
> ✔ Marmalade
>
> ✔ Molasses
>
> ✔ Popsicles and ices
>
> ✔ Sherbet
>
> ✔ Soft drinks
>
> ✔ Sugar (white and brown)

The Vegetarian Pyramid

If you don't eat meat, check out the Vegetarian Pyramid, shown in Figure 10-3. Because meat, poultry, and fish are not included in a vegetarian eating plan, the foundation of this pyramid is divided equally among fruits and vegetables, legumes such as soybeans and peanuts, and whole grains. Vegetarians should include foods from these three groups at every meal. Nuts and seeds, milk or soy milk, and oils should be consumed daily, and eggs and sugars only occasionally and in small quantities. But dieters should remember that servings of nuts, seeds, and oils should be small because they are high in fat and therefore calories.

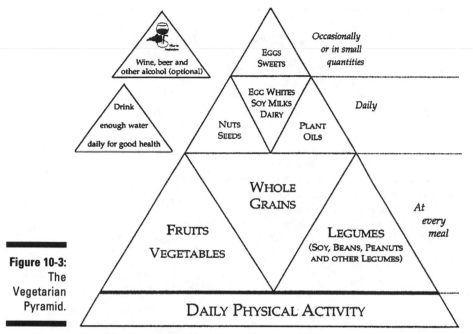

Figure 10-3:
The
Vegetarian
Pyramid.

© 1997 Oldways Preservation & Exchange Trust

Using the Pyramid for Weight Loss

Now that you have a general idea of which foods belong in which food groups, you can plan your weight-loss diet. First, revisit the material in Chapter 4 to determine your calorie needs. Then, using the information in Table 10-4, determine the number of servings from each food group that you're allowed, based on your calorie level.

Table 10-4	Food Group Servings for Various Calorie Levels		
	About 1,200	*About 1,500*	*About 1,800*
Bread group servings	5	6	8
Vegetable group servings	3	3	5
Fruit group servings	2	3	4
Milk group servings	2	2	2
Meat group	5 ounces	6 ounces	7 ounces
Fats, oils, and sweets	USE	VERY	SPARINGLY

Are vegetarian diets healthy?

There are varying degrees of vegetarianism. *Lacto-ovo vegetarians* eat dairy products and eggs and, as a group, usually meet their Daily Values for most nutrients.

Vegans eat only foods of plant origin. Because animal products are the only food sources of vitamin B₁₂, vegans must use supplements or eat breakfast cereals, soy milk products, and vegetarian burger patties that are fortified with vitamin B₁₂. In addition, vegan diets require care to ensure adequate amounts of vitamin D and calcium, which are found in dairy products. Iron and zinc are sometimes in short supply, too, because meat is a primary source of these nutrients in most people's diets.

Vegan sources of iron include

- Dry beans and peas, such as pinto beans, black-eyed peas, and canned baked beans
- Leafy greens of the cabbage family, such as broccoli, kale, turnip greens, and collard greens
- Lima beans and green peas
- Yeast-leavened whole wheat breads and rolls

Vegan sources of zinc include

- Black-eyed peas
- Miso (fermented soybean paste)
- Tofu
- Wheat germ and wheat bran
- Whole grains

Vegan sources of calcium include

- Leafy greens of the cabbage family, such as kale, mustard greens, and turnip tops; and bok choy (or pak choi)
- Tofu, if processed with calcium sulfate (read the labels)
- Tortillas made from lime-processed corn (read the labels)

Vegan sources of vitamin D include

- Fortified breakfast cereals and margarines
- Sunlight — your body makes vitamin D after sunlight (or ultraviolet light) hits your skin

The Weight-Loss Pyramid, shown in Figure 10-4, is just like the Food Guide Pyramid, except that the number of servings from each group is decreased to the minimum amount needed for good health. When you're dieting and cutting calories, it's more important than ever to choose nutrient-dense foods and not waste calories on "extras" or high fat/sugar/calorie foods that provide little in the way of vitamins and minerals.

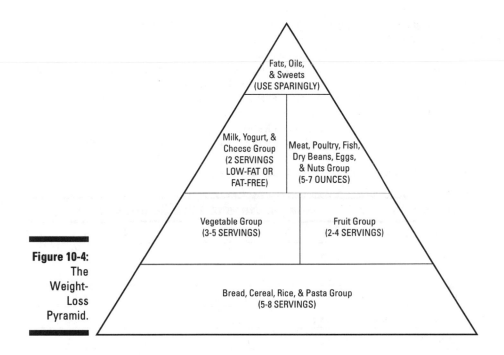

Figure 10-4:
The
Weight-
Loss
Pyramid.

For the 1,200 calorie diet, you may notice that the number of bread servings allowed is five — fewer than the usual minimum of six servings for the traditional Food Guide Pyramid. But don't worry; cutting back on a serving of bread won't put you at a loss for nutrients. You get plenty of the B vitamins and fiber that your body needs from five servings. Just make sure that your choices from this group are whole grain and high in fiber.

It's also sometimes difficult to get the 1,000 to 1,200 milligrams of calcium required from just two servings of dairy. To help boost your calcium intake from other food sources, include a serving of dark green, leafy vegetables; drink a glass of calcium-fortified orange juice as one of your fruit servings; and, for health insurance, include a calcium supplement.

Meeting all your nutrient requirements is difficult when drastically limiting calories. If your calorie intake is 1,200 calories or lower, be sure to take a multivitamin-mineral supplement.

Planning Your Meals

How do you keep all these portion sizes and food groups straight? A simple sheet of paper can help. Make a grid like the one shown in Table 10-5, placing the days of the week across the top and the food groups down the side. Next to each food group, write the number of servings that your calorie level allows. Then, each day, make Xs in the appropriate columns until you reach your daily allotment. Not only is this chart a quick visual reference for you, but studies show that dieters who track what they eat each day are more successful in losing weight and keeping it off.

Table 10-5	Sample Week at 1,200 Calories						
Food Group	*M*	*T*	*W*	*T*	*F*	*S*	*S*
Bread (5)	xxxxx						
Fruit (2)	xx						
Vegetable (3)	xx						
Meat (5 ounces)	xxx						
Milk (2)	xx						
Fats, oils, and sweets	x						

If you see that you've had all your meat and dairy for the day, for example, and you want something to snack on, try a piece of fruit or a few raw vegetables if you haven't had all your servings for the day. Here's what a sample day might look like:

Breakfast:

- ✔ 6 ounces orange juice (fruit)
- ✔ 1 slice whole-wheat toast (bread)
- ✔ Hard-cooked egg (meat)
- ✔ Jelly (fats, oils, and sweets)

"Free" foods

Certain foods are considered "free" foods because they provide almost no calories. Examples of free foods include sugar-free hard candies or chewing gum, diet soft drinks or drink mixes, club soda, sugar-free gelatin, and bouillon or broth. Using these free foods as extras throughout the day is fine, but don't overdo them. Although each one individually provides very few calories, if you go overboard with some of them, the sodium can start to add up.

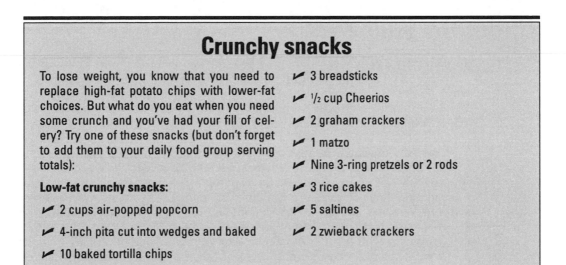

Crunchy snacks

To lose weight, you know that you need to replace high-fat potato chips with lower-fat choices. But what do you eat when you need some crunch and you've had your fill of celery? Try one of these snacks (but don't forget to add them to your daily food group serving totals):

Low-fat crunchy snacks:

✔ 2 cups air-popped popcorn

✔ 4-inch pita cut into wedges and baked

✔ 10 baked tortilla chips

✔ 3 breadsticks

✔ ½ cup Cheerios

✔ 2 graham crackers

✔ 1 matzo

✔ Nine 3-ring pretzels or 2 rods

✔ 3 rice cakes

✔ 5 saltines

✔ 2 zwieback crackers

Lunch:

✔ Turkey sandwich made with 2 ounces of meat (2 bread, 2 meat)

✔ Lettuce and tomato (vegetable)

✔ 1 cup fat-free milk (milk)

✔ One-quarter cantaloupe (fruit)

Snack:

✔ 2 cups popcorn (bread)

✔ Diet soda (free)

Dinner:

✔ 2 ounces of broiled fish (meat)

✔ 1 small baked potato (vegetable)

✔ ½ cup broccoli (vegetable)

Snack:

✔ Apple (fruit)

✔ 1½ ounces low-fat cheese (dairy)

✔ 5 saltine crackers (grain)

Planning Your Diet

To plan your diet, you could follow a printed diet sheet that offers no choice or variation regardless of your personal taste preferences. But what happens when you reach your goal weight? What have you learned? Better to use the weight-loss process as a learning experience to make healthier food choices. When you make those choices, keep these three points in mind:

- ✔ **Variety:** You can achieve a healthful, nutritious eating pattern with many combinations of foods. For the best variety, choose foods within and across food groups, because foods within the same group have different combinations of nutrients and other beneficial substances. For example, chicken, beef, pork, and fish all contain iron, but in varying amounts; pork has more B vitamins than other protein choices. Some vegetables and fruits are good sources of vitamin C or vitamin A, and others are high in folate; still others are good sources of calcium or iron. Choosing a variety of foods within each group also makes your meals more interesting from day to day.

- ✔ **Balance:** You need to balance the kinds and amounts of food on your plate as well as what you eat over the course of a day and over an entire week. The most satisfying meals are a combination of protein foods, grains, vegetables, and fruits. A lunch of only salad or a breakfast of only a bagel and coffee won't stay with you for long. But if you build balance into your meals, you'll feel more satisfied longer.

- ✔ **Moderation:** Keeping portions moderate in size and content allows for flexibility. There may be room for a small or kiddie-sized treat even on a weight-reduction diet, but probably not a super-sized one.

Chapter 11

A Matter of Taste: Using Fat Substitutes and Artificial Sweeteners

· ·

In This Chapter

▶ Finding out why calories still count

▶ Understanding fat replacers and the "low-fat" label

▶ Using sugar substitutes

▶ Changing your food preferences

· ·

*T*railer-loads of foods made with artificial sweeteners and fat substitutes are rolling down highways and into supermarkets. More than 8,000 fat-reduced foods are in supermarkets today, and an equally staggering number of foods sweetened with artificial sweeteners are available. But just as there are no free lunches, there are no free calories. This chapter tells you why some fat and sugar substitutes may help you lose weight, but also why they are not the only answer.

Why You Can Eat Only Fat-Free Foods and Still Gain Weight

A 1998 study conducted by the Calorie Control Council, an industry group that represents manufacturers of low-fat and sugar-free foods, showed that 62 percent of consumers say they always try to check the nutrition label to determine fat content in the products they buy. But only 55 percent check the label for calories. That discrepancy may be one of the reasons more people are obese today, despite the fact that total fat consumption is down.

On a gram-by-gram basis, fat has more calories than carbohydrates or protein. Therefore, eliminating fat or cutting down on the amount you eat helps you lose weight. However, if fat is replaced with carbohydrates, as it is in many fat-reduced and fat-free products, the total number of calories in a serving may not be reduced. Consequently, no weight loss occurs.

Table 11-1 shows you how reducing fat in a product doesn't always mean that its calories are reduced, too.

Table 11-1	Low-Fat Doesn't Always Mean Low-Calorie	
Food	*Portion*	*Calories*
Cool Whip	2 tablespoons	25
Lite Cool Whip	2 tablespoons	25
Franco-American turkey gravy	1/4 cup	30
Franco-American fat-free turkey gravy	1/4 cup	30
Nabisco Fig Newtons	2	110
Nabisco Fat Free Fig Newtons	2	100
Old El Paso refried beans	1/2 cup	100
Old El Paso fat-free refried beans	1/2 cup	100
Skippy peanut butter	2 tablespoons	190
Skippy reduced-fat peanut butter	2 tablespoons	190

But in some cases, a lower fat content *does* mean fewer calories, especially when it comes to dairy products. Table 11-2 gives a few examples.

Table 11-2	Where Low-Fat *Does* Mean Lower-Calorie	
Food	*Portion*	*Calories*
Cottage cheese, 4% milk fat	1/2 cup	110
Cottage cheese, 1% milk fat	1/2 cup	82
Whole milk	8 ounces	150
Fat-free milk	8 ounces	85
Yogurt, low-fat	8 ounces	155
Yogurt, nonfat	8 ounces	135
Vanilla ice cream	1/2 cup	135
Vanilla ice milk	1/2 cup	90

REMEMBER

There's more to weight loss than cutting fat

Research from the University of Vermont [published in *Obesity Research* 6(3), May 1998] proves that there's more to weight loss than counting fat grams. A group of dieters were told to restrict their fat to 22 to 28 grams per day, but nothing was said about counting calories. Another group restricted calories but wasn't given specific instructions to cut back on fat. After 6 months, the calorie counters lost more than twice as much weight as did those who restricted fat.

One reason is the incredible number of fake-fat products on the market that are not low in calories. Many people view these products as a license to overeat. Don't fall into that trap yourself!

The Role of Fat Replacers in the Foods You Eat

Fat in the diet provides calories (or energy) and important vitamins, such as vitamin E. In addition to carrying flavor and giving foods taste appeal, fat also gives foods texture — whether it's crispy or smooth and creamy. The concern about eating fatty foods is not only the number of calories they contain but also, depending on the type of fat, their potential for increasing the risk for disease. A diet high in saturated fat, for example, is often implicated in increasing blood cholesterol levels and therefore increasing the risk of heart disease.

There are two problems with eating high-fat foods. People love how fat makes foods taste. And because fat does not immediately satisfy hunger the way sugary carbohydrates do, it's easy to eat too many fat calories before realizing that you've had enough. Researchers hope that fat replacers will help people stop overeating real fat — or at least eat less of it.

Do fat replacers work?

Some fat replacers are fat-free. Others contribute calories, but fewer than they replace. Fat replacers can reduce the amount of fat you eat only if you do not consume additional fat at other meals. Research shows that test subjects who were fed fake-fat foods did not eat additional fat when only fat-reduced and fat-free foods were available. But people don't live in laboratories, and plenty of full-fat foods are always available. In theory, though, overall fat intake should go down.

However, consider this fact: Most of the fat in our diets comes from eating and cooking with fats and oils. Add red meat, poultry, fish, and dairy products to that mix, and you'll discover that all these foods account for about 90 percent of the fat we eat. Meanwhile, very few of these foods contain fat replacers. Most fat replacers are used in other foods, especially snack foods. Adding fat-reduced snack foods to an eating plan without also reducing the major sources of fat in your diet — from foods like oils, red meat, poultry, fish, and dairy products — will *add* calories, not reduce them.

What types of fat replacers are there?

Fat is complicated stuff. The kind and amount of fatty acids that make up a particular type of fat determine how the fat feels in your mouth and how it tastes, among other functions. So finding one universal fat replacer is impossible. Therefore, three basic types of fat replacers are used:

✔ **Carbohydrate-based fat substitutes** duplicate the taste and function of fat in foods but contain fewer calories than real fat. They work by combining with water to thicken and add bulk, which makes the food "feel" like fat in your mouth.

Foods that use carbohydrate-based fat substitutes include low-fat and nonfat baked goods (such as brownies, cakes, and cookies), low-fat ice creams, and fat-free salad dressings. Pureed fruits, including prunes and applesauce, are also used as fat replacers in some baked goods.

✔ **Fat mimetics** (or **fat-based replacers**) copy some or all of the properties of the fat they replace. Most are made from fat but have fewer calories per gram than fat because the chemical structure of the fat has been altered. The body is unable to fully absorb the fatty acids — and the calories they would otherwise provide.

Salatrim (brand name Benefat) is one example of a fat-based replacer. It's used in baked goods, dairy products, and candies, providing 5 calories per gram compared to fat's usual 9 calories per gram.

Olestra (brand name Olean), a calorie-free fat replacer made from vegetable oils and sugars, contributes no calories. Olestra mimics the characteristics of fat when fried. It is currently used in potato chips, tortilla chips, and other snack foods. For more information about olestra, see the sidebar "A food industry phenomenon: Olestra (Olean)."

✔ **Protein-based fat replacers** are made with egg whites or skim milk. They provide a creamy texture and an appealing appearance when fat is removed. Low-fat cheeses and ice creams made with protein-based substitutes mimic the taste and appearance of their full-fat counterparts.

Simplesse is an example of a protein-based fat replacer. It's used primarily in frozen desserts, providing 1 to 2 calories per gram.

> Protein-based fat replacers have great potential for use in many products, especially frozen and refrigerated items.

Table 11-3 lists the most commonly used fat replacers in foods.

Table 11-3	Fat Replacers That You May See on Labels	
Carbohydrate-Based	**Protein-Based**	**Fat-Based**
Cellulose (carboxy-methyl cellulose, microcrystalline cellulose)	Dairy-lo	Caprenin
Dextrin	Simplesse	Olestra (Olean)
Fiber		Salatrim (Benefat)
Gum (alginates, carrageenan, guar, locust bean, zanthan)		
Maltodextrin		
Pectin		
Polydextrose		
Starch (modified food starch)		

A food-industry phenomenon: Olestra (Olean)

It's the biggest thing to happen to the food industry since sliced bread — and the hoopla and controversy surrounding its use in our food supply has shaken up the industry. Over 150 scientific studies and 25 years of testing have made olestra (brand name Olean) the most thoroughly tested new food ingredient ever approved by the FDA.

Olestra is a specific type of fat-based fat replacer known as a *sucrose polyester.* It's made by binding a fatty acid (a fat building block) to a sugar. Because the human body doesn't have a way to separate the fatty acid from the sugar, it can't be used, and the body can't absorb the calories in it. So it passes through the body without being digested. The downside of it not being digested is that it also carries away some fat-soluble vitamins (such as vitamin A and vitamin E) with it. That's why

foods made with olestra have fat-soluble vitamins added to them.

Unlike many other fat replacers, olestra is heat stable, so it can be used in fried foods and baked goods. Currently, it is approved for use only in snack foods.

But olestra is not without its critics. The Center for Science in the Public Interest, a consumer group, is actively working to ban olestra because in some people, eating foods that contain olestra causes digestive discomfort, particularly if large amounts of an olestra-containing food are consumed. However, the FDA has deemed olestra safe for everyone, and the hope is that foods made with fat replacers will enable consumers to cut back on fat without sacrificing their favorite foods.

The Role of Nutritive and Non-Nutritive Sweeteners in Your Diet

Two kinds of sweeteners are widely used to replace sugar. Some are classified as *nutritive* because they provide calories; others are *non-nutritive* because they don't.

Everyone can relate to the story about the woman who had a huge meal and an even bigger dessert and then insisted that the waiter bring a sugar substitute for her coffee. Maybe you've even done something like this yourself! Sure, every calorie saved counts, and a sugar substitute saves you about 16 calories for every teaspoon of sugar replaced. Most people's diets include an estimated 24 teaspoons of sugar a day, and theoretically, if that sugar were replaced by non-nutritive sweeteners, this replacement would result in a deficit of 380 calories per day, or about 1 pound of weight loss in 9 to 10 days. But much of the sugar we eat isn't even visible as sugar; it's buried in our diets as ingredients in other foods.

When artificial sweeteners were introduced, everyone thought that people would eat less sugar. But evidence now suggests that people simply add the sweeteners to their diets. In reality, artificial sweeteners didn't replace anything. Just the opposite is true — consumers are eating three times the amount of sweeteners that they were 10 years ago.

Nutritive sweeteners

Most nutritive sweeteners used as replacements for sugar have just as many calories as sugar. They're simply another way to sweeten foods. Refined sugars, high-fructose corn syrup, crystalline fructose, glucose, dextrose, corn sweetener, honey lactose, maltose, invert sugar, and concentrated fruit juice are examples of nutritive sweeteners that are just as caloric as plain old sugar.

Sugar alcohols are used in many sugar-free foods and have about half the calories of sugar because the body absorbs them slowly and incompletely. You may know these sugar alcohols more specifically as *sorbitol, mannitol,* and *xylitol.* Unfortunately, in some people, a side effect of this slow absorption is diarrhea — particularly if large amounts of sugar alcohols are consumed. That's why the labels of some gums and candies that contain these sweeteners carry the statement "Excess consumption may have a laxative effect."

Non-nutritive sweeteners

Saccharin, aspartame, acesulfame potassium (or acesulfame-K), sucralose, and cyclamates are the most commonly used no-calorie sweeteners in North America. They help add sweetness to foods for people who need to limit their intake of sugar (such as those with diabetes), and they also aid in the prevention of dental cavities. They are so intensely sweet that tiny amounts can be used, so the calories they provide are undetectable. Whether or not they can help you lose weight depends on the other foods you eat. Although these no-calorie sweeteners may seem like a dream come true, most come with some warnings.

Acesulfame-K (Sunette)

Acesulfame-K, which is 200 times sweeter than sugar, is the new kid in the soft drink dispenser. It's also used as a tabletop sweetener and as an ingredient in chewing gum, desserts, candies, sauces, and yogurt in more than 15 countries. It's often used in combination with aspartame or other sweeteners in foods. Like saccharin, acesulfame-K is heat stable, so it can be used in cooked and baked goods. However, it may not work well in some recipes due to its finer texture.

Acesulfame-K doesn't provide calories because it is not metabolized by the body and is excreted in the urine.

Aspartame (Nutrasweet, Equal)

Aspartame, which is 160 to 220 times sweeter than sugar, is added to more than 6,000 foods, personal care products, and pharmaceuticals. It has 4 calories per gram, but because it is so intensely sweet and so little is needed to replace sugar, it is considered calorie-free.

Aspartame is a combination of two amino acids: phenylalanine and aspartic acid. People who have phenylketonuria, or PKU (only about 1 in 15,000 people have this condition), have adverse neurological reactions when they consume phenylalanine because they cannot metabolize it. Therefore, foods that contain aspartame are required to carry a label warning consumers that the product contains phenylalanine. In the U.S., all infants are screened for PKU at birth.

Many studies have been conducted on aspartame to evaluate the numerous claims of allergic reactions, respiratory problems, and dermatological problems that consumers have reported. However, challenge studies have failed to reproduce those reactions.

Aspartame is not heat stable and loses its sweetness in liquids over time, so it is used mostly in foods that don't require cooking or baking. Look for it in puddings, gelatins, frozen desserts, hot cocoa mixes, soft drinks, chewing gum, and tabletop sweeteners. Aspartame is approved for use in a broad variety of products in more than 18 countries, including the U.S., Canada, Japan, and the United Kingdom.

Cyclamate

Cyclamate is 30 times sweeter than sucrose and is heat stable. It's approved for use in Canada and more than 50 other countries around the world. Since 1970, however, its use has been banned in the United States based on a study suggesting that cyclamate may be related to the development of bladder tumors in rats. Although more than 75 subsequent studies have failed to show that cyclamate is carcinogenic, the sweetener has yet to be reapproved for use in the U.S.

Saccharin (Sweet'N Low)

Saccharin, which is 300 times sweeter than sugar, is the "Now you see it, now you don't" sweetener. It was discovered more than 100 years ago and has been back on the market in the United States since 1991, after having been banned in 1977 because it was found to cause cancer in rats. Its life in the U.S. is not guaranteed, however: Congress has allowed its use only until May 2002, when new studies on its safety are due. The products that contain it must carry a warning that reads: "Use of this product may be hazardous to your health. This product contains saccharin which has been determined to cause cancer in laboratory animals."

A little bit of saccharin goes a long way — just 20 milligrams provides the same amount of sweetness found in 1 teaspoon (or 4,000 milligrams) of table sugar. Saccharin is calorie-free because the body can't break it down.

Saccharin is heat-stable and, unlike aspartame, can be used in cooked and baked goods. However, because it does not have the bulk that sugar has, it may not work well in some recipes as a substitute. Saccharin is currently used in many food and beverages in more than 80 countries.

Sucralose (Splenda)

Sucralose, which is 600 times sweeter than sugar, does not contain calories. It is the only low-calorie sweetener that is made from sugar. Sucralose is heat stable in cooking and baking and can be used virtually anywhere sugar can without losing its sugar-like sweetness. Currently, sucralose is approved in more than 25 countries around the world for use in food and beverages. It is used mainly as a tabletop sweetener and in desserts and candy.

Why Depriving Yourself of "Real" Foods Is Unnecessary

One of the problems with eating "fake" foods is that you don't learn to like foods that are naturally low in fat or sugar. Continually tricking your palate with foods that taste and feel like fat and sugar may reduce the amount of fat and sugar you eat, but you're not making progress toward a naturally healthier way of eating.

Although people are born with a love of sugar and a predisposition to enjoy fat, those preferences can be unlearned over time. If you've already made the switch from whole milk to low-fat or fat-free milk, you know that the full-fat version is almost unpleasantly rich once you're accustomed to the way fat-free milk tastes and feels in your mouth. The change in preferences takes a few weeks to several months, depending on your present diet, but stick with it. Try these tricks to train your taste buds:

- ✔ **Use ingredients that are naturally low in fat or fat-free.** Try pureed fruits as a sauce for desserts or meats, low-fat yogurt to thicken shakes or fruit smoothies and dips, and evaporated fat-free milk to add body to cream sauces.

- ✔ **Add sweetness without sugar.** Instead of adding a spoonful of sugar, squeeze citrus juice over fresh fruit to enhance flavor. Cut the amount of sugar that you add to coffee or tea by half. Sprinkle fresh fruit over pancakes and waffles instead of syrup. Do the same over cereal. Add dried fruit and sweet spices such as nutmeg, cinnamon, and ginger to hot cereals to intensify sweetness without adding sugar.

You *can* learn a preference for less sweet and less fatty foods — all it takes is a little time and effort!

Chapter 12

Becoming More Active

● ●

In This Chapter

▶ Understanding the importance of exercise for weight loss

▶ Calculating your exercise prescription

▶ Balancing aerobic and muscle-building exercise

▶ Overcoming excuses for not exercising

▶ Eating smart for your workout

● ●

*I*n this book, we talk about consuming fewer calories and eating less fat to lose weight. And that's exactly what you must do if you're going to shed pounds. But if you add exercise, you speed up your weight-loss efforts by increasing the number of calories you burn. Plus, you build muscle, which keeps your metabolism in high gear to burn calories more readily. You feel better about yourself, too. This chapter tells you how to work exercise into your lifestyle — and keep at it.

Naturally, if you have any medical conditions that would make exercising difficult or dangerous for you, see your doctor. This caution is especially important if you're over 40 years old. Your physician can perform a graded exercise test, evaluate your overall health, and suggest forms of exercise that are safe for you.

Why Exercise Is Important for Weight Loss

Exercise is important for everyone. The fitter you are, the less your risk of having a heart attack or stroke or developing diabetes or some other crippling and deadly disease. But there's more: Exercise offers true, tangible benefits that are a real plus to dieters. The following sections describe those benefits.

Exercise helps you eat less

Many people eat out of boredom or habit. True hunger has little to do with why or how much people eat. Think of the mindless nibbling that you do while watching TV, for example. When you're busy and out of the house, on the other hand — or at least diverted from the call of the kitchen — you eat less.

Some people say that exercise makes them hungrier. But that's one of the greatest exercise-avoidance excuses of all time. The reasons?

- ✔ Exercise helps slow the movement of food through your digestive tract. Your stomach takes longer to empty, so you feel full longer.

- ✔ Exercise pulls stored calories — or energy — in the forms of glucose and fat out of tissues so that blood glucose levels stay even and you don't feel hungry.

Exercise increases calorie burn

The math is simple: The more calories you burn over the amount your body needs to maintain its current weight, the greater your weight loss. Another way that exercise helps burn calories is by increasing your *metabolic rate* — the pace at which your body uses calories. And exercise helps you lose fat but not muscle, which determines how fast or slow your body burns calories. Fat is relatively inert, but muscle is active and needs energy to maintain itself. So the more muscle you have, the more calories your body needs.

Exercise protects against muscle loss

Many studies have demonstrated that when a person diets, the weight that is lost is 75 percent fat and 25 percent muscle. And that ratio is not good. As muscle is lost, so is your body's ability to burn and use calories efficiently. In short, the less muscle you have, the fewer calories you need. Having less muscle and more fat is one of the reasons so many people on weight-loss diets who do not exercise reach a plateau and stop losing weight even though they are still restricting their calorie intake.

To build muscle, you need to add resistance training, such as lifting weights, to your exercise program. See the section called "Strength Training," later in this chapter, for details.

Exercise improves self-esteem

Exercise pays off physically, but its psychological benefits are dramatic as well. And we're not just talking about a runner's high or an endorphin buzz. Each time you exercise, you're doing something positive for yourself. Some psychologists even prescribe daily exercise for depressed patients and see mood improvements equal to those of prescription antidepressant drug therapy.

So much of the weight-loss process involves giving up, limiting, and cutting out. But exercise is a positive addition, not a take-away negative, and that's a powerful incentive to stick with it. When you feel good about yourself, staying with your weight-loss commitment is easy.

Active people lose weight more easily and keep it off

The National Weight Control Registry maintained at the University of Pittsburgh School of Medicine includes over 2,000 individuals who have lost more than 30 pounds and have kept it off for more than a year. But amazingly, the *average* loss is 60 pounds, and the average maintenance is 6 years. So many people actually lost more weight as time went on and have kept it off for a long period of time.

Researchers looked carefully at these success stories and found that one common thread is that they expend about 2,800 calories in physical activity a week — by engaging in a combination of walking and medium-to-heavy exercise such as cycling, running, stair climbing, aerobic exercising, and weight lifting. This activity level, researchers say, may be the most important factor in maintaining their success.

How Much Exercise Is Enough?

The current guidelines from the Centers for Disease Control and Prevention and the American College of Sports Medicine recommend 30 minutes or more of moderate-intensity physical activity on most — and preferably all — days of the week. That amount is enough for most people. But for weight loss, you need to expend a minimum of about 200 to 300 calories a day on a *minimum* of 3 days a week. (See the section "Go for the (Calorie) Burn" for a list of common exercises and the number of calories each activity burns.)

Research shows that for the best calorie-burning, greater amounts of exercise at a lower intensity are better than high intensity for shorter periods. Use the American Heart Association's "conversational pace" rule to determine whether you're setting the right pace when walking: If you can talk and walk at the same time, you're probably working at the right level. If you can sing and maintain your level of effort, you're probably not working hard enough. And if you get out of breath quickly, you're probably working too hard — especially if you actually have to stop and catch your breath.

How to Start Exercising

Expending 2,800 calories a week in exercise, as the folks in the weight-loss registry did, may sound like a tall order if you're among the 78 percent of American adults who are either totally sedentary or not active enough. So how do you go from doing very little or no exercise to developing a daily routine? Make it a habit. The easiest way to do that is to *commit to exercise every day*. That's 7 days a week! Start with 20 minutes of walking every day. You can do two 10-minute walks if you like. Just commit to 20 minutes a day.

After about 2 weeks, lengthen your walks to 40 minutes. In another 2 weeks, lengthen them to 60 minutes. Table 12-1 outlines the exercise program.

Table 12-1	Your Exercise Prescription	
Time Period	*Activity*	*Comments*
Weeks 1 and 2	Walk 20 minutes a day.	Intensity is not important.
Weeks 3 and 4	Walk 40 minutes a day.	Gradually increase the intensity.
Week 5	Walk 60 minutes a day.	Walk briskly.
Lifelong	Add recreational sports or aerobics for cardiorespiratory conditioning.	Supplement with walking on off days.

You don't have to do exercise in one lump sum. Finding a continuous 30 to 60 minutes in which to work out is difficult for almost everyone. But the day's total amount of activity is what counts — it doesn't matter how or if you break it up. For example, find three 20-minute periods in your day for exercising. Even 10 minutes here and 10 minutes there adds up to sufficient exercise quickly.

Don't try to make up for a slow day with an overly active one. But if you do go overboard with an activity that's too strenuous, still try to do something the next day, even if it means a slow walk. The important thing is to do some kind of exercise every day. That's how you make it a habit.

Keeping an Exercise Log

In Chapter 10, we ask you to keep a pyramid score sheet on the fridge. Here's another chart to add. Tape it to the bathroom mirror, your computer monitor, or wherever you're sure to see it every day.

Make a grid on a piece of paper with space to record the date along the side and 10-minute time slots along the top, as in Table 12-2. As you complete your exercise sessions, make an X in the box that corresponds to the amount of time you exercised.

Table 12-2	Sample Minutes of Walking Log						
Date	**10**	**20**	**30**	**40**	**50**	**60**	**Total**
Sunday	XX	XX					60
Monday				X			40
Tuesday		X		X			60
Wednesday	XX		X				50
Thursday	X	XX	X				80
Friday						X	60
Saturday	XX	X	X				70

Focus first on increasing the length of time you exercise, and then shift your efforts to increasing the intensity. For example, after you're comfortable with walking, you can add a variety of activities to total your 60 minutes — for example, jogging, hiking, or working out with weights. After you reach your goal of 60 minutes of daily exercise, begin jotting down the kind of exercise you do in the column that corresponds to the amount of time you're active. (Your goal, even after you've moved past the walking-only stage, is still 60 minutes a day.) Your exercise log may look like Table 12-3.

Table 12-3	Sample Exercise Log						
Day	**10**	**20**	**30**	**40**	**50**	**60**	**Total**
Sunday	jog	swim	walk				60
Monday	walk		walk				40
Tuesday			jog	walk			70
Wednesday			cycle		walk		80
Thursday	walk		jog			hike	100
Friday						walk	60
Saturday			walk			cycle	90

Going for the (Calorie) Burn

The more you weigh, the more calories you burn. It's a simple matter of physics: Moving a heavier mass takes more energy than moving a lighter one. In people terms, a 250-pound person burns twice as many calories to walk the same distance as someone who weighs only 125 pounds.

Table 12-4 shows you how many calories are burned by engaging in various aerobic activities. Notice that few of the activities require spandex or a health club membership.

Table 12-4 Calories Burned in 20 Minutes of Continuous Exercise

Activity	Body Weight of 134 Pounds	Body Weight of 183 Pounds
Aerobic dance	128	170
Ballroom dance	64	84
Basketball	172	220
Canoeing	54	74
Cleaning	76	102
Cross-country skiing	148	198
Cycling	80	106
Football	164	220
Jumping rope	204	272
Mopping floors	76	102
Mowing (push mower)	138	186
Racquetball	220	296
Raking	66	90
Running (9 minutes/mile)	240	320
Scrubbing floors	134	180
Snowshoeing	206	276
Squash	262	352
Stacking wood	110	146
Swimming, breaststroke	200	268
Tennis	136	180
Volleyball	62	84
Walking	100	134

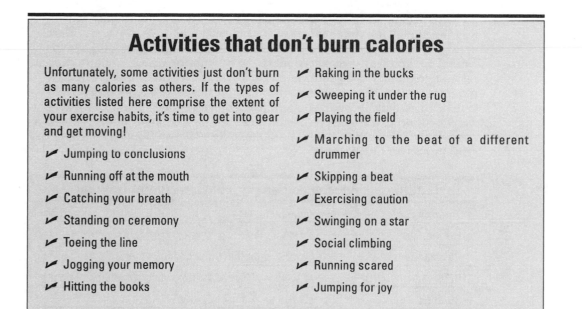

Activities that don't burn calories

Unfortunately, some activities just don't burn as many calories as others. If the types of activities listed here comprise the extent of your exercise habits, it's time to get into gear and get moving!

- ✔ Jumping to conclusions
- ✔ Running off at the mouth
- ✔ Catching your breath
- ✔ Standing on ceremony
- ✔ Toeing the line
- ✔ Jogging your memory
- ✔ Hitting the books

- ✔ Raking in the bucks
- ✔ Sweeping it under the rug
- ✔ Playing the field
- ✔ Marching to the beat of a different drummer
- ✔ Skipping a beat
- ✔ Exercising caution
- ✔ Swinging on a star
- ✔ Social climbing
- ✔ Running scared
- ✔ Jumping for joy

How frequently and intensely you exercise, as well as how long you work out, determines how much fat you burn. But don't overdo it. To burn fat, you need oxygen — get your heart and lungs pumping with aerobic activities. However, if you exercise so vigorously that you can't breathe, your workout is actually *anaerobic* (not using oxygen), which means that you're using carbohydrate and possibly protein (from your lean muscle) for energy, not fat. And that's not the point. If you want to lose weight, you want to lose fat.

Strength Training

Strength or resistance training, such as lifting weights or working out on exercise equipment, builds muscle. This type of exercise isn't just for body builders. Building muscle offers several benefits:

- ✔ It gives your body definition and firmness.
- ✔ It helps your body burn more calories.
- ✔ It strengthens bones (which helps protect against osteoporosis).

If you're new to exercise, you don't have to run to the gym; simply walking may be enough for you to increase your muscle mass. When you can walk easily for 60 minutes at a brisk pace, having followed the plan outlined in Table 12-1, you may need and want to push for more of a workout. Adding resistance training is a good way to go. Table 12-5 outlines a suggested program for weight training. Get the help of a personal trainer or gym instructor to build a routine for you that you can do at home with hand-held weights or do at the gym on the machines. Or pick up an exercise video or a copy of Liz Neporent and Suzanne Schlosberg's *Weight Training For Dummies* (IDG Books Worldwide, Inc.).

Table 12-5	Recommended Program for Weight Training
Training Factor	*Comments*
Frequency	3 days a week
Resistance	Use a weight that you can lift comfortably
Repetitions	12 to 15 in 30 seconds (the last lift should be difficult)
Stations	Work 8 to 12 muscle groups
Total time	20 to 30 minutes

Ten Inexcusable Excuses for Not Exercising (And How to Cope with Them)

We've all heard them. Most of us have used them: "justifiable" excuses for not being more active. Here are some ways to get around every "good" reason not to exercise:

✔ **Excuse:** "I don't have time."

Coping strategies: This is the number-one reason most people give for not exercising. But you must make exercise a priority. That's one reason to make your daily activity a habit — because then it becomes a priority. Get a significant other to watch the children, get up half an hour early, or walk during your lunch hour. Remember, you don't have to commit to a full hour all at once. Three 10- or 20-minute walks count.

✔ **Excuse:** "I don't feel like it."

Coping strategies: Grab a buddy or several friends and make a commitment to them. Chances are that one of you will want to keep moving even when the others don't. And don't forget to give yourself credit for every bit of exercise you do, even if you don't make your 60-minute goal on some days. Remember, some physical activity is better than none.

✔ **Excuse:** "I can't do exercises well."

Coping strategies: We're talking about walking, not jogging, running, or race walking. You can saunter, meander, or stroll. Just move. After a few weeks, you'll feel more comfortable. When you do, you can increase your speed and improve your technique.

✔ **Excuse:** "I can't get to my workout place easily."

Coping strategies: You don't have to go to a special place, although you may find it motivating to go to a school track, a mall, the woods, or some other walker-friendly environment. You can take the stairs, get off the bus a little earlier and walk the rest of the way, park at the far end of the lot, or pace instead of sitting while waiting for the train.

✔ **Excuse:** "Exercise didn't work for me in the past."

Coping strategies: Remember the little engine that could? "I think I can. I think I can. I think I can. I did!" Maybe you tried to do too much before. Maybe you were forced to be on a sports team as a child. Or you were always the last person to be chosen for a team in the schoolyard. Try to figure out why past attempts to stick with exercise failed, or why you believe that your past gets in your way. Work out your own way around the problem. It's worth repeating here: We're talking about going for a walk, not training for a marathon.

✔ **Excuse:** "I'm too fat to move."

Coping strategies: Very large people can't move easily or quickly. But eventually, as your weight comes down and your fitness level improves, your ability and enjoyment will improve. Watch for little signs of encouragement, such as walking up the stairs without huffing and puffing. Or notice that your thighs don't rub together as much as they did a few weeks earlier. The more active you become, the more progress you'll see.

✔ **Excuse:** "I have poor balance."

Coping strategies: Balance is a problem for very large people who have been sedentary. Make sure that you have comfortable footwear that has a wide sole and good support. Choose flat, paved surfaces for walking.

✔ **Excuse:** "I'm afraid."

Coping strategies: Fear stops people from doing all kinds of things, but the best antidote for fear is action. Grab a buddy to encourage you. Keep your sense of humor primed. Make exercise fun!

> ✔ **Excuse:** "Exercising hurts."
>
> *Coping strategies:* If an activity doesn't feel good, don't do it. Never exercise to the point of exhaustion. You don't want to wake up stiff. If you feel any pain at all, slow down or cut back on the exercise you do and slowly work your way back up. Learn to listen to your body. If you're new to exercise and have been very sedentary, start slowly and don't overexert yourself. But whatever you do, get up the next morning and do something again.
>
> ✔ **Excuse:** "I'm too embarrassed."
>
> *Coping strategies:* Don't worry about looking foolish. When you walk for exercise, you don't have to join a gym filled with perky, spandex-clad instructors. You can be as private or as public as you like, depending on where you walk. You can wear whatever you want, too.

Eating Smart for Your Workout

Eating 2 to 3 hours before a workout is ideal (that's how long it takes for a meal to reach your muscles), but it's not always practical. It's important not to substitute exercise for eating; you can accommodate both. The following sections offer ideas for scheduling your meals to boost your workout productivity.

Early birds

If the only time you can sneak in a workout is first thing in the morning, try to eat something before you start. Your body needs fuel constantly, and your carbohydrate stores have most likely been tapped out in the 8 to 12 hours since your last meal. Without eating, you'll feel sluggish and weak. Exercise should make you feel good. Try a bowl of cereal, a cup of low-fat yogurt, or a banana.

Lunch-hour or after-work crunchers

Split your lunch: eat half a few hours before the workout and finish the rest when you get back to your desk. If you exercise after work, plan a mini-meal (perhaps a small bowl of cereal, a piece of whole-grain bread with a dab of PB&J, or a cup of low-fat yogurt) at 3:00 or 3:30 in the afternoon.

TIP

Drink, drink, drink

Regardless of how you define "workout," you need to replace fluid losses, which tend to be great after aerobic activities. Don't wait for thirst as an indicator; by that time, you're already down half a quart of fluids.

Water is fine if your workout lasts less than an hour. But sports drinks are helpful if you're exercising longer. They're better than soda and fruit juices, which can cause stomach upset during exercise and interfere with fluid absorption because they have *too much* carbohydrate — about 12 to 15 percent by weight. Sports drinks contain 6 to 9 percent carbohydrate.

So why not water down fruit juice? Research shows that fluid and energy are better absorbed when the drink contains several carbohydrates (sports drinks contain maltodextrins, sucrose, and fructose) that use different absorption mechanisms than when the sweetener comes from a single source. In addition, the small amount of electrolytes, including sodium, that sports drinks provide can replenish those lost through sweat. And as an added bonus, the sodium helps make you thirsty, encouraging you to drink more even after you think that you've had enough. Few people drink enough fluids to replenish lost stores.

Weekend warriors

When you're doing extra exercise — a charity bike ride or a mini-marathon fun run, for example — and stay at it for more than an hour, you need to refuel during the event. The human body can store only about an hour's worth of carbohydrate; it's in the muscles in the form of glycogen. (See Chapter 4 for further explanation of metabolism.) So if you want to finish the race without dragging yourself over the finish line, you need to eat or drink some form of carbohydrate. A sports drink is one option. A small energy bar works, too.

After an especially long workout, you need to refuel to restore your energy. A small high-carbohydrate, moderate-protein, and low-fat meal is best. Reach for fruit, low-fat yogurt, and whole-wheat crackers or bread.

Chapter 13

Maintaining a Healthy Lifestyle

● ●

In This Chapter

▶ Understanding that a healthy weight is more than a number of pounds

▶ Discovering how successful maintainers keep weight off

▶ Getting the support you need

● ●

*W*e hope that you've made some good progress in your weight-loss program and are eager not to lose ground. A weight-maintenance program, which can include the tips and ideas in this chapter, should be a priority after the initial 6 months of a weight-loss diet. Weight maintenance is not a matter of "going off your diet" — it's a matter of keeping your healthy eating and activity habits a priority.

In some ways, the strategies you need for maintenance are no different from those that you used to lose weight in the first place. But in other ways, the strategies *are* different. Maintenance means keeping at it forever. Stop, and you'll slide right back up to where you started — or worse yet, even higher.

Staying at a Healthy Weight

Notice that the topic in this chapter is maintaining a healthy weight — not a supermodel's or a movie star's weight. It's not even "staying at the weight you were in high school." This chapter is about health. It's about the larger definition of health, too — not only what can be measured by tests at the doctor's office.

A healthy weight is the weight that you can reasonably attain and maintain without going crazy. For example, most people would say that a 5-foot, 4-inch woman who has gotten her weight down to 125 pounds has reached a healthy weight. But would you consider her weight healthy if you knew that she had to restrict her calorie intake so much that she couldn't relax around food for fear of losing control? And that she had to exercise vigorously for at least 2 hours a day, and sometimes more, for fear of ballooning up to her old weight? And that this lifestyle robbed her of time with her family and friends; that maintaining her weight was the sole focus of her life? That's not healthy. That's neurotic.

To maintain a healthy weight, you must maintain a healthy lifestyle — healthy eating, exercise, stress reduction, and relationships all in balance. As you work through your weight-loss plan and look forward to staying at your new, lower weight, consider the points in the following sections. They are the real measures of healthy weight.

Be realistic

Assigning a number as your "ideal" weight, based on information from a height-and-weight chart, isn't really a healthy way to judge your progress. Although the charts do serve a useful purpose as guides to a healthy weight range, specifying a number as "ideal" connotes that any number higher than that isn't good enough. Establishing an ideal weight sets you up in pass/fail mode instead of giving you credit for progress made. It's healthier to think of your weight in terms of what is *reasonable* for you.

For more information about adjusting your attitude and getting realistic about your weight, see Chapter 5.

Be adventurous

Changing your attitude about yourself and your body may be the most healthful step you can take. If your weight has kept you from enjoying activities, let the issue go. Have you ever said, "I'll go on vacation when I'm 125 pounds again" or "I'll try water-skiing when I'm thinner" or "I'll go for a hike in the woods when I'm in better shape"? Don't wait until you reach your goal weight. If you do, you're missing out on a lot of living. Don't miss out on life because you're hiding behind your weight. You can try many activities no matter what your weight — in-line skating, ballroom dancing, ice skating, skiing, hiking, or biking, just to name a few.

Have you reached a reasonable weight for you?

If you have your heart set on a particular point on the scale that is lower than you are now, ask yourself how reasonable it is for you to reach and maintain that weight. You can answer that question by looking at your current weight-loss success and your diet history. Ask yourself the following questions:

✔ What is the lowest adult weight you were able to maintain for at least 1 year?

✔ Think of a time you were at a lower weight than you are now. How difficult was it to reach that weight and stay there? How much exercise did you have to do? How few calories did you have to eat?

✔ Considering your starting weight and clothing size, what is the largest clothing size in which you feel comfortable and think that you look pretty good?

Be adventurous in your eating as well as your activities. Try a new fruit that you've never tasted. If you always eat bananas and apples but are so bored with them that you don't eat your recommended number of fruit servings, break out of your rut. Try a papaya or a kiwi. Reach for different grains, too. White long-grain rice is nice, but don't miss out on the short, medium, aromatic, and brown rice varieties. And then there's quinoa (pronounced *KEEN-wa*), barley, and cracked wheat. Experiment with recipes. Check out Chapter 24 for lots of tasty, adventuresome ideas, or pick up a copy of *Lowfat Cooking For Dummies* by Lynn Fischer (IDG Books Worldwide, Inc.).

Be flexible

You need to be flexible about what you consider to be weight-loss success. You also need to be flexible about what you consider to be a successful dieting or exercise day. Sure, you need to set goals, but you also need to accept that some days you aren't going to make them. A week's worth of healthy eating and exercise added to another week and another and another is how you build success.

If you can't work in your normal walking route one day, try to stay active in other ways. For example, park your car in the parking space that is farthest from the door. Be sure to take the stairs rather than the elevator. Any kind of exercise counts. If you're stuck at a family party or business meal and every dish in sight is a caloric disaster, don't throw in the towel and overeat. Enjoy small amounts of the foods that are offered, and then be especially diligent the next meal or the next day.

Be sensible

"I'm never going to eat another pepperoni pizza again!" Doesn't that sound silly? Ban words like *never* and *always* from your eating and exercise plans. These ultimatums put you bites away from failure. Better to have one small serving and enjoy every bit. Or share a serving with a friend, or pack half of it in a doggie bag for another meal another day.

Exercising a little every day is better than trying to make up for a missed day or week by overexerting yourself. Chances are, you won't enjoy the exercise as much if you're overdoing it, and you'll probably be so sore afterwards that you'll miss the next few days of activity as well. No pain, no gain is not our motto. Take it slow and steady and, most important, *enjoy* yourself.

Be active

Don't you just love folks who say things like "We won the baseball game," when they mean that the team they were rooting for on TV won? Or the people who say that they're going to walk the dog and then go outside and watch the dog walk around the yard while they stand in the driveway? These people are spectators, not participants.

We use many other expressions that make us sound active: "Mow the lawn" (or do we sit on the mower?); "wash the clothes" (or do we put them into the washing machine?); "shovel the snow" (or do we push the snow blower?); "run to the store" (or do we drive the car?) — you get the idea. These passive activities sound like actions, but they're really not.

If you're guilty of using more active language than actually being active, change your behavior! Look for ways — big and small — to fit activity into your day: Climb the stairs, hide the remote, don't use your kids as slaves to fetch things, walk during your lunch break instead of sitting, play ball instead of watching, walk to the school bus stop instead of driving to meet the kids.

Getting Some Tips from Losers

Lots of people lose weight. But most people don't keep it off. The number of people who regain lost weight after 5 years is as high as 95 percent. A depressing number, for sure, but don't let that statistic stop you from trying. That 95 percent figure reflects only people who have been in weight-control studies and official programs, not the vast number of people who lose weight on their own and keep it off.

The National Weight Control Registry, a database maintained at the University of Pittsburgh School of Medicine, has followed a group of people who have been successful at losing weight by using a variety of methods. The requirement for inclusion in the registry is a 30-pounds-or-greater weight loss, maintained for at least 5 years. But the actual numbers are far better. Of the 2,000 participants, the average weight loss is 60 pounds, which the participants have maintained for more than 6 years!

These people obviously can share ideas about taking weight off, but they have even more ideas about maintaining the loss. Interestingly, some of their advice flies in the face of conventional weight-loss wisdom — like weighing yourself on the scale every day. But the take-home message here is that these people have found certain strategies that work for them. What have you found that works best for you? Keeping an exercise log or food diary? Exercising in the morning versus the evening? Planning meals for the week ahead of time? People who keep their weight off have their own personal tricks. The key to successful weight maintenance is to put them into practice.

Try, try again

PRO SPEAK

The average woman goes on 15 diets in her lifetime and loses about 100 pounds. But she regains about 125! Experts call it *yo-yo dieting* or *weight cycling.* At one time, health authorities believed that each time a person's weight yo-yos, weight loss becomes more difficult in the future (he or she loses more muscle, needs fewer calories to maintain weight, and becomes more frustrated). The bottom line seemed to be that you're better off not trying to lose weight, and that going on repeated diets is dangerous.

One major study published in *The Journal of the American Medical Association* 275(5), 1994, looked at 43 studies and found no convincing evidence that weight cycling in humans has adverse health effects on body composition, energy balance, risk factors for cardiovascular disease, or the success of future efforts at weight loss. Proof positive is the fact that 90 percent of the people in the National Weight Control Registry had tried to lose weight previously — in fact, each person had lost and regained an average of 270 pounds! Yet they were able to lose weight and keep it off, once and for all — even after years of yo-yo dieting.

Weigh in

When you're trying to maintain weight loss, monitoring your weight closely is the best approach. Successful maintainers are able to catch a 5- or 10-pound weight creep and take immediate action. Many people in the National Weight Control Registry say that they weigh themselves every day. During the weight-loss phase, weighing daily can be disappointing, so experts recommend that you get on the scale no more than once a week. But when you're in maintenance, you may find it helpful to more closely monitor the scale so that you can make adjustments to your eating plan before a 1- or 2-pound gain becomes the 5 pounds you just can't seem to lose.

> ## Is yo-yo dieting a no-no?
>
> Yo-yo dieting is going on and off and on and off a diet so that weight goes up and down the scale, bouncing from one weight to another. After finding that rats who lost and regained weight had more body fat than those whose weights remained stable, researchers concluded that the more humans diet to lose weight, the less healthy we become. But a subsequent review of that study and many other studies proved otherwise. The entire body of research concludes that yo-yo dieting does *not*
>
> ✔ Make future weight loss more difficult
>
> ✔ Increase body fat
>
> ✔ Change the location where body fat is stored
>
> ✔ Lower energy expenditure
>
> ✔ Increase preference for fatty foods
>
> ✔ Change blood pressure
>
> ✔ Change blood cholesterol or triglycerides
>
> ✔ Change insulin or glucose metabolism
>
> However, the psychological effects of weight cycling can be distressing. Some research has found that weight cyclers who tend to binge, binge more when they cycle.

During your maintenance phase, continue to "weigh in," so to speak, on what you eat, too. Some successful maintainers continue to monitor what they eat by keeping food records. And they stick with a low-fat, low-calorie eating plan.

Solve problems

People who can keep their weight stable are good problem solvers. They find ways to fit exercise into their schedules. They uncover techniques to eat low-fat foods. They work balance and moderation into their eating plans and exercise routines.

Move

Physical activity is a key predictor of weight-loss maintenance success. One study showed that 92 percent of maintainers exercise regularly, but only 34 percent of regainers did. (See Chapter 12 for more information about the importance of exercise.)

Be a good team player

People are social animals. After all, what is the purpose of life if not to be in relationships with other people? Finding someone to lean on is important. But in order to get support, you must give it as well. Maybe your support person is not a fellow dieter, but he or she needs to rely on you sometimes, too. You can't take without giving, or your support will walk. Follow these tips to be a good team player:

✓ **Show up.** Whether you make plans to meet your support person at a regular time or you have a more relaxed and informal arrangement, be there. Don't have other activities planned that take away from the agenda. You're there for each other, so be there in mind, body, and spirit.

✓ **Really listen.** Listening takes effort. A phone call can work sometimes. But if possible, meet the other person and talk face to face. See the person as well as hear his or her words. Visual clues can yield lots of information. Look for expressions or body language that either supports or contradicts what you're hearing.

✓ **Don't judge.** Maybe what you're hearing sounds silly or just plain dumb. But hang in there. When your partner tells you that there's no time to exercise, the judgmental response is, "You're looking for excuses." The nonjudgmental reaction is, "What would make it easier for you to find the time?" Nonjudgmental statements are supportive and lead to discussion. Judgmental ones are conversation-stoppers.

✓ **Be supportive.** Offer moral support by showing that you understand. Share similar experiences and give constructive suggestions if you can think of ways to help.

Get support

You can't lose weight without support, nor can you maintain your loss without help. Most successful weight losers are motivated by their own personal needs, but they do have support from friends, spouses, family, or a group of like-minded dieters. They can turn to these people for help with managing the stress in their lives, solving problems, and scheduling time for exercise by handing off household or child-care responsibilities. People who lend support also can serve as cheerleaders and provide "attaboy" encouragement. Don't go it alone!

Part IV
Shopping, Cooking, and Dining Out

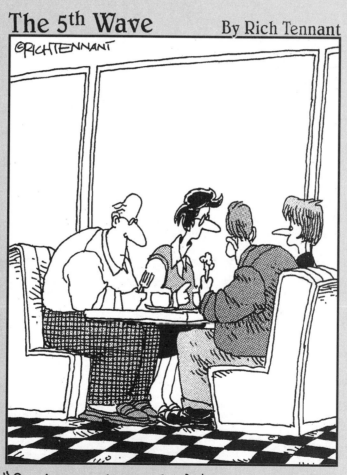

The 5th Wave — By Rich Tennant

@RICHTENNANT

"Gordon's always had trouble controlling his appetite at restaurants. I had to explain to him that you're not supposed to pull your chair up to the salad bar."

In this part . . .

You may have the best intentions to eat healthfully, but if diet-friendly foods are not within your reach, you're going to have trouble shedding pounds. This part shows you how to make the best choices at the grocery store and cook in nutritious and low-calorie ways. It also helps you navigate your way through restaurants and their often-deceptive menus, making smart choices that keep you on the right track.

Chapter 14

Healthy Grocery Shopping

- -

In This Chapter

▶ Making a grocery list of healthy foods

▶ Shopping smart

▶ Understanding food labels

▶ Purchasing lower-fat foods

- -

*T*here are more places to buy food today than at any other time in history. Just 5 years ago, people bought gas at a gas station. Today, they can buy all kinds and sizes of snacks and sodas — and lots of calories. If you don't plan ahead and do a weekly or twice-weekly grocery run, you may be forced to shop at the quick stop. That means being faced with aisles of foods screaming "Buy me! Eat me!" It's a jungle of temptation out there. To stay on the weight-loss track, arm yourself with the tips in this chapter.

Making a Healthy Grocery List

Shoppers who use lists spend slightly more money per trip to the grocery store than non-list-users, but they don't have to run back to the market as frequently to pick up forgotten items. The benefit to dieters: Fewer chances to face temptation.

Here are some tips for making sure that your grocery list is diet-friendly and that your trip to the store is as quick and painless as possible:

- ✔ Plan your menus when you're hungry (they'll be more interesting); shop when you're not (you'll have more control).

- ✔ Forget using coupons unless they're for food items that you usually buy. The savings can be tempting, but the purchase can add up to a diet disaster.

- ✔ Check your cupboards, freezer, and refrigerator in advance to avoid duplicating purchases.

✔ Learn the store's layout and write your list according to it. You'll be less apt to forget items. Or write your list according to categories: frozen foods, produce, meat, and dairy, for example.

Tips for Shopping Smart

Supermarkets are sophisticated marketing systems. Everything you see and smell in a grocery store is specifically crafted to entice you to buy more. Where items are placed in the store, whether a package is placed at your eye level or your child's, the amount of time the aroma of chickens roasting in the deli wafts under your nose, the brightness of the lights, the tempo of the music — everything is carefully chosen.

✔ Realize that the most frequently purchased foods are placed farthest from the door. That setup forces you to pass many other tempting items.

✔ Double-check the end-of-aisle displays with the usual in-aisle stock. The items featured at the ends of the aisles are not always on special.

✔ Don't forget to eat before shopping and to feed the children, too — hunger makes controlled shopping difficult for adults and nearly impossible for children.

✔ Refuse to be tempted by free samples. (If you're not hungry, you're better able to pass them by.)

✔ Look up and down. The more expensive items are generally placed at eye level. Bargains can often be found on less convenient shelves.

✔ Become a label reader and use the nutrition information. A label shows the size of a serving (it may be smaller than you think), the number of servings in the package, and the ingredients, as well as the food's nutrient profile. (See the section "Label-Reading for Dieters," later in this chapter, for more information.)

Table 14-1 lists some of the terms you see on food labels.

Table 14-1	Label Lingo
What the Food Label Says	*What It Means*
Fat-free	Less than $\frac{1}{2}$ (0.5) gram of fat in a serving
Low-fat	3 grams of fat (or less) per serving
Lean (on meat labels)	Less than 10 grams of fat per serving, with 4.5 grams or less of saturated fat and 95 milligrams of cholesterol per serving

What the Food Label Says	What It Means
Extra lean (on meat labels)	Less than 5 grams of fat per serving, with less than 2 grams of saturated fat and 95 milligrams of cholesterol
Less (fat, calories, cholesterol, or sodium)	Contains 25 percent less (fat, calories, cholesterol, or sodium) than the food it is being compared to
Reduced	A nutritionally altered product that contains at least 25 percent fewer calories, sodium, or sugar than the regular one
Lite (Light)	Contains $1/3$ fewer calories or no more than $1/2$ the fat of the higher-calorie, higher-fat version; or no more than $1/2$ the sodium of higher-sodium version
Cholesterol-free	Less than 2 milligrams of cholesterol and 2 grams of (or less) of saturated fat per serving
Low-calorie	Fewer than 40 calories per serving

Don't confuse total fat and calories with cholesterol, saturated fat, and sodium. All the nutrients that a food contains are important; however, to achieve weight loss, the total fat and calories are the most important to track. Cholesterol does not add calories, nor does sodium (or salt) — although eating too much sodium can contribute to water retention and therefore water weight. And the calories from saturated fat are included in the "calories from fat" total.

Label-Reading for Dieters

Choosing foods wisely based on the information that you can glean from Nutrition Facts labels is a key to successful dieting. At first, the label may seem awfully confusing, but if you know what to look for, interpreting a label is really pretty simple. Here's the skinny on the most important information featured on the Nutrition Facts label:

- **Calories:** The calorie total is based on the stated serving size — so if you eat more or less than what the label lists as one portion, you need to do the math.

- **Dietary fiber:** Choose the foods with the most fiber. Research shows that people who eat lots of fiber also eat fewer calories. You get the most fiber in foods made from whole grains, such as cereals and breads. Fruits and vegetables have fiber, too. A food is considered to be high in fiber if it has at least 5 grams of fiber per serving.

✔ **Serving size:** Notice how the food manufacturer's serving size compares to the size you usually eat. For example, does your normal serving of ice cream measure more than the standard ¹/₂ cup? And remember that serving amounts are given in *level* measuring cups or spoons. Servings per container can help you estimate sizes if a measuring cup or spoon is not handy.

✔ **Total fat:** For dieting, keep total fat to less than about 20 to 30 percent of calories. For someone who eats 1,500 calories a day, that's no more than 33 to 50 grams. Remember, the % Daily Value numbers on Nutrition Facts labels are based on 65 grams of fat a day (30 percent of total calories) and calculated on a 2,000-calorie-per-day diet.

TECHNICAL STUFF

USRDA versus RDA versus DV: What's the difference?

Ever wonder what happened to the % USRDA (US Recommended *Daily* Allowance) that used to be listed with the nutrition information on your cereal box? It has changed to % DV (Daily Value). The change is a bit confusing, but here's the deal.

Every 5 years or so, a group of scientists appointed by the government gets together and reviews recommendations for the amount of vitamins, minerals, and other nutrients that Americans need to stay healthy. Their recommendations, called the RDAs (Recommended *Dietary* Allowances) indicate the amount of a nutrient that you need to get in your diet each day for maintenance of good health. The USRDAs, which used to appear on food labels, were based on the RDAs for vitamins and minerals. The USRDAs provided you with the percentage of vitamins and minerals you got per serving of that food or beverage. Still with us?

The Daily Value (DV) is what you see now on food labels, expressed as % DV. These values are also set by the government and are based in part on the RDAs. Some labels list the Daily Values for 2,000 and 2,500 calories at the bottom of the Nutrition Facts Panel. The % DV gives you a general idea of a food's nutrient contributions to a 2,000-calorie-per-day diet. The values are kind of like the old USRDAs, but more expanded. % DV includes other nutrients, in addition to certain vitamins and minerals, which a serving of that particular food provides — such as fat, sodium, cholesterol, fiber, protein, and carbohydrate. Although many of the % Daily Values for nutrients are based on a 2,000-calorie-per-day diet, the DV for cholesterol, sodium, and vitamin A, vitamin C, calcium, and iron are set at a constant amount for all calorie levels.

You may wonder why you don't see the % DV listed for as many vitamins and minerals as the USRDA used to include. The reason? Most Americans get enough of certain vitamins and minerals in their diet, such as the B vitamins — thiamin, riboflavin, niacin, and so on. The vitamins and minerals that are listed on the Nutrition Facts labels are the ones that many Americans typically *don't* get enough of — vitamin A, vitamin C, calcium, and iron. However, the vitamin or mineral must be listed if the food is fortified with a specific one.

One final note: You may still see USRDA information on vitamin and mineral supplement bottles.

Sneaky Servings and Other Portion Tricks

Many dieters find portion control to be a tricky, tricky thing. Manufacturers certainly don't help in this regard. Some containers look as though they should contain one serving because that's probably how most people consume them. However, consider that

- ✔ A 16-ounce container of iced tea is 2 servings.
- ✔ A 6¹/₂- to 7-ounce can of tuna is 2¹/₂ servings.
- ✔ A 4-, 6-, and 8-ounce container of yogurt are all considered one serving.

To avoid having to pull out the kitchen scale or the measuring cups every time you want to eat, try this trick: Use your hand to estimate portion sizes. (Amounts approximate an average woman's hand.)

- ✔ **Your palm** is the size of a 3-ounce serving of meat, fish, or poultry.

- ✔ **Your cupped hand** can hold about 2 ounces of nuts or small candies, such as M&M's, but only ¹/₂ ounce of chips, popcorn, or pretzels.

- ✔ **Your thumb tip** is a teaspoon and good for tracking high-fat and often forgotten calories, such as the swipe you made through the brownie batter or the dip into the peanut butter jar. If your dunk is three times the size of the tip of your thumb, then you've had a tablespoon.

- ✔ **Your thumb** is about 1 tablespoon of liquid (or cookie dough) measured from tip to second joint. It also approximates an ounce of cheese — a food that's easy to overeat.

- ✔ **Your fist** is a cup. A cup of ice cream or frozen yogurt is 2 servings. Ditto for cereal, pasta, or rice. Half a cup of fruit or vegetables counts as 1 serving. Aim for at least 5 servings a day.

Smart Shopping Up and Down the Aisles

Your menus, shopping list, and filled grocery cart should be in the same proportion as the Food Guide Pyramid: Bread, cereal, rice, and pasta should occupy the largest space and be the foundation on which the rest is built. Fruits and vegetables come next in order of predominance, and then meat and dairy. Last are fats, oils, and sugar.

The following sections give some specifics about the Food Guide Pyramid's recommendations.

Breads, cereals, rice, and pasta

Thick-sliced, thin-sliced, with sugar or without, whole-grain or white, this category has grown to one of the most confusing and calorie-dense in the store. Shop carefully.

- ✔ When you buy breads, make sure that the first grain on the ingredient list is a whole grain, such as whole wheat, oats, or millet. Note that rye and pumpernickel breads are not whole grain, even though their color may make you think that they are. Their fiber content is similar to that of white bread, but the calorie content is often slightly higher because molasses is added for color.

- ✔ Baked goods should have 3 grams of fat or less per serving. And cereal should have at least 3 grams of fiber per serving.

- ✔ Pizza dough or crusts should be whole wheat. Search them out or ask your grocer to stock them.

- ✔ Frozen waffles and pancakes should be low-fat.

- ✔ Baked goods from the in-store bakery don't usually have nutrient labeling. Look at the ingredient list to see what kinds of flour are used. Go for the ones that list whole-grain flours first.

- ✔ Avoid giant muffins, biscuits, and scones. One has several servings' worth of fat and calories.

One store-bought Pepperidge Farms bran muffin has 160 calories and 7 grams of fat. Depending on the recipe, a homemade bran muffin may have much less. One muffin made by using the recipe in *The Joy of Cooking,* for example, has 135 calories and 4 grams of fat.

- ✔ When you read labels on packaged mixes, be sure to look at the "As prepared" column. Many mixes call for fats or eggs to be added in preparation.

- ✔ Brown rice has almost three times the fiber of white rice.

- ✔ Ramen noodle soups are flash-cooked in oil before packaging. They are high in fat.

- ✔ A sugar-sweetened cereal that has 8 grams of carbohydrate per serving has the same amount of sugar as a nonsweetened cereal to which 1 rounded teaspoon of sugar has been added.

- ✔ Seeded crackers have slightly more calories than plain ones, but they have more fiber, too.

Fruits and vegetables

No question about it: Fruits and vegetables are a dieter's delight. But there's more to healthy eating than counting calories. Vitamins and minerals are important, too. Want to get more nutrition from the fruits and vegetables you choose? Use these tips:

- ✔ In general, the darker the color, the higher the nutrient content. Dark salad greens such as spinach, watercress, and arugula contain more nutrients than pale ones such as iceberg lettuce. Deep orange- or red-fleshed fruit, such as mangoes, melon, papaya, and oranges, are richer in vitamins C and A than pears and bananas — but pears and bananas are especially good sources of potassium and fiber.

- ✔ Buy fresh fruits and vegetables that are in season for the best buy and best flavor. Otherwise, canned or frozen forms processed without added sugar, fats, or sauces are a good choice.

- ✔ Fresh produce doesn't carry nutrient labels; look for nutrition fliers or posters in the produce department for specifics. If prepared without sauces, butter, or added sugar, most fruits weigh in at less than 60 calories per $^1/_2$ cup serving. Most vegetables contain a mere 25 calories per $^1/_2$ cup cooked serving or per 1 cup raw.

- ✔ Most produce is virtually fat-free, with the exception of avocado and coconut.

- ✔ Shop the salad bar when you need ingredients for a recipe but don't want to purchase too much.

- ✔ Give prebagged salad a try if time and energy are scarce, but buy the ones packaged without dressing packets or garnishes.

- ✔ Dried fruits are a healthy, high-fiber snack food, but because most of the water has been removed from them, the nutrients are concentrated and the calories are higher. Keep an eye on serving size.

- ✔ Many dried fruits, especially bananas, cranberries, and dates, have sugar added to them.

Dairy

One of the first foods to be cut from many dieters' shopping lists and menus is dairy. What a shame! Most people, women in particular, need to *increase* their dairy consumption because they don't get enough precious bone-building calcium. Low-fat dairy products are among the best-tasting fat-reduced items in the supermarket — and they have all the calcium of the full-fat varieties. Don't cut out dairy products altogether; just cut down on the high-fat (and high-calorie) ones. Here's what to look for:

✔ Buy only low-fat (1 percent) or fat-free (skim) milk. Two-percent milk is not low-fat. Low-fat or fat-free milk is often fortified with nonfat milk protein to improve its texture. An added bonus is that it has a bit more calcium than whole milk.

✔ Buy only low-fat or nonfat yogurt and cottage cheese. Creamed cottage cheese (4% milk fat) does not have cream added to it; it's made with whole milk. The name refers to the way it's processed.

✔ Search out and buy low-fat cheeses. They are labeled "part skim," "reduced fat," or "fat free." However, strongly flavored full-fat cheeses are fine if used sparingly.

✔ Buttermilk contains no butter and is available in low-fat and fat-free varieties. Some dieters find that its thicker texture is more satisfying than that of fat-free milk.

Meat, poultry, fish, dry beans, eggs, and nuts

Many dieters make the mistake of thinking that if they cut out meat, they cut out calories. Unfortunately, they often substitute high-fat cheese, nuts, and nut butters for protein. Without meat, it's very tough to get enough zinc and iron — two nutrients that help maintain your energy and performance. Don't short-change yourself nutritionally by making unhelpful sacrifices. Shop smart instead.

✔ Some of the leanest cuts of beef are flank, sirloin, and tenderloin. The leanest pork is fresh, canned, cured, and boiled ham; Canadian bacon; pork tenderloin; rib chops; and roast. Lean lamb includes roasts, chops, and legs; white-meat poultry is lower in fat than dark.

✔ Meat labeled "select" is leaner than meat graded "choice."

✔ Ground turkey and chicken can contain the skin, which makes it high in fat and calories. Look for ground turkey or chicken *meat* for the lowest fat. Ground turkey breast is lower still.

✔ You don't have to remove the skin of chicken before cooking, which sacrifices juiciness. The meat will not absorb its fat or calories. But be sure to remove the skin before eating.

✔ Self-basting turkeys have fat injected into the meat. They are best avoided by dieters.

✔ Buy water-packed tuna and sardines rather than those packed in oil.

✔ Buy only fresh seafood or seafood that's frozen without added breading or frying.

Better burger beef

When well-done, there's virtually no nutritional difference between a burger made with regular ground beef and one made with extra lean. When broiled on a rack or grilled, about 2 ounces of fat drips out of the regular meat. Lean meat loses a similar amount of weight, but it's fat plus water. A burger made with 4 ounces of regular ground beef or chuck and cooked to well-done has only 12 calories more than a same-size, extra-lean one, and has almost the same number of calories as one made with lean ground beef. The big difference is in price and flavor — ground chuck wins on both counts.

Ground Beef	Raw		Cooked (Well Done)	
	Calories	Fat (Grams)	Calories	Fat (Grams)
Extra lean (17% fat)	264	19	186	11
Lean (21% fat)	298	23	196	12
Regular (27% fat)	350	30	198	13

- Cold cuts should be the low-fat varieties. Turkey and chicken franks don't always have fewer calories than beef or pork; check the labels.

- $1/2$ cup of beans or 3 ounces of tofu equals a serving of protein. Check the ingredient list for calcium sulfate. Tofu processed with it is a good source of calcium.

- 2 tablespoons of peanut butter counts nutritionally as an ounce of meat, but at 190 calories and 16 grams of fat, it's hardly a dieter's best bet. Even reduced-fat peanut butter has 12 grams of fat — and because it has added sugar, the reduced-fat and regular versions have the same number of calories.

Fats, oils, and sweets

At the tippity top of the Food Guide Pyramid is the tiny triangle of fats and sweets. These foods add calories without contributing much in the way of other nutrients to your diet. Use them sparingly. But do remember that when you plan carefully, you can make room for these fun foods, too.

✔ With the exception of whipped or diet spreads, all butter, margarine, and oils have about 100 calories per tablespoon. Whipped has about 70, and light varieties have 50 to 60.

✔ Sugar, syrups such as pancake and maple, and jelly beans don't add fat, but that doesn't mean that they're free foods. They still have calories. One *level* teaspoon of sugar has 16 calories — surely not enough to ruin your diet, but if you have 3 cups of coffee and a bowl of cereal a day and use 2 teaspoons of sugar in each, that's a quick 128 calories. If you substituted non-calorie sweeteners for this amount of sugar and made no other changes in the way you ate, you'd lose 1 pound in a month.

Chapter 15

Outfitting and Using Your Kitchen

*I*f you read Chapter 4, you now know how many calories you need to lose weight. And if you read Chapter 14, you know which foods make the healthiest choices in the supermarket. If you look ahead to Chapter 16, you can find out how to eat low-cal when eating out. But eventually, you'll have to go into the kitchen and actually prepare the foods you eat.

Cooking and eating low-cal and low-fat needn't be mysterious. Armed with the information in this chapter, you'll find cooking and eating low-cal and low-fat to be second nature.

Getting Well Equipped

You don't need to re-outfit your kitchen to make the switch to low-fat, low-calorie cooking techniques. In fact, you probably already own many of the most useful fat-fighting gadgets:

✔ **Nonstick skillet:** Using a skillet with a nonstick surface eliminates the need for oil, butter, or some other fat to prevent sautéed foods from sticking. If you've tried nonstick pans but gave up on them because they required special cooking spoons and spatulas and gentle washing, take another look: Nonstick coatings have come a long way since the early days of scratch-and-peel Teflon. Today, it's chip-resistant and durable.

Invest in top quality here. Look for a skillet that's heavy with a tough, textured coating. Heavy pans deliver even, high heat without hot spots because they don't warp. A ringed, circular pattern or a grid of squares on the cooking surface is a good investment because it makes deglazing easy — after you sauté meat or fish in the pan and remove the fat, you can add water, wine, or broth and make a sauce from the browned bits that cling to the bottom of the skillet.

✔ **Instant-read thermometer:** Lean meats and egg whites have very little fat, so they can be a dieter's best friend. But because they don't have fat, which also tenderizes them, cooking times must be brief. Cook pork, beef, or chicken too long and it becomes tough and chewy; overcook an egg white and it bounces. However, food poisoning from undercooked foods is really scary and, unfortunately, a fact of life. To avoid this sickening situation in your kitchen, take your food's temperature by using an instant-read thermometer, which is fast and accurate.

Minimum safe food temperatures include

- **Eggs:** 140°F
- **Beef and lamb:** 145°F for medium rare, 160°F for medium
- **Poultry:** 170°F for breast meat, 180°F for the whole bird
- **Pork:** 160°F

✔ **Measuring cups, measuring spoons, and a kitchen scale:** No, you don't need to portion out every ingredient or serving of food before it passes your lips, but watching portions is the easiest way to cut calories. So when you're starting out, keep track of how much you're eating by measuring your portion sizes. Doing so will make a difference in your weight-loss efforts. For example, you can save 75 calories by using a scale to measure your 3-ounce steak serving versus estimating and serving yourself 4 ounces instead.

✔ **Plastic bottles:** A refillable pump bottle beats cans of fluorocarbon-fortified vegetable oil cooking spray. Fill a bottle with olive oil and use it to lightly coat baking dishes and pans, or spray a shimmer of oil over vegetables before roasting. Or fill one with salad dressing to make calorie-wise serving sizes a blast.

Squeeze bottles (like the ones used for ketchup at diners) can shave calories, too, because you can put just a bit of sauce or gravy only where you need it. You just can't do that with a spoon, pitcher, or ladle. Even high-fat sauces, when dotted judiciously, are condoned in a low-fat kitchen.

✔ **Food processor:** A processor speeds up chopping, grating, and/or blending of vegetables and low-cal, low-fat sauces and marinades — jobs that seem daunting if done by hand are a snap with one of these. Mini-processors are particularly helpful for small jobs such as chopping a cup's worth of vegetables. They're more affordable than the large-sized processors, too.

✔ **Gravy strainer:** A gravy strainer is a measuring cup with a pour spout that starts at the base. It makes skimming fat from sauces, broths, and meat drippings a snap. Instead of spooning away the fat that floats to the surface, a strainer lets you pour out the nonfat portion from the bottom, leaving the fat behind. Buy a large one and use it for soups as well as pan drippings.

✔ **Sharp knives:** One of the greatest detriments to cooking, low-cal or otherwise, is not being able to quickly and safely cut and chop. The basics: a serrated-edge bread knife (which is great for tomatoes, too), a paring knife (about 3 inches in length), and a chef's knife (8 to 10 inches in length) for chopping.

✔ **Microwave oven:** If you use it for nothing else than zapping leftovers or "steaming" vegetables and fish without added fat, a microwave is worth having.

✔ **Popcorn popper:** Invest in an air popper or a popper that you can use in the microwave without added oil. After it's popped, spray the popcorn with a light mist of water before adding salt or herbs — the seasonings will stick better.

✔ **Plastic bags:** Use them to store vegetables and fruits that you've washed, trimmed, and have ready to go when you need a snack or when meal prep time is short. Plastic bags made specifically for storing vegetables and lettuce have tiny holes in them and help ready-to-eat and perishable vegetables keep for up to a week.

Healthful Cooking Techniques and Substitutions

Standard cooking methods need some reworking to make them low fat and low-calorie, and some foods can be used as substitutes, making them great, healthy stand-ins for others. Here are a few tricks that every calorie-conscious cook should use:

✔ **Sauté onion and garlic the low-fat way:** When a recipe calls for onion and garlic to be cooked in oil, use a nonstick pan and 2 tablespoons of water in place of the oil. Use low heat and cover the pan to coax the natural juices out of the onion and garlic.

✔ **Make and use yogurt cheese:** Spoon a 16-ounce container of plain, low-fat yogurt into a colander lined with cheesecloth or into a paper filter-lined coffee cone. Place it over a bowl in the refrigerator and allow the yogurt to drain for 8 to 24 hours, depending on how firm you want the "cheese" to be. Use well-drained yogurt as a cream cheese substitute; when softer, you can use it in place of sour cream or heavy cream.

✔ **Make your own vinaigrette salad dressing:** The standard vinaigrette dressing (three parts oil to one part vinegar) weighs in at about 90 calories a tablespoon. If you used more vinegar than oil, the calorie count would be great, but your salad would be unbearably pungent. Instead, use 1 part oil; 1 part flavorful yet mellow vinegar, such as balsamic; and 1 part strong black tea or citrus juice, such as orange or grapefruit.

✔ **Roast garlic:** When roasted, garlic is transformed into a rich, buttery, non-biting, non-odorous spread that makes a good substitute for mayonnaise in potato, pasta, and chicken salads. It's also delicious when spread on bread in place of butter or oil. Bake a head of garlic, trimmed to expose the cloves and sealed in foil with a scant tablespoon of water, for 45 minutes in a 400°F oven. Unwrap and cool it until it's easy to handle, and then simply squeeze the garlic from its skin.

✔ **Use aged cheese:** The stronger the flavor, the less you need. When a recipe calls for a mild cheese such as mozzarella or Monterey Jack, whose flavor often disappears when cooked, substitute aged cheddar, Asiago, imported Parmesan, or an aged and smoked cheese such as smoked Gouda. For the greatest bang for the bite, use these cheeses only where you see them, like on top of a dish, or when the recipe would suffer without the taste of cheese.

✔ **Roast vegetables:** You know that you need to eat more vegetables, but you may be bored by plain steamed ones. Roast them instead in a hot oven, and you'll caramelize the natural sugars that they contain and add a depth of flavor that naked veggies lack. Set the oven to 450°F. Slice the veggies about ¼ to ½ inch thick and arrange them in a single layer. Lightly spritz them using a pump bottle filled with olive oil to prevent them from drying.

- **Beets:** Roast for 1 to 1½ hours.

- **Winter squash:** Roast for 8 to 12 minutes.

- **Carrots:** Roast for 15 to 20 minutes.

- **Green beans and red peppers:** Roast for about 12 minutes.

- **Onions:** Roast for about 30 minutes.

- **Sweet potatoes:** Roast for 15 minutes.

- **Summer squash or zucchini slices:** Roast for 5 to 8 minutes

- **Eggplant:** Roast for 10 to 15 minutes.

To lightly and evenly coat vegetables before roasting, or to lightly dress a salad, drizzle a bit of oil or vinaigrette in an empty bowl. Then add the ingredients and toss.

✔ **Use sun-dried tomatoes in place of bacon:** You can easily duplicate the mellow richness and smokiness that fatty pork adds to soups, stews, and pizzas with chopped sun-dried tomatoes. Don't use the oil-packed ones unless you drain them well and blot them dry. You can soften up the dried ones in a bit of hot water.

✔ **Swap fruit for most of the fat in baked goods:** You can't remove all the oil or butter from baked goods and still have something worth eating. But you can reduce the fat to about one-quarter of the original amount and replace the rest with prune pie filling (sold as lekvar), apple butter, or applesauce.

✔ **Brown butter to use less:** Heat a bit of butter in a skillet until it becomes fragrant and begins to turn nutty brown. You'll punch up its flavor, so you can use less. A tiny bit drizzled over corn on the cob, eggs, or vegetables tastes like you're using lots.

✔ **Toast nuts for greater flavor bang:** Heat the oven to 350°F and toast nuts — on a cookie sheet in a single layer — for 5 minutes or until fragrant. Stir them to prevent scorching. Treat toasted nuts in a recipe as you would cheese: Use them only where the flavor really counts or where they will be seen, such as on the top of a bread.

✔ **Switch from chocolate to cocoa powder:** One ounce of chocolate (135 calories) can be replaced with 3 tablespoons of cocoa (35 calories). Dutch-processed cocoa is richer and more intense than the American varieties; dutching neutralizes the natural acidity in coca powder, making the flavor mellower and the color darker.

Table 15-1 lists a few more diet-friendly switches to consider.

Table 15-1	Calorie-Shaving Switches	
Instead Of	*Use*	*Calories Saved*
1 medium white potato	1 medium sweet potato	100
3 ounces ground beef	3 ounces ground turkey meat*	100
1 tablespoon mayonnaise	1 tablespoon low-fat mayonnaise	65
10 fried tortilla chips	10 baked tortilla chips	20
1 cup whole milk	1 cup fat-free or 1% milk	64 (fat-free) or 48 (1%)
1 flour tortilla	1 corn tortilla	50
1 cup whole-milk ricotta cheese	1 cup 1% cottage cheese whirled in a blender	268
1 whole egg	2 egg whites	46
½ cup cream	½ cup evaporated fat-free milk	145

(continued)

Table 15-1 *(continued)*

Instead Of	Use	Calories Saved
¹/₂ cup premium ice cream	¹/₂ cup regular ice cream	100
3¹/₂ ounces tuna in oil	3¹/₂ ounces tuna in water	80
¹/₂ cup canned fruit in syrup	¹/₂ cup canned fruit in juice	25

* Make sure that you select ground turkey breast meat. When the label says simply "ground turkey," skin may be included, and that means added fat.

Not all reduced-fat products are reduced-calorie. See Chapter 11 for more information about this danger.

Stocking Your Cupboard, Refrigerator, and Freezer

To cook low-calorie, you don't need to keep lots of bottled salad dressings, canned cream soups, and oils in your kitchen. Instead, stock your pantry with canned tomatoes, a very flavorful olive oil, vinegars, and herbs and spices. The following sections list good foods to keep on hand, by category.

On the shelf

You may have to dig a bit deeper into your pockets for these basics, but once you taste them, you'll agree that paying more is worth the extra flavor they deliver.

✔ **A good stock:** Use stock (or broth) in salad dressings in place of some of the oil, to cook vegetables for more flavor, to start a homemade soup, or in place of butter or oil when a recipe says to sauté in oil.

Store homemade stocks (or broths) frozen in an ice cube tray to punch out 2 tablespoons whenever needed. You also can buy canned broth. Stock bases are another alternative and are available in gourmet stores. Stock bases are super-concentrated, and you must add water to them before use. They're pricey but delish.

Seven condiments with more flavor than fat

Tired of the same old broiled chicken breast or plain potato? Reach for one of these flavor-makers to spice up your palate:

✔ Mustard

✔ Hot sauce

✔ Chili powder

✔ Aged balsamic vinegar

✔ Salsa

✔ Horseradish

Tip: Add 2 tablespoons prepared mustard to $1/2$ cup pan drippings (that you have skimmed of their fat) and heat to boiling. You get a velvety sauce without needing to add cream, butter, or flour.

✔ **A selection of vinegars:** Sherry, rice, raspberry, wine, and balsamic are all milder than pungent and acidic white or cider vinegar. To make a low-fat vinaigrette, you must cut back on oil as you do when you cook low-cal. But oil helps tame the punch of vinegar's acid, making the dressing taste more mellow. Therefore, you need a milder vinegar. Also consider using vinegar to sauté chicken breasts, or add a splash instead of fattening butter or cream sauces.

✔ **Hills of beans:** You can keep beans dry and cook them, or stock lots of different kinds in cans. Either way, beans can be pureed into sandwich spreads and dips, added to soups, and sprinkled on salads as a nearly fat-free yet protein-packed alternative to meats and cheeses.

✔ **Tomatoes galore:** Take advantage of the variety of canned tomato products sprouting in the supermarket. Many of them are already seasoned, which is a time-cutting, but not calorie-building, bonus for you. Thicken them with a little cornstarch (about 1 teaspoon to an 8-ounce can) or reduce them simply by boiling, and you have a sauce for pasta, vegetables, grilled fish, or chicken.

In the refrigerator and freezer

Of course, your fridge will be stocked with lots of fresh fruits and vegetables and plain frozen ones (which are a lot lower in calories than the frozen ones packaged in sauce or butter). But leave room for these diet-helpers, too:

✔ **Good extra-virgin olive oil:** You should use less oil on a reduced-calorie diet, so flavor counts. The earlier the press, the more flavor the olive delivers. Extra-virgin oil is made from the first press and has much more flavor than oil made from olives pressed several times.

Olive oil spoils quickly. In a hot kitchen, it can turn rancid in as little as 6 months, so keep it in the fridge. It thickens and turns cloudy when chilled, but a few minutes at room temperature returns it to a golden liquid without damaging the flavor.

✔ **Low-fat and reduced-fat cheeses:** These will help you save fat and calories. Low-fat American, Monterey Jack, cheddar, and Havarti are good bets.

✔ **Aged cheese:** Aged cheeses are typically high in fat, but because their flavor is so pungent, you can use less — a bonus in cooking. (See the section "Healthful Cooking Techniques and Substitutions" earlier in this chapter.)

✔ **Whole grains:** Whole grains don't have fewer calories than white, but they do have extra fiber, which helps fill you up. Studies show that people who eat lots of fiber have diets that are low in fat.

Because whole grains go rancid quickly, store them in the fridge. Whole-wheat flour, corn meal, cracked wheat, brown rice, and wheat germ last longer when kept in cold storage.

✔ **Fresh herbs:** Use fresh herbs for garnish and flavor. Piney herbs such as rosemary, sage, and thyme last longer than basil, oregano, cilantro, and mint. When using fresh herbs in recipes, add them at the end of cooking so that their flavors don't dissipate. (Dried herbs, on the other hand, are generally added early in cooking to coax the most flavor from them.)

Chapter 16

Eating Healthfully While Eating Out

In This Chapter

▶ Tips for eating in restaurants

▶ Menu words to watch out for

▶ The most healthful restaurant items to order

*E*ating out can pose special problems for dieters. New menu choices are tempting, portion sizes are large, and many professional kitchens don't normally use low-fat or low-calorie cooking methods as standard practice. In fact, as a rule, the less expensive the restaurant, the more apt the kitchen is to use generous amounts of fat and high-fat cooking techniques — inexpensive and easy ways to add flavor to food. A fish fillet, for example, must be of the highest quality and be cooked carefully if it's going to taste good simply broiled or baked without a coating of oil or buttery sauce.

The whole dining-out experience can cost you plenty of calories. How many times have you had to wait in the bar until your table was ready? Not only do cocktails add calories, but they also shave your diet resolve — you get to the table famished, and rarely feeling steeled against temptation. And then there's the impulse to clean your plate because you're paying big bucks for the meal. But take heart: There are ways around these predicaments.

For example, if you do dine out frequently, consider becoming a regular at one spot. That way, the wait staff and kitchen can get to know you. They can alert you to items that are especially dieter-friendly, and the kitchen won't be thrown by your special requests — a plus during the busiest dining hours.

Whether dining out is more special or a routine part of your day, keep this advice in mind:

- ✔ **Restaurant meals are often considered special occasions, which automatically sets you up for overindulging.** It's important not to go overboard. At the same time, remember to look at the meal in context of the entire day's eating, or what you'll eat over several days.

- ✔ **Restaurant meals are often loaded with fat.** Fat is an easy way to make foods taste good. Fat is also cheap compared to lean meat, so restaurants use it liberally because it makes their bottom line healthy — although it doesn't do much for the shape of *your* bottom. Be a fat detective. Ask questions about preparation and request substitutions.

- ✔ **Portions may be huge.** You often get twice the amount you really need to eat. Share an entree with a friend or order two appetizers instead of one entree. Don't be embarrassed to ask for a doggie bag.

- ✔ **Menus are organized with the focus on protein, and the servings of protein are much too large.** Meat, chicken, and fish often get the most "ink," with little attention paid to side dishes. So, cast your eye over to the side dishes section and choose from the plainer ones (that is, those without sauces). Another way to create a better balance may be to order your entree from the appetizer section.

- ✔ **Most meals eaten out include alcohol.** Not only is alcohol calorie-heavy and nutrient-poor, but it also lowers your resolve to eat healthfully. If you enjoy a cocktail or wine when eating out, plan to limit your intake of wine, beer, and spirits to one, and drink it with, not before, the meal.

These are important tactics to keep in mind wherever you dine. They're a start. But menus are written to entice and seduce you into ordering more than you intend. If you can learn to read between the lines and spot the red flags for dieters, you'll rarely be duped into ordering and eating more than you want. And when you eat ethnic, try to learn a little about the cuisine, the ingredients, and the typical methods of cooking so that foreign phrases don't throw you.

Menu Sleuthing

Don't be fooled. If you know how to translate the code, menu descriptions can yield clues to the fat and calorie contents of a dish. For example, "Grande taco salad served in a crispy tortilla shell, topped with lean sautéed ground beef" may at first read like a good choice. But the words *grande, crispy,* and *sautéed* tell you that this is no low-cal salad. In fact, it contains about 700 calories! If you're restricting your intake to 1,200 calories a day, do you really want to get more than half your calories from a single dish?

These are the most commonly used menu words that speak volumes — calorically, that is.

Lots of fat:

- ✔ Alfredo
- ✔ Basted
- ✔ Batter-dipped
- ✔ Breaded
- ✔ Buttery
- ✔ Creamy
- ✔ Crispy and crunchy (except when describing raw vegetables)
- ✔ Deep-fried
- ✔ Marinated
- ✔ Pan-fried
- ✔ Rich
- ✔ Sautéed

Huge portion size:

- ✔ Combo
- ✔ Feast
- ✔ Grande
- ✔ Jumbo
- ✔ King size
- ✔ Supreme

Saner sizes:

- ✔ Appetizer
- ✔ Kiddie
- ✔ Luncheon
- ✔ Petite
- ✔ Regular
- ✔ Salad size

FYI

A portion to a restaurant may not be a portion to you!

Restaurant portion sizes have more to do with controlling operation expenses than with balancing nutrients. Most restaurants use standardized ladles, spoons, cups, and scoops, and their capacity is generally larger than what you would use at home. Here are some typical institutional measures:

- ✔ Salad dressing ladle = ¼ cup
- ✔ Pat of butter = 2 teaspoons
- ✔ Scoop of ice cream = 1½ to 2 cups

- ✔ Burger = 6 to 8 ounces
- ✔ Meat, poultry, or fish = 8 to 12 ounces
- ✔ Beverages: small = 2 cups, medium = 4 cups, large = 6 cups
- ✔ Theater popcorn: small = 4 cups, large = 10 cups, jumbo = 15 to 20 cups
- ✔ Wine = 6 to 8 ounces

A Dieter's Tour of Restaurants

You may think that you must avoid certain types of restaurants or cuisines while you're dieting. Not true! The following sections guide you through various cuisines and food scenarios and tell you what's "safe" and what's not.

Chinese

Depending on your order, you can get a healthy low-cal meal or a calorie nightmare in a Chinese restaurant; foods are either very lean or very fatty. Generally, the protein foods used in Chinese cuisine — duck, spare ribs, and pork — are extremely fatty, although you can also find chicken, shrimp, and lean beef.

Much of the food is deep fried — even items that may surprise you, such as vegetables used in a simple stir-fry, are sometimes blanched in hot oil instead of water. And the amount of oil used in stir-fries can be staggeringly large.

"Family style" dining, where the dishes are placed on the table for guests to help themselves, offers another temptation to eat too much simply because the food is there. So start with small portions and have seconds only if you're *really* hungry.

Dieter's aid: Eat the way the Chinese do. Rice is the centerpiece of the meal, and diners eat from their rice bowls, not from plates. Meat and vegetables are selected from the serving dishes, almost one bite at a time, added to the bowl, and eaten with rice. Also, if you can't pass up an especially fatty dish, be sure to balance it with very lean ones.

Choose more of these:

- ✔ Bean curd (unless fried)
- ✔ Fish, shrimp, and scallops
- ✔ Hot and spicy
- ✔ Served on a sizzling platter
- ✔ Vegetables
- ✔ Velvet sauce

Eat less of these:

- ✔ Anything served in a bird's nest
- ✔ Batter-fried foods
- ✔ Breaded and fried foods
- ✔ Crispy noodles on the table
- ✔ Sweet and sour dishes
- ✔ Sweet duck sauce
- ✔ Twice-cooked dishes

Delis and sandwich shops

True delicatessens are overly generous on servings, piling sandwiches so high with meat that you need a knife and fork to eat them. What delis do vertically, sub shops (those that sell grinders and hoagies) do horizontally. Therefore, portion control is a must. Menus are usually very flexible, so this is one type of restaurant where you can exercise your calorie-smart creativity.

Dieter's aid: Go to lunch with a friend, split a sandwich, and order an extra roll or bread to make two sandwiches out of the meat in one. Or if you're by yourself, order half a sandwich and extra bread and create two sandwiches for the price of one — taking one home for later, of course. Most restaurants that serve sandwiches also have soup. Order a bowlful of a soup made without cream and eat it with an unbuttered roll, and you have a lower-calorie meal.

Choose more of these:

- Bagels
- Baked or boiled ham
- Beet salad
- Bread, especially one made with whole grains
- Carrot and raisin salad
- Extra tomato, lettuce, and veggies for sandwiches
- Mustard (not mayo)
- Pickles
- Roast or smoked turkey
- Sliced chicken (not chicken salad with lots of mayo)
- Tuna

Eat less of these:

- Bologna
- Corned beef
- Eggplant or chicken Parmigiana
- Extra cheese
- Hot pastrami
- Knockwurst
- Liverwurst
- Meatballs
- Mortadella
- Rueben sandwiches (grilled corned beef, sauerkraut, and Swiss cheese with Thousand Island dressing)
- Salami
- Sausage and peppers
- Tongue

Fast food

You can swear never to eat another burger, fry, or shake again, but get real. Often, the one and only option on America's interstates is fast food. And certainly, a trip to the mall usually means passing the food court, with its aromas seducing you to stop for just a little something. Ever noticed where they put the restrooms in shopping malls? Other than the ones located within department stores, the men's and women's rooms are stacked near the food court. It's no accident — mall designers plan it that way.

Dieter's aid: Along with all the grim news about fast foods, here are a few happy thoughts to consider:

- ✔ There are no surprises. You know what will be on the menu. With few exceptions, the menus are the same from coast to coast, so you can choose a restaurant that you know offers items that fit into your diet.
- ✔ Except for beverages, portions are generally small, especially if you stick to the regular or kids' sizes.
- ✔ Most restaurants post nutrition information or will provide it when asked, so you can make informed choices.

Even a small soda is a generous portion, so be sure to order a diet one or a seltzer and drink it all before going back for more food — it will fill you up.

Choose more of these:

- ✔ Baked potato
- ✔ Grilled chicken
- ✔ Fat-free or low-fat milk
- ✔ Fat-free salad dressing
- ✔ Salad with the dressing on the side
- ✔ Single burger (regular or kid-size)
- ✔ Small fries

Eat less of these:

- ✔ Cheese sauce
- ✔ Chicken nuggets (they often include the skin)
- ✔ Croissants
- ✔ Fish sandwich (it's fried)
- ✔ Fried chicken or fish
- ✔ Large and jumbo-size fries
- ✔ Onion rings
- ✔ Salad dressing (unless it's fat-free)
- ✔ Sauces and high-fat add-ons such as cheese, chili, and tartar sauce

French

Fat is the pitfall when it comes to French cuisine, from the butter on the table to the cream sauces, rich salad dressings, and desserts. Even lean meats and fish have added fat. Unless the restaurant specializes in *nouvelle cuisine* (the updated style of cooking that relies more on fresh ingredients and less on classic butter-enhanced sauces), you'll be hard-pressed to find diet-friendly foods.

Dieter's aid: Start with an appetite-taming green salad (easy on the dressing) or a clear soup.

Choose more of these:

- *Au vapour* (steamed)
- *En brochette* (skewered and broiled)
- *Grillé* (grilled)

Eat less of these:

- *A la crème* (in cream sauce)
- *A la mode* (with ice cream)
- *Au gratin* or *gratinée* (baked with cheese and cream)
- *Crème fraîche* (similar to sour cream)
- Drawn butter
- *En croûte* (in a pastry crust)
- Hollandaise
- Puff pastry
- *Remoulade* (a mayonnaise-based sauce)
- Stuffed

Indian

Some styles of Indian cooking are vegetarian, but don't let that lull you into thinking that these foods are low-cal. Plenty of fat is used in Indian cooking — usually clarified butter called *ghee.* Roasting tandoori style (in a clay oven called a *tandoor*) is a good low-fat cooking method, but other dishes are often stewed and fried. Indian breads are many and varied, ranging from *chapati* to high-fat, deep-fried *poori.* Often, the chef gives the breads a shimmer of butter before serving them.

Dieter's aid: Indian cuisine doesn't focus on meat; rather, it uses carbohydrates such as basmati rice (an aromatic long-grain variety) and lentils as its foundation. Vegetables are a part of almost every dish, and the sauces are enriched with yogurt, not cream.

Choose more of these:

- ✔ Chutney
- ✔ *Dahl* (lentils)
- ✔ *Masala* (curry)
- ✔ *Matta* (peas)
- ✔ *Paneer* (a fresh milk cheese)
- ✔ *Pullao* or *pilau* (rice)
- ✔ *Raita* (a yogurt and cucumber condiment)

Eat less of these:

- ✔ Chickpea batter used to deep-fry
- ✔ *Ghee* (clarified butter)
- ✔ *Korma* (cream sauce)
- ✔ *Molee* (coconut)
- ✔ *Poori* (a deep-fried bread)
- ✔ *Samosas* (fried turnover appetizers)

Italian

Most Americans think of heavy southern Italian food when they think of high-cal items: meatballs, eggplant Parmigiana, veal Parmigiana, and lasagna. However, the food of northern Italy, while it may appear less caloric, also has its detractors: butter, olive oil, and cream.

Dieter's aid: Portions are overly generous in most Italian restaurants, so this may be a good place for sharing — particularly important when you consider that an antipasto of cheese, marinated vegetables, salami, and garlic bread can use up a day's calorie budget before the main course arrives. Bread on the table served with butter or olive oil can be a diet buster. Ask for tomato sauce for dipping if you must fill up on bread, and have the fats removed. Or, better yet, out of sight, out of mouth; have the bread removed, too. Order vegetables à la carte as long as they are not cooked with lots of fat or deep-fried. And instead of a creamy dessert, order a low-fat cappuccino with fruit.

Choose more of these:

- ✔ Light red sauce
- ✔ Marinara sauce
- ✔ Pasta (other than those stuffed with cheese)
- ✔ *Piccata* (lemon-wine sauce)
- ✔ White or red clam sauce (but ask the wait staff; some clam sauces are made with cream)
- ✔ Wine sauce

Eat less of these:

- ✔ Alfredo
- ✔ *Alla panna* (with cream)
- ✔ Butter
- ✔ *Carbonara* (butter, eggs, bacon, and sometimes cream sauce)
- ✔ Fried eggplant or zucchini
- ✔ *Frito misto* (fried mixed vegetables or seafood)
- ✔ Olive oil
- ✔ *Parmigiana* (baked in sauce with cheese)
- ✔ Prosciutto
- ✔ Salami

Japanese

Japanese can be one of the healthiest cuisines, with only a few fattening dishes, such as tempura, teriyaki, katso, and sukiyaki. If eaten in the balance that the Japanese apply — heavy on the vegetables and light on the fats and meats — Japanese food can be a dieter's dream.

Dieter's aid: Portions are small, and rice and noodles are the foundation. Cooking techniques are most often broiling, steaming, braising, or simmering — all of which generally produce low-cal and low-fat dishes.

Choose more of these:

- ✔ Clear broth
- ✔ *Miso* (fermented soy)
- ✔ *Miso* dressing

- ✔ *Mushimono* (steamed)

- ✔ *Nabemono* (a one-pot dish)

- ✔ *Nimono* (simmered)

- ✔ Sashimi

- ✔ Sushi

- ✔ *Udon* (noodles)

- ✔ *Yaki* (broiled)

- ✔ *Yakimono* (grilled)

Eat less of these:

- ✔ *Agemono* (deep fried)

- ✔ *Katsu* (fried pork cutlet)

- ✔ *Sukiyaki* (a one-dish meal made with fatty beef)

- ✔ *Tempura* (batter-fried)

Mexican

The good news is that Mexican cuisine places minimal emphasis on meat protein. The bad news is that most Mexican food is fried or cooked in lots and lots of fat.

For example, a flour tortilla is fine on its own, but roll it around a filling and deep-fry it, and you have a caloric disaster. Many of the national Mexican food chains don't use lard or animal fat drippings, which is typical in many independent restaurants, but they do use plenty of vegetable oil. As far as calories are concerned, there's no difference between animal fat and vegetable fat.

Dieter's aid: Use salsa instead of salad dressing, guacamole, or sour cream on entrees. Ask for cheese toppings to be omitted, or ask if low-fat sour cream and cheese are available.

Choose more of these:

- ✔ Black bean soup

- ✔ *Ceviche* (fish or scallops marinated in lime juice)

- ✔ Chili

- ✔ Enchiladas, burritos, or soft tacos (skip the sour cream, guacamole, and most of the cheese)

- Fajitas
- Gazpacho
- Mexican salad minus the fried taco shell

Eat less of these:

- Chimichangas
- Extra Cheese
- Refried beans
- Sour cream
- Tortilla shells

Pizza

The trend toward newfangled pizza is a real plus for dieters. You can add or subtract ingredients to fit your particular tastes. Meat choices have moved from extra pepperoni, sausage, and bacon to grilled chicken and shrimp. You can specify the kind of cheese you like and replace high-fat, low-flavor mozzarella for a smaller amount of full-flavored goat cheese or feta. Even a traditional pizzeria can be diet-friendly if you order selectively.

Dieter's aid: If you can, start with a small salad to take the edge off your appetite. Order it with the dressing on the side, or extra vinegar to thin it. Also, don't leave your naked pizza crust ends on your plate — that's not where the bulk of the calories are, and the crust is a good source of low-fat, filling carbohydrate.

Choose more of these:

- Canadian bacon
- Grilled chicken
- Part-skim cheeses, or strongly flavored ones
- Shrimp
- Tuna
- Vegetable toppings, especially broccoli and spinach

Eat less of these:

- Bacon
- Extra cheese

- ✔ Extra olive oil
- ✔ Meatballs
- ✔ Olives
- ✔ Pepperoni
- ✔ Sausage

Thai

Light on fats, most Thai dishes are stir-fried, steamed, braised, or marinated. The one exception is Thai curry, which is made with coconut milk. It's loaded with calories — 1 cup of the milk contains 445 calories.

Dieter's aid: Rice and noodles are staples. Ask the chef to substitute leaner scallops, shrimp, or skinless chicken for fatty duck. The ingredients in many Thai dishes are interchangeable, so asking for substitutions shouldn't pose a problem.

Choose more of these:

- ✔ Basil sauce
- ✔ Bean thread noodles
- ✔ Fish sauce
- ✔ Lime sauce
- ✔ *Sâté* (skewered and grilled meats)
- ✔ Sizzling
- ✔ Thai salad

Eat less of these:

- ✔ Anything topped with nuts or ground peanuts
- ✔ Coconut milk soup
- ✔ *Mee-krob* (crispy noodles)
- ✔ Peanut sauce
- ✔ Red, green, and yellow mussman curries (they contain coconut milk)

Low-calorie by law

You can be sure that you're getting a low-calorie meal when you order one. The Food and Drug Administration (FDA has ruled that all restaurants (including airlines) must demonstrate that special menus comply with the same federal regulations as those used on the labels of packaged foods. The only difference is that restaurateurs are not held to the same grueling standards applied to food manufacturers. They are not required to do laboratory nutrition analysis — they can use computer programs to do their calculations and show that the menu items are prepared from recipes that comply with the standards. They don't have to post the nutrient contents of their food, but they must have it available if you ask.

If you see these terms on a menu, they must comply with FDA standards.

- ✔ **Low-calorie** means that the item contains 120 calories or less per 100 grams (about 3½ ounces).

- ✔ **Low-fat** means less than 3 grams of fat per 100 grams.

- ✔ **Low-cholesterol** items must contain less than 20 milligrams of cholesterol per 100 grams and no more than 2 grams of saturated fat.

- ✔ **Low sodium** means that the item has 140 milligrams or less of sodium per 100 grams.

- ✔ **Light** can mean that the item is low in fat or calories. (Restaurants may continue to use the term *light* as in "Lighter Fare" to mean smaller portions, as long as they make it clear how they're using the word.)

- ✔ **Healthy** means that the item is low in fat and saturated fat, has limited amounts of cholesterol and sodium, and provides significant amounts of one or more key nutrients: vitamin A, vitamin C, iron, calcium, protein, and fiber.

Airline Food

There are few standards for airline food. First-class servings are larger than those offered in coach; international flights are catered differently than domestic ones; meal service varies with the time of day. One thing is sure, though: If you fly coach, portions are tightly controlled, and that may be the best thing about eating on board.

Your larger challenge is probably the wait between connecting flights. Making sane, low-calorie choices from all the fast food available in terminals is tough, but it is getting easier because the variety of restaurants is enormous. A word of caution: Don't use food and eating as a way to kill time. Visit the magazine stand. The long corridors make great walking space if you stay off the moving sidewalks. Use them.

You can order a special meal for a flight as long as you give the airline 24 hours' notice. Each airline's selection of special menus varies, so call and ask what's offered. What you get to eat when you order a special meal varies, too, but rest assured that if you request a low-calorie tray, it will be low-calorie. Low-cholesterol is indeed low. Low-sodium is salt-restricted, and diabetic conforms to standards. That's because the feds are watching. Menus that make health claims must comply with standards set and regulated by the Food and Drug Administration.

Vegetarian meals, which are ordered more frequently than any other type, are not regulated. Although many are low-cal and low-fat, don't bet on it. Make sure to ask.

Part V
Enlisting Outside Help

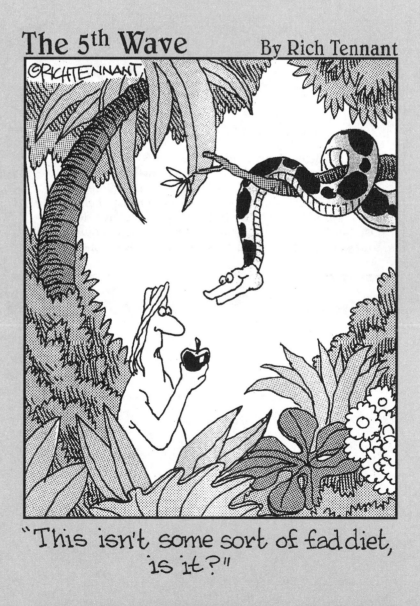

The 5th Wave   By Rich Tennant

"This isn't some sort of fad diet, is it?"

In this part . . .

Some dieters have more success when they enlist outside help, whether it comes from a weight-loss program, a doctor-prescribed medication, or a dietitian. This part explains how the various options can help you, and helps you spot sources that may be best avoided. It also talks about some of the most popular diets out there today and points out the pros and cons of each one.

Chapter 17

Getting Help from a Weight-Loss Professional

. . . .

In This Chapter

▶ Finding a weight-loss expert

▶ Knowing what to expect from professional counseling

▶ Searching for qualified help

▶ Spotting a quack

. . . .

*R*eading this book is a good way to get started toward your weight-loss goal. But sometimes going it alone isn't the best route. That's especially true if

- ✔ You're involved in competitive sports and would like to enhance your performance.

- ✔ You've tried to lose and maintain your weight many times and have regained it (and more).

- ✔ You have health problems and need to modify your eating habits both to lose weight and to control your condition.

If you look up "Nutritionist" in the Yellow Pages, you're apt to find a hodgepodge of qualifications. How do you know whether a person you find is qualified to help you? This chapter helps you sort the pros from the charlatans. Knowing the difference is important — your health depends on it.

(For information about weight-loss centers, which also may be listed in the phone book under "Nutrition" or "Diet," turn to Chapter 19.)

Who Are the Professionals?

No nationwide law mandates who can be called a "nutritionist," "diet counselor," or "health advisor." However, the majority of states license or certify qualified nutritionists and dietitians. (In Canada, dietitians must be registered in the province in which they practice.) Unfortunately, a few states have no requirements or standards of practice yet. So it's easy to be fooled into thinking that the advisor you meet is qualified to dispense accurate weight-loss information.

Table 18-1 lists some abbreviations that you're apt to encounter in your search for a nutrition specialist. But be sure to ask the counselor to explain his or her degree.

Table 18-1	Abbreviations for Nutrition-Related Degrees and Other Related Designations
Abbreviation	*Degree or Designation*
C.D. or C.N.	Certified Dietitian or Certified Nutritionist (granted by some states)
C.D.E.	Certified Diabetes Educator
C.D.N.	Certified Dietitian/Nutritionist (granted by some states)
C.E.P.	Certified Exercise Physiologist (available soon)
C.S.P.	Board Certified Specialist in Pediatric Nutrition
D.T.R.	Dietetic Technician, Registered
L.D.	Licensed Dietitian (granted by some states)
M.D.	Doctor of Medicine
M.Ed.	Master of Education
M.S.	Master of Science
M.P.H.	Master of Public Health
N.D.	Naturopathic Doctor
Ph.D.	Doctor of Philosophy
R.D.	Registered Dietitian
Sc.D.	Doctor of Science

The following sections tell you more about these nutrition professionals.

Registered dietitian

One way to ensure that you receive accurate nutrition and diet information is to search out a *registered dietitian,* or R.D. — a professionally trained authority in the role that food and nutrition play in health. R.D.s are a reliable source for information about nutrition and can provide sound advice on eating and health.

To earn an R.D., an individual must have a bachelor's degree in nutrition or a related field from a regionally accredited college or university. The program of study must be accredited by the Commission on Accreditation and Approval of Dietetics Education of the American Dietetic Association. Courses include food science, nutrition, biochemistry, anatomy, physiology, biology, organic chemistry, and management. The individual must also complete a dietetic internship or supervised practice experience and pass an extensive examination to become registered.

All R.D.s are required to stay current by completing a minimum of 75 hours of continuing education every 5 years. Only dietitians who have passed the exam and maintain their continuing education are considered registered. Many R.D.s go on to earn additional degrees, such as master's (M.S. or M.P.H. or M.Ed.) or doctorates (Ph.D. or Sc.D.) in nutrition or a nutrition-related specialty.

Registered dietitians can also hold additional certifications in specialized areas of practice, such as pediatrics (C.S.P.) and diabetes (C.D.E.). These individuals must not only pass an extensive exam in their specialty but also accumulate a specific number of practice hours in their specialty.

Forty states either certify or license dietitians and/or nutritionists who meet specific criteria established by the state agency that regulates health professionals. Certification entitles professionals to use either "dietitian" or "nutritionist," depending on how the law is written within an individual state. The initials C.D. or C.N. appear after the name of a dietitian who is also state-certified as a dietitian or nutritionist. Licensure protects the title "dietitian" or "nutritionist" and defines how they practice. The initials L.D. appear after the name of a licensed dietitian or nutritionist. In some states, dispensing nutrition advice without a license is against the law.

Dietetic technician, registered

The initials D.T.R. stand for *dietetic technician, registered.* A person who is a D.T.R. is qualified to be part of the nutrition care team, which may include teaching nutrition classes, diet counseling, and nutritional assessment. To become a D.T.R., an individual must earn an associate degree from a regionally accredited U.S. college or university, complete a dietetics practice program accredited by the Commission on Accreditation and Approval of Dietetics Education of the American Dietetic Association, pass a registration exam, and maintain at least 50 hours of continuing professional education every 5 years.

Exercise physiologist

Exercise physiologists can help you plan an exercise program to aid in your weight-loss efforts, but they should not dispense diet advice. An exercise physiologist holds a bachelor's degree with an emphasis in exercise physiology. In addition to basic science courses, exercise physiologists study human anatomy and physiology, biomechanics, cardiopulmonary rehabilitation, exercise physiology, sports nutrition, electrocardiography, stress tests, and research and statistics. They also take a variety of specialized courses.

In the near future, the American Society of Exercise Physiologists Board of Certification will adopt a national certification test for all graduates of an approved exercise physiology curriculum. A certified exercise physiologist will then be allowed to use the initials C.E.P. after his or her name. In the meantime, the American College of Sports Medicine (ACSM) certification is available to any professional within the preventive and rehabilitative exercise field who meets the established prerequisites.

Exercise physiologists go through six progressive levels of ACSM certification. Each requires a written exam to test knowledge and a practical exam to measure hands-on skills. After earning ACSM certification, an exercise physiologist must participate in continuing education and maintain a current CPR certification.

Physician

Medical doctors (M.D.s) offer medical weight-loss programs, which may include the use of prescription drugs and very low calorie diets (VLCD). Although any licensed physician can offer this kind of treatment, a *bariatrician* (from the Greek word *barros,* meaning heavy or large) specializes in treating obesity and has received special training and extensive continuing medical education. Often, a physician refers a patient to a registered dietitian for help in working out specific food issues.

VLCD, which stands for *very low calorie diet,* describes a plan — usually liquid — of 800 or fewer calories per day. These diets are generally considered safe when supervised by a health care team. Medifast, Optifast, and New Direction are examples of a medically supervised VLCD. (See Chapter 19 for more information about these programs.)

What Professionals Can Do for You

A nutritionist, dietitian, exercise physiologist, or physician can tailor an exercise and weight-loss program to meet your needs. The program should include personal, ongoing care. You attend an evaluation session, during which the health care professional assesses your history, preferences, and needs. He or she then gives you a personalized plan to follow and schedules follow-up appointments to check your progress and make adjustments to your program as needed.

 Medical nutrition therapy, which is what insurance companies call diet counseling, may be covered by your health plan if it is provided by a registered dietitian. Be sure to ask your physician or insurance provider for information.

Assessing your situation

A dietitian or other medical professional will want to know your health status before making dietary recommendations. He or she will assess your blood pressure, plus information from a blood test, including your cholesterol, glucose, hemoglobin, and hematocrit levels. These measurements are helpful for determining the best diet recommendations for you.

An exercise physiologist will also need to know whether any health concerns would limit your ability to exercise. Therefore, before you discuss your diet and exercise habits with the physiologist, it may be necessary to have a medical check-up.

Your dietitian may ask you to fill out a food diary for several days before your first visit so that no details will be missed. Bring this diary, along with any vitamin and mineral or herbal supplements that you're taking, too. These supplements figure into your daily nutrient needs; in some cases, taking very large doses of one nutrient or a combination of large doses can throw an otherwise healthy eating plan out of balance. Your dietitian may want to make adjustments or recommendations.

Expect to spend at least an hour at your first visit with a dietitian. Be prepared to answer questions — lots of them. The dietitian will want to know whether you have food sensitivities or allergies, what foods you like and dislike, what you usually eat, how much you eat at one time, when you eat, and where you eat — the whole ball of wax. Your weight history is also important.

You will be asked about your family as well. Who does the cooking? Who does the food shopping? What is your normal routine? Do you work out of your home? What kind of employment do you have? Be honest in your answers; trying to paint a rosy picture of your habits serves neither you nor the dietitian.

The dietitian will record your starting weight and help you set realistic weight-loss goals. He or she may do skin-fold measurements (see Chapter 2) as well to determine what percentage of your weight is fat and what percentage is muscle. (You can expect the same from an exercise physiologist.) All these factors help you and the dietitian build a diet that meets your individual needs.

From the information that the dietitian gathers from your interview, he or she determines your normal calorie intake and expenditures and, with your input, designs a weight-loss plan.

You may want to bring your spouse, parent, or child with you to your first meeting, especially if one of these people does the food shopping and cooking. Support is important throughout your weight-loss program, so consider starting out by taking your "team" along.

Creating a plan

A dietitian focuses on lifestyle and food choices, not quick results, so don't expect miracle cures. Nor should your weight-loss success depend on your buying and taking expensive supplements. (See the sidebar "Ten red flags that signal bad nutrition advice.") A qualified exercise physiologist should not expect you to purchase special equipment or a health club membership, nor should he or she recommend dietary supplements.

If you don't understand something about a plan that a dietitian or exercise physiologist creates for you, ask. You may hear nutrition or sports lingo that throws you, and it's important that you understand exactly what's being said. Remember, the only dumb question is the one you *don't* ask. You can comply with the diet and exercise recommendations only if you understand what's expected.

Following up

The dietitian will ask you to commit to follow-up visits while you work toward your goal weight. Not only will you get moral support, but the dietitian can adjust your plan, answer questions, and record progress. Positive changes take time, encouragement, and most likely some tweaking. Plan your schedule to allow time for follow-up appointments.

WARNING!

Ten red flags that signal bad nutrition advice

How do you know whether the nutrition advice you receive or the weight loss materials provided to you are reliable? Consider any combination of these ten red flags a signal of questionable nutrition advice:

1. Recommendations that promise a quick fix

2. Dire warnings of dangers from a single product or regimen

3. Claims that sound too good to be true

4. Simplistic conclusions drawn from a complex study

5. Recommendations based on a single study

6. Dramatic statements that are refuted by reputable scientific organizations

7. Lists of "good" and "bad" foods

8. Recommendations made to help sell a product

9. Recommendations based on studies published without peer review

10. Recommendations from studies that ignore differences among individuals or groups

Source: Food and Nutrition Science Alliance (FANSA), of which the ADA is a member.

Finding a Health Care Professional Who Specializes in Weight Loss

The following sections provide resources for finding a health care professional who can help you with weight loss. You can contact the organizations that we include or consult your local Yellow Pages to locate health care professionals in your area.

American Dietetic Association (ADA)

The American Dietetic Association (ADA) is the world's largest organization of food and nutrition professionals. For recorded food and nutrition information and a referral to a registered dietitian in your area, call the American Dietetic Association/National Center for Nutrition and Dietetics Consumer Nutrition Hotline at 800-366-1655. For customized answers to your nutrition questions, call 900-CALL-AN-RD (900-225-5267). The cost is $1.95 for the first minute and 95 cents for each additional minute. For more information, including a referral to an R.D., visit the ADA's Web site at www.eatright.org.

American Society of Exercise Physiologists (ASEP)

The American Society of Exercise Physiologists (ASEP) is a national non-profit professional organization committed to the advancement of exercise physiologists. The society sets standards for exercise physiologists through ASEP-approved curricula in universities and colleges in the United States.

To locate an exercise physiologist in your area, contact

ASEP National Office
College of St. Scholastica
1200 Kenwood Avenue
Duluth, MN 55811
Phone: 218-723-6297
Fax: 218-723-6472
www.css.edu/users/tboone2/asep/toc.htm

American College of Sports Medicine (ACSM)

The American College of Sports Medicine (ACSM) is the largest sports medicine and exercise science organization in the world, with more than 16,500 members in more than 70 countries. The ACSM is dedicated to promoting and integrating scientific research, education, and practical applications of sports science and exercise science to maintain and enhance physical performance, fitness, health, and quality of life.

To locate a certified exercise specialist in your area or for more information, contact

ACSM National Center for Certification Department
P. O. Box 1440
Indianapolis, IN 46206-1440
317-637-9200
ACSM.org

American Society of Bariatric Physicians (ASBP)

The American Society of Bariatric Physicians (ASBP) is a national professional medical society of licensed physicians who offer specialized programs in the medical treatment of obesity. ASBP members receive additional training in the field of obesity.

To locate a physician who specializes in treating overweight and obese patients, call 303-779-4833. By following the instructions of the ASBP automated system, you can obtain a list of all the physician members in your state. Enter the state's two-letter postal abbreviation (for example, NY for New York) and your fax number. Within seconds, a list of names starts printing from your fax machine.

For more information, contact

American Society of Bariatric Physicians
5600 South Quebec Street, Suite 109-A
Englewood, CO 80111
303-770-2526
www.asbp.org/bariatrics

Tracking down a dietitian

To find a registered dietitian in your area who can provide scientifically based nutrition guidance on weight loss, contact

✔ Your doctor or health maintenance organization (HMO) for a referral

✔ Your local dietetic association, the nutrition department of an area college or university, or the extension service at the nearest state university

✔ The chief clinical dietitian at your local hospital

✔ The American Dietetic Association/National Center for Nutrition and Dietetics (Ask for a referral to a registered dietitian in your area by calling 800-366-1655 or by visiting the ADA's Web site at www.eatright.org.)

Chapter 18

Using Medications for Weight Control

● ●

In This Chapter

▶ Determining whether medication can help you

▶ Evaluating prescription drug choices

▶ Considering over-the-counter medications

▶ Knowing the risks and limits of drug use for weight loss

● ●

*U*sing drugs to lose weight is nothing new. In the 1950s and 1960s, people swallowed lots of diet pills, mostly amphetamine derivatives (speed). Addiction and abuse were common, so physicians gradually stopped prescribing drugs for weight loss.

For a long time after that, diet and exercise, not drug therapy, were the preferred forms of treatment. But in 1973, the Food and Drug Administration (FDA) approved a new drug for weight loss. Its name was fenfluramine (trade name Pondimin). Next came dexfenfluramine (trade name Redux) in 1996. Some physicians prescribed phentermine (a different kind of weight-loss medication in use since 1959) in combination with fenfluramine, and the medication became known as fen-phen. Phentermine has also been used in combination with dexfenfluramine (known as dexfen-phen). But in September 1997, after reports of serious heart valve disease, the manufacturers of fenfluramine and dexfenfluramine withdrew the drugs from the market. Prescriptions were no longer written for Redux, Pondimin, or fen-phen.

A new medication called sibutramine (trade name Meridia) is the newest weight-loss drug currently being prescribed, and a conga line of others is in development or waiting for FDA approval. But you don't need a prescription to find medications that claim to help in weight loss — plenty of over-the-counter medications are available. Can they help you lose weight? This chapter gives you the scoop.

Redux, redux

During the year and a half that fenfluramine (trade name Pondimin) and dexfenfluramine (trade name Redux) were being used as weight-loss drugs, 14 million prescriptions were written. The drugs worked by increasing serotonin levels in the brain. *Serotonin* is a brain chemical, a neurotransmitter, that's associated with improved mood and has a role in the feedback system of appetite and satiety.

People did lose weight on these medications. But in September 1997, the FDA requested that they be removed from the market because it was becoming clear that taking the drugs, either alone or in combination, was associated with fatal heart valve problems. In fact,

patients who took the drug had a 30 percent chance of developing heart valve abnormalities, often without symptoms.

The FDA advises that anyone who took Pondimin or Redux or fen-phen should have an echocardiogram (ECG) — even if he or she shows no symptoms of heart or lung disease, such as a heart murmur or shortness of breath. Undergoing an ECG is particularly important before having an invasive procedure that may release bacteria into the bloodstream — even dental work — to determine whether antibiotic treatment is necessary to prevent *bacterial endocarditis,* a potentially fatal infection of the heart's lining.

How Do the Current Weight-Loss Drugs Work?

Most drugs approved by the FDA for use in weight loss work by decreasing appetite. But the mechanism of action of today's available medications is far more complex than that of the old pep pills and diet pills of the 1950s and 1960s, most of which were amphetamines. (Amphetamines can still be prescribed, but because of the potential for abuse and addiction, they are rarely used for weight loss anymore.)

The new generation of appetite-regulation drugs works on brain chemicals (called *neurotransmitters*) to partially suppress appetite and thereby reduce how much you eat. Another class of obesity drugs, known as *lipase inhibitors,* exert their effect on fat directly in the gastrointestinal tract. Lipase inhibitors work by blocking the absorption of fat. And then there are over-the-counter (OTC) diet preparations, which act as stimulants to decrease your appetite.

Weight loss drugs don't work without lifestyle changes. Appetite-suppressant medications must be combined with physical activity and a calorie-reduced diet. Think of these medications as aids in — not substitutes for — your weight-loss program.

Are Prescription Weight-Loss Drugs for You?

Before prescribing a medication to aid in weight loss, your physician will take a careful medical history and perform a physical exam. He or she will ask whether any of your relatives has heart disease or diabetes. Your physician will also calculate your Body Mass Index (BMI). (For an explanation of BMI and to find out how to calculate your own, See Chapter 2.) The result of this calculation is the primary guideline used to determine whether you are a candidate for prescription drugs. If you have a BMI of 30 or greater (or 27 or greater if you have heart disease, diabetes, or other factors that would make your weight a health risk), you are a potential candidate for weight-loss drugs. Diet counseling from a registered dietitian should always be provided along with weight-loss medication.

Weight-loss medication may *not* be for you if . . .

✔ You are pregnant or breast-feeding.

✔ You have a history of drug or alcohol abuse.

✔ You have a history of an eating disorder.

✔ You have a history of severe depression or manic-depressive disorder.

✔ You are taking a monoamine oxidase (MAO) inhibitor or any other type of antidepressant medication.

✔ You get migraine headaches and take medication for them.

✔ You have an unstable medical condition such as glaucoma, diabetes, high blood pressure, or heart disease or a heart condition such as an irregular heartbeat.

✔ You are having surgery that requires general anesthesia.

After you've been on your medication for about 4 weeks, your doctor will schedule another visit to see whether the prescription is working and evaluate its effects on your overall health. A weight loss of 1 pound a week is considered "working." If the medication doesn't work in the first 3 to 6 weeks of treatment despite adjustments in dosage, chances are good that the diet drug will never work for you. Your physician will tell you to stop taking the drug you're on and may suggest that you try another.

For weight-loss drugs to be effective, you must be sure to take them. Just as your car slows down when you take your foot off the gas pedal, your weight loss slows down when you stop taking the medication. Also keep in mind that only one of the drugs (Meridia) has been approved for long-term use.

Few severely obese people reach their ideal body weights by using the currently available medications alone. But for these individuals, even a modest weight loss of 5 to 10 percent of their starting body weights can improve health and reduce risk factors for disease. The current weight-loss medications are *not* recommended for use by people who are only mildly overweight unless they have health problems that their weight makes worse. These drugs should not be used solely for cosmetic reasons.

Using Prescription Medications

In the following sections, we offer some information about specific prescription medications for weight loss.

People who used some appetite-suppressant medications for more than 3 months have a greater risk for developing primary pulmonary hypertension (PPH) — a rare but potentially fatal disorder that affects the blood vessels in the lungs. Forty-five percent of PPH victims die within 4 years of contracting the disorder, which affects about 1 in 22,000 to 1 in 44,000 patients per year.

If you took Pondimin, Redux, or fen-phen or dexfen-phen (fenfluramine or dexfenfluramine in combination with phentermine) and you experience symptoms such as shortness of breath, chest pain, faintness, or swelling in your lower legs and ankles, contact your doctor. The vast majority of PPH cases were related to fenfluramine or dexfenfluramine (both were taken off the market), either alone or in combination, but a few cases of PPH have been reported in people taking phentermine alone. No cases of PPH have been linked to the use of sibutramine.

Orlistat (trade name Xenical)

Orlistat, which is currently under FDA review, works in the intestinal tract. It does not suppress appetite, but it reduces the amount of fat that can be absorbed during digestion by about 30 percent. Studies show that people who use Orlistat can lose about 10 percent of their initial weight over the course of a year, but because fat can't be digested, diarrhea is common if you don't follow a low-fat diet. Orlistat is expected to be available in the U.S. in 1999.

Sibutramine (trade name Meridia)

Sibutramine is FDA-approved for both weight loss and weight maintenance. It works on brain chemicals to reduce appetite and give a sense of fullness. Studies have shown that sibutramine can help people lose weight and maintain the loss, but the weight loss tends to plateau after about a year, with a loss of about 10 percent of starting weight. That's enough to produce measurable health benefits, but probably not a sufficient loss to satisfy an "ideal" body image.

Like all medications, sibutramine can cause side effects. The drug may elevate both blood pressure and heart rate.

Other appetite suppressants

The following appetite suppressants are currently available by prescription:

- ✔ Diethylpropion (trade names Tenuate and Dospan)
- ✔ Mazindol (trade names Sanorex and Mazanor)
- ✔ Phendimetrazine (trade names Bontirl, Plegine, Prelu-2, and X-Trozine)
- ✔ Phentermine (trade names Apidex-P, Fastin, Ionamin, and Oby-trim)

In studies that combined these drugs with diet and exercise in long-term tests (longer than 6 months), about three-quarters of the participants lost about 5 percent of their starting weight, about half lost about 10 percent, and about a third lost 15 percent. But because all medications come with side effects, the FDA has approved these appetite suppressants only for short-term use — generally, only a few weeks to a few months. However, some physicians do prescribe them for off-label use (see the following paragraph for an explanation of this term). As with all drugs, weight loss stops when you discontinue use unless diet and exercise are part of the treatment.

The FDA regulates how a manufacturer can advertise or promote a medication. These regulations restrict a doctor's ability to prescribe the medication for different conditions, in larger doses, or for different lengths of time. The practice of prescribing medication for periods of time or for unapproved conditions is known as *off-label use*. Using more than one appetite-suppressant medication at a time (combined drug treatment) or using a currently approved appetite-suppressant medication for more than a few weeks is also considered off-label use. (Meridia *is* approved for long-term use, however.)

Antidepressants

Some antidepressants (particularly fluoxetine — trade name Prozac) have been studied as appetite-suppressant medications. Although these drugs are FDA-approved for the treatment of depression, their use in weight loss is an off-label use.

In studies, patients taking antidepressants to suppress appetite lost modest amounts of weight for up to 6 months. But most reached a plateau after about 4 months and tended to regain weight while they were still on the drugs. Antidepressant therapy *has* been effective in the treatment of eating disorders. (See the sidebar "Drug use in eating disorders.")

Drug use in eating disorders

Hundreds of double-blind studies have shown that treatment with antidepressants can help reduce bulimic behavior and binge eating by about half. Doctors first started using antidepressants to treat eating disorders when they realized that many people with bulimia are depressed. And as with depression, many kinds of medications can be effective.

Only a doctor can prescribe the correct dose and type of medication by evaluating a patient's history, current medications (if any), and how quickly and thoroughly symptoms are relieved. Close monitoring until the drug of choice is determined is crucial. The medication often takes several weeks to take effect.

Taking Over-the-Counter (OTC) Drugs

Most over-the-counter (OTC) medications act as stimulants to decrease your appetite.

Few long-term studies have been conducted on the safety or effectiveness of over-the-counter drugs. Herbs packaged for weight loss are crowding the shelves and leaving less room for other OTC drugs, such as those made with the chemical phenylpropanolamine (PPA). Unfortunately, few herbal preparations are labeled with amounts of active ingredients, so knowing how much of a drug you're getting is nearly impossible. Remember that just because a product is herbal doesn't mean that taking a lot of it is safe. Many preparations combine several of the ingredients that we describe in the following sections.

5-hydroxytryptophan (5-HTP)

5-HTP is a compound formed during serotonin synthesis from tryptophan. Serotonin is associated with feelings of calm and fullness. Studies using this metabolite in humans are inconclusive, but some experts are concerned that any drug that elevates serotonin levels may be associated with the same kind of risks seen with prescription appetite suppressants.

The FDA has found impurities in supplements of 5HTP. One of those impurities is similar to one found in L-tryptophan supplements that was linked to eosinophilia-myalgia syndrome (EMS), a serious illness that can result in death. L-tryptophan was removed from the market because of the contamination.

The bottom line: Not recommended.

Chromium picolinate

Chromium is needed for insulin metabolism and plays a small role in energy production. It's found in mushrooms, broccoli, and potatoes. But chromium picolinate is a synthetic compound. There's no recommended dietary allowance for chromium, and deficiencies are extremely rare. Supplements increase chromium levels significantly, which may lead to chromosomal damage and may be linked to kidney failure.

The bottom line: Not recommended.

Ephedra (ma huang)

Ephedrine, which is structurally similar to amphetamines, is the active ingredient in ephedra, which is commonly known as ma huang. You may see either ephedrine, ephedra, or ma huang listed on the labels of some herbal weight-loss drugs and fat burners. Doses of ephedrine that are sufficient to cause weight loss also can cause tremors, induce severe headaches, and make your blood pressure soar — especially when combined with caffeine, as it often is in over-the-counter diet preparations.

Ephedra has been linked to more than 800 incidents, including high blood pressure, severe headaches, heart rate abnormalities, seizures, heart attacks, and even deaths. Ephedra derivatives also have been reported to produce acute hepatitis and other unexplained liver injuries. The FDA has little power to regulate the sale or use of ephedra because it falls under the Dietary Supplement Act, which allows the sale of such preparations as foods. However, the FDA recommends that no more than 8 milligrams a day of ephedra should be used for no more than 7 consecutive days, and that labels disclose all potential side effects, including death. Unfortunately, many preparations are sold without comprehensive ingredient labels, so you have no way of knowing how much ephedra the product includes.

The bottom line: Not recommended for use in doses larger than or for periods longer than what the FDA recommends.

Guarana

Guarana is sold as a fat burner and a metabolism booster, but its active ingredient is basically caffeine — 100 milligrams of guarana has about the same caffeine content as a cup of black coffee. Taken by itself, guarana is probably not dangerous.

Guarana is often used in herbal preparations in combination with ephedra, making the ephedra even more powerful and dangerous. This combination increases the risk of high blood pressure, stroke, and death.

The bottom line: No more effective for weight loss than caffeine.

Phenylpropanolamine

Over-the-counter weight-loss drugs, including Acutrim and Dexatrim, generally contain the active ingredient phenylpropanolamine (PPA). PPA works by decreasing appetite. Most studies (and there aren't many) show that using PPA may increase weight loss, but not by much. When compared to an 8-week diet and exercise plan without PPA, a program that included PPA produced an average additional weight loss of only 3 pounds.

Taking more than the dosage recommended on the drug's label can cause heart palpitations and elevate your blood pressure, possibly putting you at greater risk of stroke. Seventy-five milligrams is the maximum recommended daily dose. PPA is also used in over-the-counter nasal decongestant cold remedies, so check the labels — you may take too much PPA because you're getting it from two sources.

The bottom line: Diet and exercise are the keys to weight loss. If you use any OTC drug, including any drug that contains PPA, use it with care.

Pyruvate

This compound occurs naturally in the body and can be found in foods such as beer, red wine, and cheese. Proponents claim that pyruvate can increase metabolism and speed up carbohydrate digestion. Many athletes believe that it can increase their performance and endurance. However, the studies on weight loss and exercise performance have not shown a connection.

The bottom line: Probably not harmful, but not effective, either.

St. John's Wort

You can find St. John's Wort in many herbal diet preparations. It has been used to treat depression in Germany for many years and may increase the brain's serotonin levels, which boosts mood and possibly curbs the depression sufferer's tendency to eat.

Extended use may cause eye and skin sensitivity to sunlight.

The bottom line: May help relieve overeating due to depression.

Senna

Senna, an herbal laxative, is often an ingredient in herbal "diet teas." It stimulates the colon and can result in extreme diarrhea, nausea, and dehydration. The weight loss is apt to be due to water loss, not fat loss. And drinking tea made with this herb can be as habit-forming as regularly using laxatives, making it impossible to have a bowel movement without it.

The bottom line: More harmful than helpful.

The idea that a pill or potion can make losing weight easy is seductive — that's why dieters spend billions of dollars buying them and drug companies spend billions of dollars developing new ones. But while drug therapy offers hope of thinness to many people, study after study shows that weight-loss medications work only when used in combination with a low-calorie diet and exercise plan.

Chapter 19

Joining a Weight-Loss Program

. . . .

In This Chapter

▶ Determining what you need from a weight-loss program

▶ Sorting out the differences among programs

▶ Deciding whether a particular program is for you

. . . .

Several types of weight-loss programs are available. Some require more
visits than others, some cost more than others, and some are more
restrictive than others. You can find self-help groups that offer only support,
not concrete diet or exercise advice. Others require membership and the
purchase of special foods. Still others, run by physicians, are generally
based in hospitals (although you don't have to stay at the hospital) and
restrict daily food intake to a few liquid meals.

This chapter shows you how these programs compare and gives you the
background ammunition that you need to sort through the maze of options.
Start by completing the quiz on what you need to know before signing up in
the following section. Then evaluate the information that we provide on
some of the most popular diet programs out there. We've collected the same
crucial statistics for each program, so comparing is easy.

We adapted this list based on information collected by Shape Up America!
(www.shapeup.org), the National *Initiative* to Promote Healthy Weight and Physical Activity (Guidance for Treatment of Adult Obesity — Shape Up America!,
6707 Democracy Blvd., Ste. 306, Bethesda, MD 20817, and American Obesity
Association, 1250 24th Street NW, Ste. 300, Washington, DC 20037, 1996).

Questions to Ask Before Enrolling in a Diet Program

An educated consumer is the best customer. So before you sign up for a
weight-loss program, ask yourself the following questions. You may not be
able to answer all of them with certainty, but do keep these points in mind
as you weigh your options:

✔ Do I need the peer pressure of a group to keep me going?

✔ Do I have the time to commit to attending weekly sessions or meetings for up to a year?

✔ Can I afford to join a club or program?

✔ Does the program require special foods, and can I afford them? If so, will my eating special foods interfere with my family's lifestyle?

✔ Am I willing to follow a program's instructions, guidance, and skill-building techniques to learn to eat in a more healthful way and, whether or not the program requires it, be physically active for the long term?

Self-Help Programs

If you could use some peer support while trying to lose weight — but don't require a regimented plan structure or the services of program-provided weight-loss professionals — one of the organizations in this section may be your best choice.

Overeaters Anonymous (OA)

Approach/method: This nonprofit international organization provides volunteer support groups, which are modeled on Alcoholics Anonymous and other 12-step programs. Members are encouraged to seek professional help for individualized diet and nutrition plans and for emotional or physical problems.

Clients/staff: Members are individuals who define themselves as compulsive overeaters. The staff are nonprofessional volunteers who meet specific criteria, sit on the board, lead meetings, and conduct activities.

Expected weight loss/length of program: The program makes no claims about the weight loss of members or the length of time needed to reach a goal.

Healthy lifestyle component: The group recommends emotional, spiritual, and physical recovery changes. It makes no exercise or food recommendations.

Comments: This program is inexpensive and provides group support. You don't need to follow a specific diet plan to participate. Minimal organization exists at the group level, so groups vary in approach. No health care providers are on staff.

Cost: The group supports itself with members' contributions and sales of publications (including workbooks, tapes, newsletters, and sponsor outreach programs). Its international monthly journal, *Lifeline,* costs $12.99 per year within the United States, and $17.99 per year outside the United States by surface mail or $24.99 per year via air mail.

Availability: 9,000 groups meet in more than 50 countries. See the Overeaters Anonymous listing in your local telephone directory.

Headquarters: The organization is located at World Service Office (WSO), 6075 Zenith Court NE, Rio Rancho, NM 87124; phone 505-891-2664; Web www.overeatersanonymous.org.

TOPS Club, Inc. (Taking Off Pounds Sensibly)

Approach/method: TOPS is an international, nonprofit, noncommercial weight-loss support group. You bring your own exercise and food plan and a goal weight from your personal physician. TOPS merely provides a supportive environment in which you can make the slow, steady, permanent lifestyle changes that are necessary to reach and maintain your goal.

Clients/staff: Chapters are run on a local level by members who elect a volunteer leader. Each chapter varies in its approach according to the needs of its members, but all chapters address the complex issues involved in weight loss. Chapters frequently invite health professionals to speak at meetings, and are supported by trained field staff. Headquarters provides educational materials and a monthly magazine. A strong incentive plan with awards and recognition is woven into the program at all levels. Activities include rallies, workshops, and recognition days, as well as low-cost, week-long retreats.

Expected weight loss/length of program: TOPS recognizes that your hopes, dreams, and weight-loss goals are unique, personal, and dependent on your health, so the group doesn't set a timetable for reaching a goal. After you reach your weight goal, the focus changes to maintaining that weight. The group invites and encourages you to remain a part of TOPS as long as you need support.

Healthy lifestyle component: TOPS offers programs and addresses issues related to maintaining healthy lifestyles. People who have achieved their goals are an integral part of helping those in TOPS who are trying to do so. (People at their goal weight report that they receive satisfaction from helping others.) TOPS members who have reached and maintained goal weight are called KOPS (Keep Off Pounds Sensibly) and are honored accordingly.

Cost: Annual membership is $20 in the United States and $25 in Canada. This amount includes the monthly magazine. Local chapters charge a small weekly fee (usually no more than $5 a month).

Availability: Almost 300,000 members meet weekly in 12,000 meetings in the United States, Canada, and military bases around the world.

Headquarters: The organization is located at 4575 South Fifth Street, Milwaukee, WI 53207. For information about local chapters, call 800-932-8677 or 414-482-4620. You can find TOPS on the Web at www.tops.org.

Commercial Weight-Loss Programs

Commercial weight-loss programs can be good options for people who have trouble sticking to a weight-loss plan on their own. These programs offer a variety of services, from special foods and custom-designed exercise programs to plain old moral support. There are many different plans to choose from, so you should be able to find a program that suits your needs.

Having so many choices can be confusing, however — and sitting in the office of a recruiter for one of these programs can be intimidating. (Recruiters are often salespeople, well trained at closing a deal.) By carefully evaluating the programs in this section, you can avoid signing up and then not showing up because you hate the foods that you must eat or because the plan doesn't provide enough supervision.

Diet Workshop

Approach/method: The program consists of diet, exercise, and behavior modification. Diets range from 1,600 to 2,600 calories and 27 to 40 grams of fat per day. Menus follow the Food Guide Pyramid. The purchase of special foods is optional.

Clients: Members are mostly female (80 percent) and range in age from 25 to 65 years.

Staff: The weight-loss program was developed by a team of registered dietitians, a registered nurse, a physician, and a licensed psychologist. The program is delivered by Diet Workshop graduates. Leaders must complete a 3-week training program that covers nutrition, weight-loss dynamics, customer service, and presentation. Ongoing training for the staff involves 96 to 100 hours per year.

Expected weight loss/length of program: A client can expect to lose 1 to 2 pounds per week. The amount of weight that a client needs to lose determines the length of the program. You must participate in the program for a minimum of 3 months.

Healthy lifestyle component: The program involves an exercise and behavior modification component. Group and individual counseling are available.

Comments: Vitamin and mineral supplements are optional.

Cost: The 3-month behavior modification program costs $169. A 1- to 3-month extension is available for $49 per month. There's no charge for a maintenance program; when a client reaches his or her goal weight, attendance is free.

Availability: 10,000 clients are served weekly at 15 franchises, with 100 locations in the northeastern United States.

Headquarters: The organization is located at 50 Cummings Parkway, Woburn, MA 01801; phone 800-488-3438; Web www.dietworkshop.com.

Jenny Craig, Inc.

Approach/method: The program is based on exercise, lifestyle modification, and a low-calorie diet. Diets range from 1,000 to 2,300 calories a day, depending on the client's energy needs. All menus are based on the Food Guide Pyramid. Jenny Craig food purchases are required at first and are gradually eliminated as the client transitions to self-planned menus.

Clients: Most members are females over the age of 18. Programs are available for adolescents aged 13 to 17 (with parental permission).

Staff: Registered dietitians and psychologists direct the weight-loss programs, with active participation by the Medical Advisory Board, consisting of physicians, psychologists, and exercise physiologists. The maintenance program is directed by psychologists. All programs are delivered by trained employees, who complete 40 hours of training and pass a certification exam. Staff also participate in weekly meetings and monthly continuing education sessions.

Expected weight loss/length of program: Anticipated weight loss is 1 to 2 pounds per week. The amount of weight the client wants to lose determines the length of the program.

Healthy lifestyle component: Both group and individual counseling are available. The program provides information about aerobic exercise and resistance training and encourages members to use these activities to aid in weight loss and maintenance. Behavior modification is a part of the program's overall goal.

Comments: Vitamin and mineral supplements are available.

Headquarters: The organization is located at the University of California, San Francisco, Department of Family and Community Medicine, AC-9, Box 0900, San Francisco, CA 94143-0900; phone 415-457-3331.

Weight Watchers

Approach/method: The program is based on a low-calorie diet, exercise, and lifestyle modification. Diets range from 1,225 to 1,745 calories per day and are individualized for the client's energy needs. Commercial Weight Watchers food products can be purchased but are optional for program participation. (The labeled food products are produced and sold independently of the weight-loss program.)

Clients: Members are mostly female (95 percent), ages 10 and older.

Staff: The program was developed by registered dietitians, exercise physiologists, and clinical psychologists. Leaders (who are Lifetime Members) deliver the program; their initial training requires at least 46 hours of classroom instruction.

Expected weight loss/length of program: The individual client determines the length of the program. Individuals must enter the Maintenance program when their Body Mass Index (BMI) reaches 20. (For an explanation of BMI and to find out how to calculate your own, see Chapter 2.) Expected weight loss is up to 2 pounds per week.

Healthy lifestyle component: The program includes group counseling sessions. It provides information about both aerobic exercise and resistance training and encourages members to use these activities to aid in weight loss and maintenance. Lifestyle modification is a component of the overall program structure.

Comments: Vitamin and mineral supplements are available.

Cost: For weight loss, there is a one-time registration fee of $16 to $20 and a weekly fee of $10 to $14. For maintenance, the fee is $10 to $14 weekly for about 6 weeks until Lifetime Member status is reached. Lifetime Members don't pay a fee.

Availability: About 600,000 clients are served in North America weekly. There are 19,000 weekly meetings.

Headquarters: The organization is located at 175 Crossways Park West, Woodbury, NY 11797; phone 800-651-6000 or 516-390-1400. Web www.weight-watchers.com.

Clinical/Medically Supervised Programs

If you have a lot of weight to lose and haven't had success with commercial plans, you may find a clinical setting more hopeful. This section offers some options. These programs use liquid meal replacements (in other words, fortified liquid formulas that you blend with a low- or non-calorie liquid such as fat-free milk or water) for all or some of your food.

Health Management Resources (HMR)

Approach/method: This program for moderate or high-risk weight-loss patients combines a nutritionally complete diet with intensive lifestyle education. Options include

- A very low calorie liquid diet (VLCD) under medical supervision (500 or 800 calories per day)
- Healthy Solutions, a moderate weight-loss option that includes packaged entrees and regular foods in addition to liquid meal replacements (1,000 to 1,600 calories per day)

Health risk evaluations are provided at the beginning of the program. Either option is available with or without prescription appetite-suppressing medication. Mandatory weekly 90-minute group classes focus on teaching specific skills for overall health management. A long-term maintenance program and individual counseling are also available.

Clients: Patients with heart disease, diabetes, high blood pressure, or other obesity-related illnesses need a physician's written approval to join the program. People who are pregnant, lactating, or have active substance abuse are not allowed to participate.

Staff: The program was developed by physicians, registered dietitians, registered nurses, and psychologists. Each location has at least one physician and another health educator on staff. Participants are assigned personal coaches (registered dietitians, exercise physiologists, and health educators) who help dieters learn and practice weight-management skills. Dieters on a VLCD see a physician or a registered nurse weekly.

Expected weight loss/length of program: Weight loss averages from 1 to 5 pounds weekly. The reducing phase varies according to weight-loss goals but averages 12 to 20 weeks. A maintenance program is recommended for up to 18 months.

Healthy lifestyle components: The program recommends that clients burn a minimum of 2,000 calories in physical activity weekly and advocates consuming a diet with no more than 30 percent of calories from fat and at least 35 servings of fruits and vegetables per week (or 5 a day). The plan emphasizes lifestyle issues during weekly classes and provides personal coaching.

Comments: The program emphasizes exercise as a means for weight loss and weight maintenance. Participants make few decisions about what to eat and are supervised by a health professional. The program requires a strong commitment to physical activity. The side effects of a very low calorie diet may include intolerance to cold, constipation, dizziness, dry skin, and headaches. The diet is very high in protein, even at higher calorie levels.

Cost: Fees vary depending on the client's medical condition and the diet required. Healthy Solutions program fees average $20 per week. (Shakes and entrees are additional and average approximately $80 per week.) Counseling for the very low calorie liquid diets averages from $80 to $150 per week, depending on the amount of supervision required. (Some insurance plans will reimburse this fee.) The liquid meal replacements cost approximately $60 per week. Maintenance costs average $80 per month.

Availability: The program is available at more than 200 hospitals and medical settings in the United States.

Headquarters: The organization is located at 59 Temple Place, Suite 704, Boston, MA 02111; phone 617-357-9876 or 800-418-1367; Web www.yourbetterhealth.com.

Medifast

Approach/method: Medifast offers a physician-supervised very low calorie diet (VLCD) program of fortified liquid meal replacements containing 450 to 500 calories per day. Lifestyles — the Medifast program of patient support — prepares patients to maintain their goal weight after completing the VLCD. Medifast also provides a low-calorie diet of approximately 850 calories per day and a moderately low-calorie plan of 1,200 to 1,500 calories a day for those not indicated for the VLCD. Medifast also offers Take Shape, a line of food products that can be used as part of a weight-loss or weight-maintenance program.

Clients: The VLCD program is limited to individuals who have a Body Mass Index (BMI) of 30 or more, who have reached sexual and physical maturation, and who are not pregnant or lactating. People who recently suffered a stroke or who have conditions such as bulimia nervosa, unstable angina, type 1 diabetes, thrombophlebitis, active cancer, and uncompensated renal or hepatic disease are not admissible to the program.

Staff: The program is supervised by a physician. At the corporate level, a medical advisory group of physicians, Ph.D.s, and registered dietitians is consulted on program and product development.

Expected weight loss/length of program: The physician and patient arrive at an individualized goal weight by using BMI guidelines and weight history. Weight loss varies with the individual; the average weight loss is 3 to 5 pounds per week. The weight-reduction phase lasts 16 weeks, and return to eating lasts 4 to 6 weeks. Maintenance is strongly encouraged for up to a year.

Healthy lifestyle components: The Medifast plan includes a comprehensive education program called Lifestyles that includes behavior modification, a recommended physical activity program, and nutrition education. Instruction booklets and patient guides, including a quarterly newsletter, are provided.

Comments: The program offers close contact with one or more health professionals. The low calorie level promotes rapid weight loss. An extensive product line is available. Participants must rely on company products during the reducing phase. The maintenance program assists with the transition to regular foods. Company products and regular foods are incorporated into the diet for people who do not qualify for the VLCD diet.

Cost: The cost for office visits, laboratory tests, and Medifast products varies from individual to individual. The program fee ranges from $65 to $85 per week. Insurance may cover the cost of lab work and office visits.

Availability: The program is available from 15,000 physicians in the United States, primarily in office-based settings, and in 6 foreign countries.

Headquarters: The organization is located at Healthrite, Inc., 11445 Cronhill Drive, Owings Mills, MD 21117; phone 800-638-7867.

New Direction

Approach/method: New Direction offers two program methods:

- ✔ New Direction's low-calorie diet program is a medically supervised low-calorie liquid meal replacement diet of 600 or 800 calories per day.

- ✔ The Outlook program is a moderate program of 1,000 or 1,500 calories per day, including fortified nutritional bars and liquid meal replacements as well as traditional foods.

All patient materials are included as part of both New Direction programs. Their goal is to give the patient complete support — medical, nutritional, behavioral, lifestyle, and educational.

Clients: New Direction's low-calorie liquid diet does not allow the following individuals to participate: those who are less than 18 years of age, pregnant and lactating women, and those who have conditions such as metastatic cancer, recent myocardial infarction, liver disease requiring protein restriction, insulin-dependent diabetes mellitus, and renal insufficiency. The company offers a special program for people with type 2 diabetes that includes special educational materials and medical monitoring.

Staff: Weekly sessions, covering a variety of subjects in both New Direction programs, are led by health professionals who are knowledgeable in dietetics, exercise, and behavior. One-on-one interaction is part of each program. Both programs are headed by a physician who serves as medical director.

Expected weight loss/length of program: In the New Direction low-calorie liquid diet program, the average weight loss is 3 pounds per week; the New Direction Outlook program weight-loss rates vary with each individual. The length of the program participation for the Low Calorie Program: 12 to 16 weeks in reducing, 5 to 10 weeks in adapting (the transition to regular food), and 6 to 12 months in sustaining (maintenance). Ongoing participation in each phase is strongly encouraged.

Healthy lifestyle component: Weekly classes concentrate on problem solving, lifestyle development, nutrition education, and a dieter-friendly light exercise program.

Comments: Each program emphasizes individualized care and consistent contact with health professionals. Program support includes a comprehensive treatment approach that's easy for patients to understand and follow. Patients make few decisions about what to eat while on this type of low-calorie diet. The Outlook program includes regular food with a strong emphasis on lifestyle modification.

Cost: The average cost for the New Direction low-calorie liquid diet program averages from $110 to $120 per week. Medical monitoring is about $45 to $60 of the fee and is usually covered by insurance. The Outlook program costs about $45 to $60 per week for the nutritional bars and liquid meal replacements. Maintenance, which varies from patient to patient, generally runs 3 to 12 weeks and costs about $100 per week.

Headquarters: The organization is located at 8295 Glenmill Court, Cincinnati, OH 45249; phone 800-310-6359.

Optifast

Approach/method: This medically supervised program of fortified liquid meal replacements and/or fortified food bars eventually includes more regular foods. Each dieter is assigned to an 800-, 950-, or 1,200-calorie plan depending on starting weight and intended weight loss. Staff provide one-on-one counseling and weekly group sessions on how to change eating behavior.

Clients: Optifast does not allow the following individuals to participate in the program: those who are less than 30 percent or 50 pounds over desirable weight, corresponding to a BMI of approximately 30 to 32; those who are less than 18 years of age; those who are pregnant or lactating; and those who suffer from a recent acute myocardial infarction, unstable angina, insulin-dependent diabetes mellitus, or advanced liver or kidney disease.

Staff: Physicians, registered nurses, registered dietitians, and psychologists regularly see each dieter at most locations; exercise physiologists are used on a consulting basis. Group meeting leaders and one-on-one counselors are psychologists, licensed counselors, or dietitians.

Expected weight loss/length of program: The program limits weekly weight loss to 2 percent of body weight. The weight-loss portion of the plan lasts about 13 weeks. The transition phase lasts about 6 weeks. Maintenance, which begins at the 20th week, is part of the program and continues on an ongoing basis. Maintenance has no time limit.

Healthy lifestyle components: The emphasis in group and individual counseling is on modifying behavior, developing problem-solving and stress-management skills, and choosing a healthy diet and activity plan. An exercise physiologist is available to help design personal exercise plans.

Comments: The program offers close contact with a physician and other health professionals. Controlling the calorie level promotes quick weight loss, which is beneficial for people with certain health problems. Clients make few decisions about what to eat. Participants must rely on Optifast products during the reducing phase.

Cost: The expense varies with the type of diet and the length of the program. Costs range from $1,500 to $3,000, depending on the patient's health status and the amount of weight that he or she needs to lose. The price may include maintenance at some centers. Insurance may cover a portion of the cost.

Availability: The program is available in numerous hospitals and clinics in the United States and abroad.

Headquarters: The organization is located at Novartis Nutrition, 1441 Park Place Blvd., Minneapolis, MN 55416; phone 800-662-2540; Web www.optifast.com.

Which Program Is Right for You?

After you consider the different types of weight-loss programs and find one that you think may work for you, make an appointment to visit one of that program's centers for a personal interview. Take along this list of questions and demand satisfying answers. (You may already know some of the answers based on the information given in this chapter, but having the program reconfirm that information certainly doesn't hurt.) How truthfully and in how straightforward a manner the answers are given can help you decide whether a particular program is right for you.

- What data proves that the program actually works? What has been written about the program's success, besides individual testimonials?

- Do customers keep off the weight after they leave the diet program? (Ask for results over 2 to 5 years. The Federal Trade Commission requires weight-loss companies to back up their claims.)

- What are the program's requirements? Are special menus or foods, counseling visits, or exercise a part of the program?

- Does the plan include physical activity recommendations? Will the program include guidance on physical activity for the long term? How?

- What are the approaches and goals of the program?

- What are the health risks?

- If I don't need to purchase special meals, does the plan take into account my personal food preferences? Will I have to give up all my favorite foods? Are the foods available at the supermarket? Will the program help me learn to live with its eating plan for the long term? How?

- What are the costs of membership, weekly fees, food, supplements, maintenance, and counseling? What's the payment schedule? Are any costs covered under health insurance? Will the organization give a refund if I drop out, or give rebates for successful weight loss and maintenance?

- Will the staff monitor my success at 3- to 6-month intervals and then modify the program if needed?

- Does the plan have a maintenance program? Is it part of the package or does it cost extra?

- What kind of professional support is provided? What are the credentials and experiences of these professionals? (Detailed information should be available on request.)

Chapter 20

Sorting Fact from Fiction: Fad Diets and Dieting Scams

. . . .

In This Chapter

▶ Evaluating diet research

▶ Reviewing the hottest diets

▶ Spotting gimmicks

. . . .

*P*ounds of diet books are published every day. Check out any online or traditional bookstore and you'll be amazed — literally hundreds of these books are for sale.

A closer look at the contents of these diets reveals that almost every book is a rehash of a previous one — in most cases, the pitch has not changed since dieting became an industry. But based on the way these diets are written and promoted, you may believe that the author has uncovered a heretofore unheard-of formula that assures weight loss once and for all. But despite these claims, diet success is still a matter of calories in versus calories out.

Scientists now have a much better understanding of why people get fat and how they get thin. They know what happens at the cellular level in DNA, not only what happens on plates and scales. It's technical stuff involving hormones, enzymes, and compounds so newly discovered that many don't have names yet. Unfortunately, the new science behind weight change is not well understood by the public. And diet purveyors count on that lack of knowledge. They take old diet programs and market them by using the current scientific weight-loss vocabulary and a little technical-sounding mumbo jumbo. The old diets become "New" and "Revolutionary," when in fact they are the same plans that failed in the past.

This chapter explains some of the most common diets and scams — many making encore appearances dressed in new names. It would be easy for us to tell you that none of these diets works, and that they have no redeeming health value. But we don't entirely believe that. Some have merit. And when you analyze the thinking behind the plans, you can learn some valuable lessons about healthy eating.

Evaluating the Most Common Fad Diets

The current crop of weight-loss advice making the rounds in bookstores and locker rooms generally falls into one of several categories. Some tout or ban specific foods; others suggest that food can change body chemistry; and still others blame specific hormones for weight problems. This section explains and evaluates the most common fad diets and gives you the facts behind the fibs.

Just because a diet-book author is a medical doctor and uses the initials M.D. after his or her name, or has a Ph.D., doesn't mean that all the advice in the book is good nutrition science or nutrition advice. See the sidebar "Is the research legit?" to evaluate whether the research on which a diet is based is legitimate.

Food-specific diets

The premise of food-specific diets is that some foods have special properties that can cause weight loss. But no food can. So why do some people swear by these diets? Because any food eaten to the exclusion of others — even eating hot fudge sundaes and only hot fudge sundaes — can result in weight loss. Eventually, you get bored and stop eating the allowed food, or at least enough of the allowed food to maintain your weight.

But these diets don't teach healthy eating habits; therefore, you won't stick with them. Sooner or later, you'll have a hankering for something else — anything else, as long as its texture and flavor are not that of the allowed food. You may even have a strong urge (dare we say *craving?*), for celery sticks, but it also may be for steaks.

Nutritionists call the human appetite for a variety of foods *food-specific satiety.* It's nature's way of assuring that you eat a diverse diet and therefore get the full spectrum of nutrients. You don't have to eat only hot fudge sundaes to see the dynamic at work. Think of last Thanksgiving's dinner, for example. After eating a full savory, salty meal of turkey, stuffing, gravy, mashed potatoes, rolls, and so on, we bet that you were still tempted to have a slice of sweet pecan or pumpkin pie. That desire for dessert was because your palate was looking for the full complement of flavors. Unless you ate lots of marshmallow-topped sweet potatoes, sweet had not been satisfied. Sour, salty, and bitter — the other components of flavor in the Western diet — probably were featured in the main course. Sweet comes from dessert.

Is the research legit?

One common feature in recent diet-book writing has been to quote experiments, studies, and research. How do you know whether the research to which an author refers is scientifically valid? Understanding the lingo helps. Look for these terms in the text:

✔ **Associated with:** There may be a connection or an occurrence more frequent than can be explained by mere coincidence, but a cause has not been proven.

✔ **Blind, single-blind, or double-blind study:** A single-blind experiment includes subjects who do not know whether they are part of the treatment or are receiving a *placebo* (fake treatment). In a double-blind experiment, neither the researchers nor the participants know which subjects are receiving the treatment or placebo while the study is being conducted.

✔ **Control group:** The subjects — usually the group not receiving the treatment — in a study to whom a comparison is made in order to determine whether the treatment is effective.

✔ **Correlation:** An association that is often defined statistically. It may not prove cause and effect.

✔ **Meta-analysis:** A technique in which the results of several individual studies are pooled to yield an overall conclusion.

✔ **Probability:** There is a chance that the event will occur. Probability can be high or low but does not indicate certainty.

✔ **Prospective study:** Research that follows a group of people over a period of time to observe the effects of diet, behavior, or other factors. Generally, a prospective study is considered a more valid research design than a retrospective study, which relies on the recall of past data or information.

✔ **Random sampling:** A method of selecting subjects for a study in which all the potential subjects have an equal chance of being selected.

✔ **Reliable:** A reliable test gives reproducible results when performed on the same person several times.

✔ **Risk factor:** Anything that shows a relationship to the incidence of disease. It does not necessarily imply cause and effect. It is important to understand what the risk is. If the original risk is 1 in 1 million, then double the risk is only 1 in 500,000. But if the risk is 1 in 100, then double would be 1 in 50, which may be a cause for concern.

✔ **Statistically significant:** Sometimes this phase is simply written "significant." It implies that there is a very small chance that the results would have occurred if there had been no real effect or association.

High-protein, low-carbohydrate diets

These plans have been around since Dr. Stillman's Quick Weight Loss Diet made its first appearance in 1967 — although we imagine that even Dr. Stillman started with someone else's promise of easy weight loss. These diets are based on the idea that carbohydrate is bad, that many people are "allergic to it" or are insulin-resistant and therefore gain weight when they eat it. So by eliminating or severely limiting carbohydrate, you can force your body to use the fat it already has in storage for energy instead of adding to those fat stores. The authors of these diets are quick to point out that because people are eating lots of carbohydrates — which most mainstream nutrition professionals recommend — they are heavier than ever before. What the advocates of these diets *don't* tell you is that people are eating more total calories, too, and *that's* the real reason they're gaining weight.

The Carbohydrate Addict's LifeSpan Program

The authors: Rachael Heller, Ph.D., and Richard Heller, Ph.D.

The premise: The authors believe that you can break your carbohydrate cravings (which are why you're overweight) by limiting the amount of carbohdrate you eat. Two meals each day are made up of high-protein foods with very little carbohydrate. You can eat high-carbohdrate foods at the third meal as long as you balance them with more high-protein foods.

The truth: There's no magic to eating high- or low-carbohydrate foods other than the fact that they contain different amounts of calories. Most experts agree that giving in to cravings is better than trying to eat around them, because you eventually eat too many calories in trying to avoid the one food you truly want to eat. Plus, if you follow this diet, you *must* eat a second serving of a protein food if you eat a second serving of a high-carbohydrate food; therefore, eating too many calories is easy. And fat can creep up to dangerously high levels even if you select lean protein foods.

Lessons to learn: Because of its emphasis on protein, this diet reminds dieters to eat some protein at every meal to keep hunger at bay. Adding protein to meals gives them more staying power than high-carbohydrate foods alone can.

Dr. Atkins New Diet Revolution

The author: Robert C. Atkins, M.D.

The premise: You can eat as many calories from fat and protein as you want as long as you eat very little carbohydrate. This diet consists of four phases. Phase one is the most dramatic, allowing no more carbohydrate than you'd get in 3 cups of salad — about 4 grams. Phase four allows no more than 40 to 60 grams of carbohydrate a day. But most nutritionists recommend that 55 to 60 percent of your calories come from carbohydrate, which translates into about 234 to 255 grams on a 1,700-calorie weight-loss diet.

The truth: Eating high-fat foods, such as burgers, cheese, bacon, butter, and mayonnaise, may sound dreamy, but you can't eat a bun with your double bacon cheeseburger or eat rye bread with your ham sandwich. Beyond the starch cravings that dieters may experience, the body can't burn fat efficiently without the carbohydrates that bread, potatoes, pasta, and other starches provide. As a result, the body produces compounds called *ketones* that accumulate in the blood. Ketones put a strain on the kidneys and can make kidney disease worse. Those who follow this diet often experience constipation, nausea, headache, fatigue, and bad breath. Eating high-fat foods day after day is a sure way to increase your risk of heart disease and cancer, too.

Lessons to learn: The goal of losing weight should be to improve your health, not make it worse. Unfortunately, this diet offers very little information of value other than that eating fat can help make you feel full.

Protein Power

The authors: Michael R. Eades, M.D., and Mary Dan Eades, M.D.

The premise: The hormone insulin is a monster that, if released in great quantities, can cause health problems such as heart disease, high blood pressure, elevated cholesterol and other blood fats, diabetes, and excess fluid retention, as well as excess weight. The authors claim that eating carbohydrates releases the monster. Therefore, by keeping consumption of carbohydrate foods very low — to as little as 30 grams a day during the initial phases of the diet — your body will burn its fat stores instead of feeding them, and your risk of health problems is reduced. The diet and theory are very similar to The Zone (described later in this chapter) in that protein requirements are based on lean body mass.

The truth: Another example of putting the cart before the horse. The authors confuse the scientific evidence demonstrating that being overweight is not the result of insulin being out of whack. Rather, being overweight often *causes* problems with insulin. The diet is extremely low in carbohydrate; the 30 grams a day allowed during the initial phase is about 205 to 225 grams less than what is considered healthy even during weight loss. (Nutritionist experts recommend that 55 to 60 percent of your calories come from carbohydrates. Therefore, on a 1,700-calorie diet, which is low enough for most people to lose weight, daily carbohydrate intake should be approximately 234 to 255 grams.) Also, this diet minimizes the importance of reducing fat intake.

Lessons to learn: Many overweight adults eat too much carbohydrate because they concentrate too much on reducing fat while ignoring total calorie intake. Many of these folks are heavy consumers of foods that have been engineered to be low in fat, which usually means that they're eating too much carbohydrate in the form of sugar. (When fat is removed from a product, sugar is often added to make up for the loss in taste and texture.) Because many foods that contain a lot of sugar supply calories but few or no nutrients, everyone should keep sugar consumption low, and those who are trying to lose weight should eat it sparingly.

Sugar Busters!

The author: H. Leighton Steward, editor

The premise: Sugar, not fat, is the cause of extra weight. Foods that cause a spike in insulin supposedly increase the likelihood that their calories will be stored as fat rather than used for energy. Foods to avoid are classified according to their *glycemic index,* a measure of how fast they appear as glucose in the blood. Foods with a high glycemic index, such as white bread and pasta, refined grains, carrots, beets, and bananas, are to be avoided. High-fiber carbohydrates do not promote an insulin surge and therefore may be eaten.

The truth: High insulin levels increase the risk of heart disease, but no evidence shows that they cause people to store fat. And although it's true that some foods cause a more rapid glycemic response than others when measured independently under laboratory conditions, in the body the composition of the entire meal influences how quickly the foods enter the bloodstream. And for most people who do not have a metabolic disorder such as diabetes, if bread, pasta, or any other "off-limits" food is eaten alone, the insulin response — even a dramatic rise — is temporary, and the body accommodates it easily.

Lessons to learn: Many people eat too much sugar and refined grains and not enough high-fiber foods. Many foods that contain a lot of sugar supply calories but few or no nutrients. Most healthy people should use sugars in moderation, and anyone who wants to lose weight should use sugars sparingly. Although most people eat only about 11 grams of fiber a day, health authorities recommend consuming 20 to 35 grams of fiber per day. And remember, eating excess calories from fat, carbohydrate, or protein makes you gain weight — not just from carbohydrate alone.

The Zone

The author: Barry Sears, Ph.D.

The premise: To stay within the healthy zone for maximum calorie burn, every meal and snack must be 40 percent carbohydrate, 30 percent protein, and 30 percent fat. That's where the diet's other name, "the 40-30-30 diet," comes from. (Most nutritionists recommend 50 to 55 percent carbohydrate, 15 to 20 percent protein, and no more than 30 percent fat.) The diet, says the author, is based on hormones, not on calories. He claims that most people are insulin-resistant, so eating carbohydrates makes them fat. Insulin is a hormone that takes glucose (the product of carbohydrate digestion) from the blood and delivers it to the cells. The author claims that when people eat carbohydrate foods, their bodies produce too much insulin, which causes too many calories to be stored as fat. Therefore, he says, carbohydrates must be kept low, and some are banned all together.

Not only are carbohydrates kept to a minimum, but they must be matched by perscribed amounts of protein (which are calculated on your lean body mass) and fat to keep eicosanoids *(eye-KOH-suh-noids)* in balance. The author claims that eicosanoids are the chemical moderators that control all hormonal reactions, and the closer you get to your ideal protein-to-carbo-hydrate ratio, the better you'll balance your good and bad eicosanoids. Supposedly, bad eicosanoids increase insulin production. Good ones moderate hunger.

The truth: The pseudo-science on which this diet is based is complicated and unsubstantiated, and has been strongly disputed by the scientific community. Only 20 to 25 percent of adults are insulin-resistant, usually because they have some other health problem that causes the condition. Further, insulin resistance often *results from* being overweight. It does not cause it. And although eicosanoids are involved in blood clotting and in the immune system, no evidence shows that this diet (or any other, for that matter) affects their synthesis. Any weight loss that you achieve on this diet is due to the 700- to 1,200-calorie plan, not a hormonal shift. And with so much focus on eating protein, which usually comes bundled with heart-damaging fat, it's easy to get more than 30 percent of your calories from fat — the amount that most health professionals consider healthy.

Lessons to learn: Many people, especially women, give up meat to cut calories. Instead, they fill up on carbohydrates. But carbohydrates are not particularly satisfying by themselves, and they don't satisfy for long. Therefore, eating too many calories from carbohydrates is easy. By adding protein and a bit of fat to every meal, including snacks, you feel satisfied longer.

High-fiber, low-calorie diets

The thinking behind these diets is that because fiber cannot be digested, it doesn't have calories (true). And because it takes up so much room in the stomach, it's filling, too (also true). Therefore, if a diet is very high in fiber, weight loss should be easy. But although some fiber is necessary and a good thing, eating too much is not always better. Too much fiber — more than 50 or 60 grams a day — can cause bloating, cramping, and diarrhea. Eating lots of fiber will not cause weight loss; only eating fewer calories will.

Eat More, Weigh Less

The author: Dean Ornish, M.D.

The premise: By keeping fat to no more than 10 percent of daily calories and eating basically a high-fiber vegetarian diet, you can reverse heart disease and lose weight.

The truth: Studies published in scientific journals have shown that this diet keeps its promises. However, many people find such a low-fat, vegetarian diet too stringent and difficult to stick with for long. Many nutritionists believe that this diet is too low in fat and that meals provide little satiety or long-term satisfaction.

Lessons to learn: We can recommend some aspects of this diet. For example, it has some good ideas for healthier food choices. However, it may not be a promising lifelong plan for many people because it is so restrictive. But if you can incorporate some of the low-fat, high-fiber strategies into your normal eating style, you can make positive health changes.

Dr. Bob Arnot's Revolutionary Weight Control Program

The author: Robert Arnot, M.D.

The premise: Foods are drugs and can be used to enhance mood and aid in weight loss. Light therapy can reduce carbohydrate cravings, and negative ion therapy can help in weight loss as well. Hard foods that require a lot of chewing, such as high-fiber foods, resist digestion and can promote the transport of the amino acid tryptophan into the brain. Tryptophan is a precursor to serotonin, the brain's feel-good and antihunger chemical.

The truth: Light therapy can help depressed people by boosting serotonin levels in the brain, and it has been shown to improve mood in people who are affected by seasonal affective disorder (SAD). These people suffer most in the low-light months of winter. However, light therapy has not been shown to help people lose weight. As for the diet's other claim, hard foods do not raise serotonin levels in the brain any more than mush does.

Lessons to learn: This diet is basically a high-fiber, low-calorie one, and exercise is encouraged. But putting too much stock in light therapy is probably unwise.

Liquid diets

Two kinds of liquid diets are available: over-the-counter liquid meal replacements and very low calorie diets that require medical prescription and supervision. Neither plan should be used for long-term weight loss. In fact, weight loss tends to plateau after about 3 months on either regimen.

Liquid meal replacements

The premise: Drink two liquid replacement meals (such as Slimfast or Sweet Success) and eat a "sensible" dinner for a total of about 1,500 calories a day. The beverages are fortified with vitamins and minerals, and some varieties have added fiber.

The truth: These diets can backfire by teaching your body to hoard the very few calories that the beverages provide (about 200 per serving). When you don't give your body enough food, it switches to starvation mode and uses calories at a slower rate. Plus, depriving yourself of food for most of the day leaves you feeling tired and weak and more likely to splurge later on.

If you have a lot of weight to lose, using meal replacements does not ensure success. Data published by the Slimfast company in the *Journal of the American College of Nutrition* 13(6), 1994, a well-respected scientific publication, showed that after more than 2 years on the program, women lost a total of 13 pounds and men lost 14 — not a lot of weight for 116 weeks of dieting! And despite being paid $25 a week to stay on the plan, only 51 percent of the people enrolled stayed on the plan for the entire study. We call that guaranteed failure.

Lessons to learn: When time is short and eating a well-balanced, low-calorie meal is nearly impossible, these beverages can stand in a pinch. But they are no way to learn to eat healthfully because they can become a crutch.

Very low calorie diets (VLCDs)

These medically supervised diets, such as Optifast and Medifast, allow only 300 to 800 calories per day. The liquids-only regimens are fortified with vitamins, minerals, and high-quality protein. People who use these plans must be closely supervised by doctors and other highly trained professionals because the diets present a real health risk if not monitored carefully. (See Chapter 19 for information about medically supervised liquid diets.)

Fasting

Fasting to cleanse the body and jump-start a weight-loss diet has been recommended for years. But the reality is that fasting deprives the body of nutrients. The result is low energy, weakness, and lightheadedness, not real weight loss. Any loss is water and muscle, not fat, and you will regain the weight when you start eating again. Fasting does not clear toxins from the body, either — just the opposite: Ketones can build up when carbohydrates are not available for energy, and that massing of ketones stresses the kidneys and can ultimately be harmful to your health.

Considering Gimmicks, Gadgets, and Other Scams

Diet scams, including weight-loss products and gadgets, often rely on unscrupulous but persuasive combinations of message, program, ingredients, and mystique. The following sections describe a few of the currently popular ones. Also see Chapter 18 for a look at over-the-counter weight-loss drugs.

Chitosan

Chitin, the compound from which chitosan is derived, is found in the skeletons of shrimp, crabs, and lobsters. It can bind four to six times its weight in grease, oils, and toxic substances, and has been used in water filtration systems for years. Because it can bind fatty acids, chitosan has been promoted for weight loss. It may be effective in reducing blood cholesterol, but it has not been shown to aid in weight loss. People who are allergic to shellfish may react negatively to it.

Inhalers

Imagine that simply smelling chocolate cake could keep you from eating it. That's the premise behind The Scentsational Weight Loss Plan. The theory is that the sense of smell triggers the portion of the brain responsible for satiety. When you feel hungry, you sniff an odor from an inhaler (available in banana, apple, and peppermint); then, when you sit down to eat, you'll eat less. However, the research that tested the theory was conducted for a short time and has never been duplicated.

If the inhalers really work, why wouldn't smelling a food wrapper or the food itself accomplish the same result? The author claims that people are too tempted to eat the real food after smelling it.

Spirulina

Enthusiasts claim that spirulina, also called super blue green algae, suppresses hunger pangs and is effective in treating diabetes, hepatitis, cirrhosis of the liver, anemia, stress, pancreatitis, cataracts, glaucoma, ulcer, and even hair loss. They also boast that it's protein- and vitamin-packed. The algae does contain protein composed of a good balance of amino acids and offers certain B vitamins, but neither is difficult to find in the American diet.

Does spirulina suppress appetite? In theory, because it contains carbohydrate, spirulina could cause an increase in blood sugar and a corresponding reduction in hunger as any carbohydrate food does. However, the recommended doses of the supplement have too little carbohydrate to have such an effect. An average of about $25 for a 20-day supply is a hefty price to pay for something that may not produce the same result as your normal diet.

Is a product or service worth the money?

Before you plunk down your hard-earned cash for a product or service that makes weight-loss promises, consider the following points. Your cash is better left in your wallet if the product or service

✔ Claims or implies a large (more than 1 to 2 pounds a week) or fast weight loss — often promised as easy, effortless, guaranteed, or permanent. (The exception is medically supervised VLCD programs.)

✔ Is described as miraculous, a breakthrough, exclusive, secret, ancient, from the Orient, an accidental discovery, or doctor developed.

✔ Declares that the established medical community is against this discovery and refuses to accept its miraculous benefits.

✔ Relies heavily on undocumented case histories, before and after photos, and testimonials. By law, weight-loss claims must be typical of all clients or include a disclaimer.

✔ Implies that weight can be lost and maintained without exercise and other lifestyle changes.

✔ Professes to be a treatment for a wide range of ailments and nutritional deficiencies as well as for weight loss.

✔ Includes gadgets such as body wraps, sauna belts, electronic stimulators, passive motion tables, and cellulite creams.

✔ Makes a drug claim not allowed by the Food and Drug Administration for any ingredient, food supplement, or nonprescription drug. Claims that ingredients surround calories, starch, carbohydrate, or fat and remove them from the body are illegal drug claims. The only drugs that are allowed to claim that they suppress appetite are phenylpropanolamine (PPA) and benzocaine.

✔ Is sold by self-proclaimed health advisors or "nutritionists," often door-to-door or by a pyramid sales organization.

✔ Is distributed through a mail-order advertisement, television informerical, or ad listing a toll-free number but not an address.

Part VI
The Part of Tens

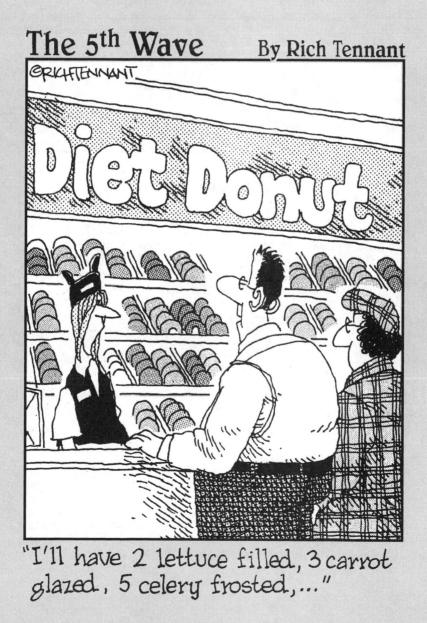

The 5th Wave   By Rich Tennant

"I'll have 2 lettuce filled, 3 carrot glazed, 5 celery frosted,..."

In this part . . .

*E*very *...For Dummies* book includes a Part of Tens, full of quick tips and tidbits of useful information. In this part, you'll find tips for cutting calories and living health-fully. You'll also find out the truth about ten dieting myths, plus a variety of diet-friendly recipes to inspire you in the kitchen.

Chapter 21

Ten Myths about Dieting

We've all heard them: the little tricks and "wisdoms" that people say can make or break a diet. In this chapter, you can find some of the most common beliefs — and the truth behind the hype.

Eating Late at Night Is Sure to Pack on the Pounds

Your body doesn't process calories differently after dark. However, the foods that people tend to go for in front of the TV after dinner — chips, ice cream, chocolate treats, and the like — are usually high in fat and calories. The *kinds of foods you're eating* are the concern, not the clock.

You Can Break Through a Weight-Loss Plateau by Eating Fewer Calories

Eat fewer than 800 to 1,000 calories a day, and your body will turn down its thermostat to conserve every calorie it can get. It doesn't know whether you're a prisoner of war suffering from starvation or a prisoner in your head. The only way to keep your metabolism purring is to exercise. When weight loss slows, walk a little longer or work out more frequently or intensely — and don't forget to eat.

Never Have Seconds

Instead of using a plate of food or a predetermined serving size as a yard-stick for how much you should eat, try taking hunger and fullness clues from your body. Eating according to your appetite is much healthier. And when you eat slowly, recognizing when you've had enough is much easier.

Keep in mind that there's a difference between appetite and hunger. *Appetite* has more to do with flavor preferences and craving; *hunger* is a biological manifestation of the body's real need for food. If it's been a while since you and your appetite have seen eye to eye on how much to eat, try this: Serve yourself only half of what you think you want to eat. If you're still hungry after eating at a leisurely pace, go for it — in moderation, of course.

 Also recognize that you're hungrier on some days than on others. So when you're really, truly hungry, it's fine to eat more. Remember that one meal does not define healthy eating. What you eat over the course of a day, or actually over several days, does.

Deny Your Cravings; They're All in Your Head

Sometimes, the faster you give in and have a small portion of the food you're craving, the better off you are. You can pack on lots of calories by trying to eat around the one thing you truly want. Have a small serving of the food you crave and get over it.

Don't Eat Between Meals

Most people need to eat every 3 to 4 hours to avoid a feast-or-famine mental-ity and risk overeating because you're overhungry. Dividing your calories into three meals and two or three snacks, instead of only three meals, can keep you well fueled for the day. Try planning two or three snack-sized portions (for example, a piece of fruit or a couple of Fig Newtons plus low-fat or fat-free milk or yogurt) into your day's food choices. Doing so may help lessen your hunger pangs so that you're less likely to overeat at the next meal.

Eating Breakfast Makes You Hungry All Day

Many typical breakfast foods — Danish, toast with jelly, and bagels, for example — are mainly carbohydrates in their simplest form. These foods, while initially satisfying, are out of your system in about 30 minutes, and you need (and want) to eat again. That's why many people say that breakfast kicks off nonstop eating throughout the day.

Breakfast foods that have some protein and a little fat, in addition to complex carbohydrates and sugars, stay with you longer and give you the energy you need to make it through the morning. Whole-grain cereal with low-fat or fat-free milk, an egg on toast, and even a fruity breakfast shake made with low-fat or fat-free milk are good choices.

To Lose Weight, Become a Vegetarian

Being vegetarian doesn't ensure that you'll lose weight. Like any way of eating, a vegetarian diet can be high in fat and cholesterol, low in fiber, or both. Many vegetarian foods, including cheese and nuts, are high in fat and calories. So cutting out meat and replacing it with other equally fatty (or even more fatty) vegetarian foods is not only a bad diet move, but it may also increase your chances for nutritional deficiencies — especially if you don't plan your diet well.

Fasting for a Few Days Drops the Pounds Quickly and Shrinks Your Stomach

If you fast, you may drop pounds, but some of that weight will be muscle, and most of it will be water. You need to eat protein foods such as lean meat, eggs, low-fat or fat-free milk, or legumes (beans and peas), or you'll be thin and flabby, not thin and shapely.

There's a misconception that fasting cleans out your system. But actually, the opposite is true. When the body doesn't get food, body chemicals called *ketones* build up over time. That process puts a burden on the kidneys, which can be harmful to your health. Not to mention that it gives you really bad breath, too!

You Can Eat Anything You Want as Long as It's Fat-Free

Fat-free foods are not calorie-free foods; check the Nutrition Facts panel on the food label. Many have just as many calories as the original versions, and a few have even more, because lots of sugar (among other ingredients) is needed to replace the way fat tastes and feels in your mouth. In the end, the total number of calories in a food is what's important.

A little fat is a good thing because it can help you eat less by giving a meal staying power, which keeps you from feeling hungry too quickly. Instead of a sandwich made with fat-free mayonnaise and fat-free cold cuts, make one with a teaspoon of real mayonnaise and low-fat meat; it will stay with you longer than a fat-free meal.

Chapter 22

Ten Ways to Cut Calories

In This Chapter

▶ Reading food labels

▶ Remembering that portion size is key

▶ Eating slowly and off of plates

▶ Using lower-fat products and avoiding high-fat ones

▶ Using healthy cooking techniques

A food's fat content is important, but when it comes to weight loss, total calories are *more* important. So many of the low-fat products on the market are not calorie-reduced. For example, 2 tablespoons of reduced-fat peanut butter has the same number of calories as the regular kind. And replacing a tablespoon of butter on a bagel with 2 tablespoons of jelly eliminates the fat but doesn't change the number of calories.

In this chapter, you can find some calorie-cutting tricks to live by.

Pay Attention to the Nutrition Facts Panel on Food Labels

Seemingly healthy foods can be surprising sources of calories and fat, so make sure to check out the details on the Nutrition Facts panel on the food label. A container of ramen noodles, for example, packs 15 grams of fat and 400 calories; a bran muffin can top 10 grams of fat and 250 calories. Portion sizes can be deceptively small, too. A serving of sugar-sweetened iced tea contains 60 calories, but there are often two servings per bottle. And a serving of ice cream or other frozen dessert is a skimpy 1/2 cup.

Limit Alcohol

Alcohol, although fat-free, packs 7 calories per gram, or about 70 calories per ounce (2 tablespoons). The higher the proof, the more calories alcohol has: 80-proof alcohol averages 65 calories per ounce, and 100-proof alcohol comes in at 85 calories per ounce. The average light beer or 5-ounce glass of wine contains about 100 calories. A typical regular beer has about 150 calories.

In addition to the calorie wallop, alcohol whittles away your resolve to stay in control of your eating. And any cardiac benefits you may derive from drinking, such as that seen in men who drink a daily glass of red wine, are not nearly as important as those you derive from weight loss and exercise.

Switch to Smaller Plates

Serve yourself on a salad-sized plate, about 8 inches in diameter, rather than on a dinner plate, which is typically 10 to 12 inches in diameter. Your portion sizes will be closer to those suggested in the Food Guide Pyramid (see Chapter 10), and more in tune with the number of calories you should be eating.

Kid-Size; Don't Super-Size

It may seem like a bargain, but is an extra 240 calories for 39 cents really a good way to spend your calorie budget? That's the difference between a small order of fries and a large one. A kid-size popcorn at most movie theaters contains 150 calories, but a large can top 1,000 (*without* the butter-flavored topping!). A child-size soda (8 ounces) has about 95 calories; a large soda measuring 36 ounces or more contains at least 400.

Serve in the Kitchen; Eat in the Dining Room

When you bring plates to the table already filled, you won't be tempted to pick from serving bowls and plates of food in front of you. You're also forced to go out of your way for seconds and have the chance to reconsider. An added benefit: Because you don't have to dirty serving bowls and plates, you have fewer dishes to wash.

Eat Slowly

It takes 20 minutes for your brain to register the fact that your stomach is full. Try putting your fork down and taking a sip of water between bites. Chew your food well, and don't load up your fork or spoon until you swallow what's in your mouth. Doing so enables you to more easily recognize when you're full.

Eat Off of Plates

Nibbling from packages of crackers and shaving "tastes" from the brownie pan or forkfuls of cake from the platter can add up to plenty of calories, and more than you think you've eaten. Portion out everything you eat onto a plate or into a small bowl and put the package or pan away.

Use measuring cups and spoons to portion out a serving onto your dinnerware. Study and memorize how it looks. What does $1/2$ cup of ice cream look like in your dessert dishes? A cup of whole-wheat cereal in your breakfast bowl? A cup of pasta on your dinner plate? Five ounces of wine in your stemware? You can mark your dinnerware and glassware with a dot or dash of nail polish to remind yourself.

Fill Up on Plant Food

Fruits, vegetables, and whole grains without butter, dressings, or sauces take up stomach space, leaving less room for more dense, high-calorie foods. They also take more time to chew and eat. Consider the fact that a teeny little pat of butter has as many calories as 3 cups of broccoli, or that a 1-inch cube (1 ounce) of cheddar cheese has the same number of calories as 1 cup — that's 8 ounces — of bran flakes.

Switch to Lower-Fat Dairy Products

Dairy is one place where going with the reduced-fat, low-fat, or fat-free variety makes sense, because the calories are significantly reduced in the lower-fat version. For example, an 8-ounce glass of whole milk contains 150 calories, but the same amount of fat-free (skim) milk has only 85. One ounce of regular cheddar cheese has 114 calories, but reduced-fat and low-fat varieties contain 80 and 49 calories, respectively.

Note one exception, however: Dairy products such as ice cream and flavored yogurt that are marketed as reduced-fat, low-fat, or fat-free often contain added sugar to make up for the loss of flavor and texture that fat provides. Don't be fooled into thinking that they provide fewer calories, too. Always check the calorie content on the Nutrition Facts panel of the food label.

Remember That Dull Is Better

Not dull as in "boring," but dull as in "not the shiny stuff." At the salad bar, shiny means a thick coating of oily (meaning high-calorie) salad dressing. Vegetables that shimmer usually have butter added to them. Muffins that leave a grease slick on your napkin have more calories than ones that don't. Bread or rolls that are slick with butter . . . you get the idea.

Cook Meats Using Methods That Start with the Letter B

Broil, barbecue, bake (on a rack), or braise meats, and you save lots of calories over frying, sautéing, and stewing, because the fat (and therefore its calories) has a chance to drip away from the meat.

Cooking chicken and other poultry with the skin on and removing it after it has been cooked is fine, because the meat absorbs little of the fat but stays moist.

Chapter 23

Ten Rules for Healthy Living

*E*ating low-cal is definitely a healthy habit. But there's more to good living than just counting calories. The nutrients in the foods you eat can make or break your healthy living efforts, so choose your calories by the company they keep. In this chapter, you can find ten easy guidelines to remember.

Eat a Minimum of 3 Servings of Vegetables and 2 Servings of Fruit Each Day

Most people don't eat enough vegetables — especially the leafy-green and deep-orange ones. On average, Americans eat the equivalent of only about one-quarter of a serving a day. About half eat no fruit at all on some days.

Vitamin pills can't replace the vitamins, minerals, and other nutrients in produce. But not to worry, because servings are actually quite small: $^1/_2$ cup of most cooked vegetables, 1 cup of salad, or a piece of fruit qualifies as one serving.

Don't drink all your fruits in the form of juice. You'll miss out on fiber if you do, and you'll easily consume too many calories. A mere 4 ounces of juice equals one serving of fruit, and most people drink much more than that at a time.

Eat at Least 3 Servings of Whole Grains Each Day

Only 20 percent of the bread sold in the United States is whole-grain. That's too bad, because you get more fiber, vitamin E, vitamin B$_6$, magnesium, zinc, copper, manganese, and potassium in whole-wheat bread than in white. These nutrients help protect against heart disease, diverticulosis, cancer, and diabetes. The fiber difference between a single slice of whole-wheat bread and one of white is 2 grams.

Twenty to thirty-five grams of fiber a day are recommended.

Eat at Least 4 Servings of Beans, Lentils, or Peas Each Week

Like most vegetables, beans, lentils, and peas are good sources of fiber and *phytochemicals* (plant nutrients) that help cut the risk of cancer, heart disease, and diabetes. But unlike other vegetables, they have enough protein to substitute for a serving of meat, poultry, or fish.

Eat 3 Meals and 2 or 3 Small Snacks a Day

You generally need to eat every 3 to 4 hours. Research has shown that people who snack are often less likely to overeat than those who restrict their eating. The body is also better able to absorb and use the nutrients in a meal than it can when presented with the feast-or-famine scenario of the typical three-meals-a-day, no-snacks pattern.

Eat Breakfast

Missing this meal is a big mistake. After an overnight fast, your body needs fuel to move. Otherwise, metabolism slows, which reduces how many calories you burn. Many studies have shown that children who skip breakfast have difficulty concentrating during the day. It's true for adults, too.

Limit Soft Drinks

Sure, you may prefer swigging soft drinks to water, juice, or milk. But cola-type soft drinks (as well as many citrus-flavored sodas) pack a dose of caffeine with lots of sugar and calories without contributing nutrients, except perhaps water. Sugar-free versions don't add empty calories, at least, but when soft drinks replace fat-free milk in your diet, you're missing out on one of the best sources of calcium you can get. That's a shame, because most adults don't get enough of that bone-building mineral.

Drink Water

Humans are 55 to 75 percent, or 10 to 12 gallons, water. How much water your body contains depends on your age, sex, and lean body mass. The leaner you are, the more water you have, because muscle holds greater amounts of water than fat. Therefore, men have more water than women. And the younger you are, the greater your percentage of water.

Studies show that when you think you're hungry, often you're actually thirsty, because dehydration is a major contributing factor to fatigue, which leads some people to seek food for energy. The rule is 1 liter (about 4 cups) per 1,000 calories. That translates to about eight 8-ounce glasses a day for people who eat about 2,000 calories.

The average adult loses about 2½ quarts of water a day: 4 to 6 cups in the urine, 2 to 4 cups as perspiration, 1½ cups through breathing, and about ⅔ cup in the feces. Roughly 3 to 4½ cups of your daily water comes from solid food.

Limit Caffeine to 2 Servings or Less a Day

Coffee is the main source of caffeine in the American diet, although chocolate, tea, cola and some citrus-flavored soft drinks (such as Mountain Dew), and some over-the-counter pain relievers contribute to a day's total. Caffeine speeds up your heart rate and can make you feel jittery and anxious. It also can contribute to dehydration due to its diuretic effect, which causes your body to lose water.

Table 24-1	Compare and Save		
Nutrient	*1,200 Calories*	*1,500 Calories*	*1,800 Calories*
Protein	30 grams	37 grams	45 grams
Carbohydrate	180 grams	225 grams	270 grams
Fat	< 40 grams	< 50 grams	< 60 grams
Saturated fat	13 grams	16 grams	20 grams
Cholesterol	< 300 milligrams	< 300 milligrams	< 300 milligrams
Fiber	At least 20 grams	At least 20 grams	At least 20 grams
Sodium	< 2,400 milligrams	< 2,400 milligrams	< 2,400 milligrams

It helps to know how much of your daily nutrient needs a particular recipe supplies so that you can plan the rest of the day's meals accordingly. Therefore, you'll find a nutrient analysis for each recipe in this chapter, listing the amount of each of these nutrients that the recipe provides, at the end of the recipe. The analysis does not include optional ingredients, such as salt to taste or parsley for garnish.

Appetizers, Snacks, and Sauces

Hummus

Use this recipe for a dip with a selection of raw vegetables or as a sandwich spread — it's great in a pita topped with lots of shredded lettuce and chopped tomato. Or turn it into a wrap and roll it in a tortilla with a sprinkle of hot sauce, a dusting of sesame seeds, and sprouts. Because it's made with beans, hummus makes a good meatless source of protein.

Preparation time: 15 minutes

Cooking time: None

Yield: 2 cups

2 garlic cloves, peeled

1¹/₂ cups cooked chickpeas, or 1 15¹/₂-ounce can chickpeas, rinsed and drained

¹/₄ cup tahini (sesame paste) or smooth peanut butter

3 tablespoons freshly squeezed lemon juice

1 teaspoon extra-virgin olive oil

¹/₄ teaspoon ground cumin

¹/₄ teaspoon salt, or to taste

¹/₃ cup chopped fresh flat-leaf parsley

(continued)

1. Mince the garlic by dropping it through the feed tube of a food processor or blender while the motor is running.

2. Stop the motor and add the chickpeas, tahini or peanut butter, lemon juice, olive oil, cumin, and salt. Process until smooth, stopping the motor occasionally to scrape down the sides of the bowl. Add the parsley and pulse just until combined.

Nutrient analysis per 2 tablespoons: *50 calories, 2 grams protein, 5 grams carbohydrate, 3 grams fat, 0.5 grams saturated fat, 0 milligrams cholesterol, 1 gram fiber, 35 milligrams sodium.*

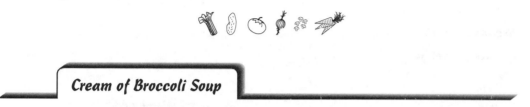

Cream of Broccoli Soup

This recipe is basic but hardly boring. In the summer, use zucchini or summer squash in place of the broccoli when gardens and stores are overrun with them. Carrots work well, too; be sure to cook them thoroughly. And adjust the seasoning if you vary the vegetable: Tarragon is nice with zucchini or squash, and dill marries well with carrots.

Preparation time: *15 minutes*

Cooking time: *10 minutes*

Yield: *6 servings*

4 cups chicken broth

1 bunch fresh broccoli, coarsely chopped, or 2 10-ounce packages frozen chopped broccoli

1 tablespoon butter

1 pear, peeled and chopped

1 medium onion, peeled and chopped

1 teaspoon chili powder

1 cup nonfat yogurt

Orange zest for garnish

1. Heat the chicken broth to boiling in a large saucepan over high heat. Add the broccoli and return to boiling. Cook until tender, about 10 minutes for fresh or 5 minutes for frozen.

2. Melt the butter in a large skillet over medium heat. Sauté the pear, onion, and chili powder in the butter until the pear is tender, about 5 minutes. Stir the sautéed ingredients into the chicken broth and broccoli.

3. Remove from the heat, cool slightly, and then puree in a blender or food processor until smooth. Garnish each serving with a dollop of yogurt and a little orange zest.

Nutrient analysis per serving: *115 calories, 8 grams protein, 13 grams carbohydrate, 4 grams fat, 2 grams saturated fat, 7 milligrams cholesterol, 4 grams fiber, 595 milligrams sodium.*

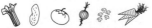

Caesar Dressing

Sure, you can buy a bottle of Caesar dressing, but you won't get the fresh taste that this recipe produces. Another bonus is that this dressing is a good way to sneak soy into your diet. Soy is showing promise in the fight against breast and prostate cancers and heart disease, and it may even reduce the symptoms of menopause. One serving of this dressing doesn't guarantee you good health, but it's a start. This dressing is best if made one day in advance because the flavor intensifies with time. Serve it over romaine lettuce.

Preparation time: *10 minutes*

Cooking time: *None*

Yield: *2 cups*

¹/₂ pound soft tofu	*¹/₃ cup red wine vinegar*
1 tablespoon anchovy paste	*1 tablespoon Worcestershire sauce*
1 garlic clove, peeled and minced	*1 tablespoon Dijon mustard*
Juice of 1 lemon	*Freshly ground black pepper to taste*
¹/₄ cup water	

Combine all the ingredients in a blender jar and process until smooth.

Nutrient analysis per 2 tablespoons: *15 calories, 1 gram protein, 1 gram carbohydrate, 1 gram fat, 0 grams saturated fat, 0 milligrams cholesterol, 0 grams fiber, 44 milligrams sodium.*

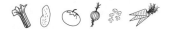

Mango Salsa

If you think of a plain, broiled chicken breast as the little black dress of the kitchen, then salsa is the pearls, taking the dish from boring to stunning with just a garnish. This recipe features mango or papaya, but you can substitute tomatoes, tomatillos, or even pears or peaches. Experiment!

Preparation time: *15 minutes*

Cooking time: *None*

Yield: *About 2 cups*

(continued)

1 mango (or papaya), peeled and cubed (about 1³/₄ cups)

1 to 2 jalapeño peppers, seeded and minced

1 scallion, minced, or 2 tablespoons minced white onion

2 tablespoons chopped fresh mint or coriander

2 tablespoons freshly squeezed lime juice

1 garlic clove, peeled and minced

Salt and freshly ground black pepper to taste

Combine all the ingredients and mix well.

Nutrient analysis per ¹/₄ cup: *20 calories, 0.5 grams protein, 5 grams carbohydrate, 0 grams fat, 0 grams saturated fat, 0 milligrams cholesterol, 1 gram fiber, 2 milligrams sodium.*

Main Dishes and a Few Sides

Tuna and White Bean Salad

Here's a way to turn tuna salad into a hearty meal. Serve it on a bed of salad greens and garnish it with tomato wedges.

Preparation time: *15 minutes*

Cooking time: *None*

Yield: *6 servings*

1 16-ounce can white beans, rinsed and drained

2 6¹/₂- to 7-ounce cans water-packed light tuna, drained

2 tablespoons extra-virgin olive oil

2 tablespoons freshly squeezed lemon juice

2 tablespoons grainy mustard

1 tablespoon red wine vinegar

1 tablespoon balsamic vinegar

1 garlic clove, peeled and minced

1¹/₂ teaspoons sugar

Salt and freshly ground black pepper to taste

¹/₄ cup finely chopped fresh basil leaves

(continued)

1. Combine the beans and tuna in a large bowl and set aside.

2. In a small bowl with a whisk, or in a small jar with a tight-fitting lid, combine the oil, lemon juice, mustard, vinegars, garlic, sugar, salt, and pepper and beat or shake until well blended. Pour the mixture over the tuna and beans.

3. Just before serving, fold in the basil.

Nutrient analysis per serving: *200 calories, 19 grams protein, 20 grams carbohydrate, 5 grams fat, 0.5 grams saturated fat, 15 milligrams cholesterol, 4 grams fiber, 231 milligrams sodium.*

Surprisingly, a can of water-packed white-meat tuna has about 30 more calories and 4 grams more fat than the same amount of water-packed light tuna. Even after being drained, oil-packed light tuna has about 145 more calories than water-packed, and oil-packed white tuna has about 110 more calories than the water-packed varieties.

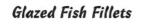

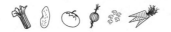

Glazed Fish Fillets

You can use the glaze in this recipe for marinating pork tenderloins or chicken breasts, too. Even slices of eggplant, dressed with the glaze before grilling, are a tasty option. Don't serve the leftover marinade; it contains uncooked fish or meat juices that can make you very sick if you eat them. If you want to use the leftover marinade, boil it for about 5 minutes first.

Preparation time: *5 minutes*

Marinating time: *20 minutes*

Cooking time: *10 minutes*

Yield: *6 servings*

3 tablespoons sugar

¹/₃ cup soy sauce

1 teaspoon roasted sesame oil

¹/₂ teaspoon coarsely ground black pepper

¹/₄ teaspoon crushed red pepper flakes

1¹/₂ pounds salmon fillets

3 tablespoons finely chopped mint, basil, and/or cilantro

(continued)

1. Measure the sugar, soy sauce, sesame oil, and peppers into a resealable bag. Swish to blend. Add the fish and set aside for 20 minutes.

2. Heat the oven to 450°F. Lightly coat a baking pan with vegetable oil cooking spray. Place the fillets skin-side down on the pan. Roast the fish for 5 to 7 minutes, or 10 minutes per inch of thickness. The fish is done when it is barely opaque and flakes when tested with a fork.

3. Remove from the oven and immediately sprinkle the minced herb(s) over the top.

Nutrient analysis per serving: *215 calories, 26 grams protein, 2 grams carbohydrate, 11 grams fat, 2 grams saturated fat, 82 milligrams cholesterol, 0 grams fiber, 406 milligrams sodium.*

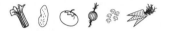

Spicy Vegetable Couscous

Here's a meatless entree that will become a favorite in your house. It's a delicious and healthy way to eat more vegetables. In fact, one serving almost fulfills your daily recommendation of five or more fruits and vegetables.

Preparation time: *15 minutes*

Cooking time: *15 minutes*

Yield: *4 servings*

3 teaspoons olive oil

1 medium onion, peeled and coarsely chopped

1 garlic clove, peeled and minced

¹/₂ medium turnip, scraped and cubed (about 2 cups)

2 large carrots, scraped and thinly sliced diagonally

1 8-ounce can tomatoes, drained

¹/₂ teaspoon salt

¹/₂ teaspoon ground cumin

¹/₄ teaspoon crushed red pepper flakes

2 cups chicken broth

1 small zucchini, thinly sliced

1 cup canned chickpeas, rinsed and drained

1 cup instant couscous

Fresh cilantro leaves and sesame seeds for garnish if desired

1. Heat 2 teaspoons of the oil in a large skillet over medium-high heat. Add the onion and garlic and sauté until tender but not browned, about 5 minutes.

2. Add the turnip, carrots, tomatoes, salt, cumin, red pepper, and ¹/₂ cup of the chicken broth.

(continued)

3. Turn the heat to high and bring the vegetable mixture to a boil. Reduce the heat to low, cover, and simmer for 10 minutes or until the vegetables are tender but firm when tested with a fork.

4. Add the zucchini and chickpeas and cook just until the zucchini is tender.

5. Meanwhile, bring the reserved 1 teaspoon olive oil and 1½ cups chicken broth to a boil in a medium saucepan. Stir in the couscous and cover. Remove from the heat and set aside for at least 5 minutes.

6. To serve, divide the couscous among four plates and top with the vegetables and some of their broth. Garnish with cilantro and sesame seeds if desired.

Nutrient analysis per serving: 280 calories, 11 grams protein, 47 grams carbohydrate, 5 grams fat, 1 gram saturated fat, 0 milligrams cholesterol, 7 grams fiber, 746 milligrams sodium.

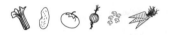

Chicken in Mustard Sauce

Looking for something new to do with chicken breasts? Try this rich-tasting, creamy recipe. The secret ingredient that makes the sauce so velvety without cream is the mustard. And the combination of its pungent bite and the sweetness of the apples is sublime.

Preparation time: 15 minutes

Cooking time: 15 minutes

Yield: 4 servings

4 chicken breast halves, boned and skinned	*1 garlic clove, peeled and minced*
1 tablespoon olive oil	*1½ teaspoons fresh thyme leaves, or ½ teaspoon dried*
1 cup apple juice	*2 tablespoons Dijon mustard*
1 medium onion, peeled and thickly sliced	*1 apple, cored and very thinly sliced*

1. Place the chicken breast halves between two sheets of waxed paper. With the broad side of a heavy knife, pound the chicken breasts to flatten them to about ½ inch thick.

2. Heat the oil in a large skillet over high heat until hot. Add the chicken and sauté for about 3 minutes on each side or until golden.

(continued)

3. Add the apple juice, onion, garlic, and thyme. Cover and cook for 10 minutes or until the chicken is fork-tender.

4. Remove the chicken and keep it warm. Heat the liquid remaining in the skillet to boiling. Blend in the mustard. Add the apple slices and cook until heated through. Pour the sauce over the chicken.

Nutrient analysis per serving: 245 calories, 27 grams protein, 16 grams carbohydrate, 7 grams fat, 1.5 grams saturated fat, 73 milligrams cholesterol, 1 gram fiber, 256 milligrams sodium.

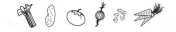

Asparagus-Goat Cheese Lasagna

Diet lasagna? You betcha! This one tastes very fattening but isn't. It's made in the classic Italian way, without lots of stringy cheese or beef. When asparagus is no longer in season or affordable, you can find a variation using winter squash at the end of this recipe, or you can substitute cooked ground turkey for the asparagus in the master recipe for equally delicious results.

Preparation time: 25 minutes

Cooking time: 30 minutes

Yield: 8 servings

4 pounds asparagus, trimmed

2 tablespoons olive oil

Salt to taste

3 tablespoons butter

$^1/_4$ cup all-purpose flour

$1^1/_2$ cups chicken broth

6 ounces mild goat cheese, such as Montrachet

1 teaspoon freshly grated lemon zest, or to taste

6 7-x-6$^1/_4$-inch sheets instant (no-boil) lasagna, or equivalent amount of another size sheet

1 cup freshly grated Parmesan cheese

1. Heat the oven to 450°F. Cut the tips off the asparagus spears and reserve them. Cut the remaining spears into $^1/_2$-inch pieces and place them in a large baking pan. Toss with the oil.

2. Roast the asparagus, shaking the pan every few minutes, for 5 to 10 minutes or until tender-crisp. Sprinkle the asparagus with salt to taste and let cool. Reduce the oven temperature to 400°F.

(continued)

3. In a medium saucepan over medium heat, melt the butter. Add the flour and cook over moderately low heat, stirring, for 5 minutes or until the sauce thickens. Blend in the chicken broth and ¹/₂ cup water and cook, stirring constantly, until the sauce comes to a boil. Reduce the heat to low and simmer, stirring, for 5 minutes or until the sauce thickens. Blend in the goat cheese, lemon zest, and salt to taste until the sauce is smooth.

4. Spray the bottom and sides of a 13-x-9-inch baking dish with vegetable oil cooking spray. Arrange two sheets of lasagna in the bottom (the lasagna will not cover the bottom of the dish completely); spread with one-third of the sauce. Top the sauce with half the roasted asparagus and sprinkle it with one-third of the Parmesan cheese. Top with two more sheets of pasta and repeat the layering, ending with a top layer of pasta.

5. Arrange the reserved asparagus tips on the top of the pasta. Spoon on the remaining sauce and then the remaining Parmesan cheese. Cover the dish with foil and bake for 20 minutes. Remove the foil and bake for 10 more minutes or until golden and bubbling. Let stand for 10 minutes before serving.

Nutrient analysis per serving: 235 calories, 16 grams protein, 18 grams carbohydrate, 12 grams fat, 6 grams saturated fat, 19 milligrams cholesterol, 5 grams fiber, 462 milligrams sodium.

Variation: Winter Squash Lasagna: Substitute 5 pounds winter squash, such as butternut, for the 4 pounds asparagus. Peel and dice the squash and toss with the oil, plus add 1 tablespoon fresh or dried rosemary. Roast until tender, about 10 minutes. Proceed as above but substitute ²/₃ cup low-fat milk for the goat cheese when making the sauce.

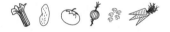

Meatloaf

Here's a homey dish that's normally loaded with calories. In this recipe, we stretch the calories by adding bulghur (or bulgur), which is similar to cracked wheat. And to assure a good, meaty flavor, we add dried mushrooms.

Preparation time: 20 minutes

Cooking time: 60 minutes

Yield: 10 servings

(continued)

1¹/₂ ounces dried mushrooms (about 1 cup)

³/₄ cup bulghur

2 teaspoons olive oil

1 small onion, peeled and chopped

2 garlic cloves, peeled and minced

3 ounces tomato paste

1 tablespoon Worcestershire sauce

1 large egg

2 large egg whites

1 cup fine dry bread crumbs

³/₄ cup evaporated skim milk

1¹/₂ pounds lean ground beef

¹/₄ cup chopped fresh parsley

1 teaspoon dried thyme leaves

¹/₂ teaspoon salt

1. Soak the mushrooms in enough warm water to cover them for 30 minutes or until softened. Drain the mushrooms and coarsely chop them.

2. Meanwhile, in another bowl, combine the bulghur with 1 cup boiling water and set aside for 30 minutes or until the water is absorbed.

3. Heat oven to 350°F. Coat a baking sheet with vegetable oil cooking spray.

4. In a small skillet over medium heat, heat the oil, onion, and garlic and cook, stirring occasionally, until translucent, about 5 to 7 minutes. Stir in the tomato paste and cook for 3 minutes. Blend in the Worcestershire sauce.

5. In a large bowl, beat the egg with the egg whites. Stir in the bread crumbs, evaporated skim milk, sautéed onions and garlic, and the soaked mushrooms and bulghur. Use your hands to gently work in the ground beef, parsley, thyme, and salt.

6. Turn onto the prepared baking sheet and shape into a loaf. Bake for 50 to 60 minutes or until a meat thermometer inserted into the center of the loaf reads 160°F. Remove from the oven and cool for 10 minutes before slicing.

Nutrient analysis per serving: 280 calories, 20 grams protein, 30 grams carbohydrate, 9 grams fat, 3 grams saturated fat, 45 milligrams cholesterol, 4 grams fiber, 672 milligrams sodium.

Shaping meatloaf or burgers is easier if you moisten your hands first.

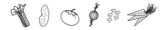

Oven-Fried Chicken

You can use corn flakes or bread crumbs to coat chicken, but we found the nuttiness of whole-wheat crackers to be a nice change.

Preparation time: *20 minutes*

Cooking time: *35 minutes*

Yield: *6 servings*

5 ounces low-fat, unsweetened, whole-wheat crackers, such as melba toast

1 tablespoon paprika

$^1/_2$ teaspoon dried thyme leaves

$^1/_2$ teaspoon crushed rosemary leaves

$^1/_2$ teaspoon salt

2 large egg whites

$^1/_2$ cup nonfat ranch dressing

6 chicken breast halves, skin (but not bones) removed

1. Heat the oven to 425°F. Set a wire rack on a baking sheet and lightly coat it with vegetable oil cooking spray.

2. In a blender or food processor, combine the crackers, paprika, thyme, rosemary, and salt and process to make coarse crumbs. Transfer the crumbs to a shallow bowl.

3. Whisk the egg whites in a bowl until frothy; then blend in the ranch dressing.

4. Dip the chicken breast halves in the eggs and dressing and then in the crumbs. Set them bone-side-up on the prepared rack. Lightly coat the chicken with vegetable oil cooking spray. Turn and lightly spray the other side.

5. Bake for 30 to 35 minutes or until the crumbs are browned and crisp and the chicken juices run clear when tested with a fork.

Nutrient analysis per serving: 190 calories, 17 grams protein, 23 grams carbohydrate, 2 grams fat, 0.5 grams saturated fat, 36 milligrams cholesterol, 2 grams fiber, 606 milligrams sodium.

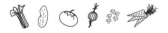

Barbecued Pork Tenderloin

You can grill this pork over a wood or charcoal fire, or you can broil it. Either way, you'll get that real Southern taste because the homemade sauce has a North Carolina pig-pickin' flavor. Use it for your next chicken cookout (or roast-in), too.

Preparation time: *20 minutes*

Marinating time: *2 hours*

Cooking time: *15 minutes*

Yield: *6 servings*

1 cup white vinegar	*3 teaspoons freshly ground black pepper*
1 tablespoon salt	*2 ³/₄-pound pork tenderloins*
1 tablespoon red pepper flakes	*1 tablespoon Worcestershire sauce*
1 teaspoon ground red pepper	

1. In a jar with a tight-fitting lid, combine the vinegar, salt, red pepper flakes, ground red pepper, and 2 teaspoons of the black pepper. Shake until well combined. Refrigerate for at least 2 hours or overnight.

2. Rub the tenderloins with the Worcestershire sauce and the reserved teaspoon of black pepper. Cover and refrigerate for 2 hours or overnight.

3. Light the outdoor grill or broiler. Cook the tenderloins over medium heat or 6 inches from the broiler, turning once or twice and basting with the vinegar-pepper sauce until the outside is browned and a meat thermometer inserted into the meat reads 150°F. Let the meat rest for 5 minutes before slicing.

Nutrient analysis per serving: *190 calories, 32 grams protein, 0 grams carbohydrate, 5 grams fat, 2 grams saturated fat, 90 milligrams cholesterol, 0 grams fiber, 90 milligrams sodium.*

This barbecue sauce gets better over time and will keep for up to 2 months in the refrigerator. To prevent illness, never use barbecue sauce that has come in contact with raw meat or fish unless you boil it first.

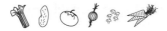

Roast Turkey with Gravy

You used to make turkey gravy by blending flour with the pan drippings and adding water or stock. But that meant lots of fat and calories, and a bad rap for gravy. This new method for making gravy will convince you that cooking healthier tastes better.

Preparation time: *45 minutes*

Cooking time: *About 3 hours*

Yield: *10 servings*

1 12- to 14-pound turkey (not self-basting)	*2 carrots, chopped*
Salt and freshly ground black pepper to taste	*2 teaspoons olive oil*
6 garlic cloves, peeled	*5 cups reduced-sodium chicken broth, fat removed*
3 apples, quartered	*2 or 3 sprigs fresh parsley*
¹/₂ cup apple cider	*¹/₂ teaspoon black peppercorns*
Wings, neck, and giblets (but not the liver) from the bird	*¹/₂ cup white wine or apple cider*
1 large onion, peeled and chopped	*3 tablespoons cornstarch*

1. Heat the oven to 325°F.

2. Remove any visible fat from the turkey cavity. Liberally salt and pepper the cavity. Place the garlic and apples in the bird and tie the drumsticks together. Set the turkey breast-side up on a rack in a large roasting pan.

3. Roast the turkey, basting it every 45 minutes or so with the ¹/₂ cup apple cider and pan drippings, until golden, about 2 hours. Cover with a tent of aluminum foil and continue roasting and basting for 1 hour longer, or until a meat thermometer inserted into the thickest part of the thigh reads 180°F. Place the turkey on a large platter to rest for 30 minutes before carving.

4. Meanwhile, make the stock for the gravy. Place the wings, neck, giblets, onion, and carrots in a large saucepan with the olive oil and brown, stirring frequently, for about 15 minutes. Add the broth, parsley, peppercorns, and 2 cups water and heat to boiling. Reduce the heat to low; partially cover, and simmer for 1 hour. Strain through a fine sieve into a clean sauce-pan and refrigerate until the fat comes to the surface. Remove and discard the fat.

5. When the turkey is done, pour the drippings from the roasting pan into a chilled metal bowl and place in the freezer to chill so that the fat can be skimmed off the top quickly and easily. Or use a gravy strainer (see the tip at the end of the recipe).

(continued)

6. Place the roasting pan on the stovetop and add the white wine or apple cider. Cook, stirring to scrape up the browned bits from the pan. Add to the saucepan with the stock. Skim and discard the fat from the pan drippings and add the drippings to the stock. Heat to boiling; then reduce the heat to low to maintain a simmer.

7. In a small bowl, dissolve the cornstarch in ¼ cup water and whisk into the simmering stock. Season with salt and pepper to taste.

8. Remove the skin from the turkey and carve. Serve with the gravy.

Nutrient analysis for 4 ounces of light and dark meat plus 5 tablespoons gravy: *235 calories, 35 grams protein, 6 grams carbohydrate, 8 grams fat, 2.5 grams saturated fat, 88 milligrams cholesterol, 0 grams fiber, 135 milligrams sodium.*

 A gravy strainer (it looks like a measuring cup with a spout that comes from the bottom) makes easy work of skimming the fat from gravy and stock. Because fat floats, the spout enables you to pour off the fat-free part of the gravy or stock and leave the fat behind.

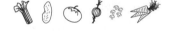

Chili Burgers

You can trim the fat off a steak, but removing the fat from ground beef is not always easy, so making burgers leaner and lower in calories requires a bit of kitchen wizardry. Here, we add beans to reduce the calories and season the burgers with Southwestern flavor. Serve them with some toe-tingling salsa instead of plain old ketchup.

Preparation time: *25 minutes*

Cooking time: *10 minutes*

Yield: *6 servings*

1 teaspoon olive oil	*2 tablespoons tomato paste*
1 small onion, peeled and finely chopped	*¾ pound extra-lean ground beef*
1 jalapeño pepper, seeded and minced	*½ teaspoon salt*
1 garlic clove, peeled and minced	*½ teaspoon freshly ground black pepper*
1½ teaspoons ground cumin	*6 sandwich rolls*
¾ cup black beans, rinsed, drained, and slightly mashed	*6 lettuce leaves*
1 slice firm white bread, torn into crumbs	*2 tomatoes, sliced*
1 egg white	

(continued)

1. Heat the grill or broiler.

2. In a small skillet, heat the oil. Cook the onion, jalapeño, garlic, and cumin in the oil until fragrant, about 3 minutes. Remove from the heat.

3. Combine the beans, bread, egg white, and tomato paste in a medium bowl. Mash into a paste with a fork or potato masher. Add the ground beef, salt, pepper, and sautéed ingredients. Mix thoroughly.

4. Shape into four $^3/_4$-inch-thick burgers. Grill or broil until the burgers reach 160°F in the center (test the temperature with a meat thermometer), about 5 minutes per side. Serve on rolls with lettuce and tomato.

Nutrient analysis per serving: *350 calories, 19 grams protein, 28 grams carbohydrate, 9 grams fat, 3.8 grams saturated fat, 14 milligrams cholesterol, 5 grams fiber, 636 milligrams sodium.*

Chili peppers can burn you. The oils that reside in the white membrane where the seeds are attached are powerful. Be sure to wash your hands well with soapy water before touching sensitive body parts! Or wear rubber gloves while you handle chilies.

To prevent food poisoning, always cook ground beef until it is no longer pink inside. An instant-read thermometer inserted in the center of the meat should read 160°F.

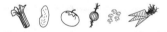

French (Un)fries

Even if you bake frozen french fries in the oven, you get more fat than a serving of these fries delivers, minus the sweet flavor and healthy dose of beta carotene that sweet potatoes provide.

Preparation time: *10 minutes*

Cooking time: *35 minutes*

Yield: *4 servings*

1¹/₂ pounds sweet potatoes	*¹/₂ teaspoon salt*
2 teaspoons olive oil	*¹/₂ teaspoon chili powder*

(continued)

1. Heat the oven to 450°F. Lightly coat a baking sheet with vegetable oil cooking spray.

2. Scrub the potatoes well and cut them lengthwise into about 10 wedges.

3. In a large bowl, combine the oil, salt, and chili powder. Add the potatoes and toss until well coated.

4. Spread the potatoes on the prepared baking sheet and roast for 20 minutes. Loosen the potatoes from the sheet with a spatula, turn, and roast for 10 to 15 minutes longer or until golden.

Nutrient analysis per serving: *195 calories, 3 grams protein, 41 grams carbohydrate, 3 grams fat, 0.5 grams saturated fat, 0 milligrams cholesterol, 5 grams fiber, 287 milligrams sodium.*

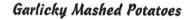

Garlicky Mashed Potatoes

One of the secrets to making mashed potatoes low-calorie is to use naturally buttery-tasting yellow potatoes. Another trick is to use lightly browned butter, which boosts its flavor.

Preparation time: *15 minutes*

Cooking time: *15 minutes*

Yield: *6 servings*

2 pounds Yukon Gold or baking potatoes, peeled and cut into chunks

4 garlic cloves, peeled and halved

2 teaspoons butter

1 cup buttermilk

Salt and freshly ground pepper to taste

1. Place the potatoes and garlic in a large saucepan with enough lightly salted water to cover. Heat to boiling over high heat. Reduce the heat to low; cover and simmer until fork-tender, about 10 to 15 minutes.

2. Meanwhile, in a small skillet or saucepan over low heat, heat the butter, swirling the skillet until the butter begins to brown, about 1 minute. Stir in the buttermilk and heat through, but do not boil or the milk will curdle.

(continued)

3. Drain the potatoes well and mash them with a potato masher or electric mixer. When smooth, blend in the buttermilk and browned butter and add salt and pepper to taste.

Nutrient analysis per serving: 170 calories, 4 grams protein, 35 grams carbohydrate, 2 grams fat, 1 gram saturated fat, 5 milligrams cholesterol, 2 grams fiber, 63 milligrams sodium.

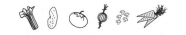

Desserts

Lemon Cake

Remember this recipe for picnics, pot-luck dinners, or whenever you need a dessert that travels well. This cake also makes a tasty after-school or mid-afternoon snack with a dollop of vanilla yogurt and a spoonful of berries.

Preparation time: 15 minutes

Cooking time: About 35 minutes

Yield: 12 servings

2 tablespoons butter	*3 lemons*
²/₃ cup buttermilk	*2 large eggs*
1¹/₂ cups all-purpose flour, plus more to dust the pan	*1 cup granulated sugar*
2 teaspoons baking powder	*1 tablespoon canola oil*
¹/₂ teaspoon baking soda	*1 teaspoon vanilla extract*
¹/₂ teaspoon salt	*1¹/₄ cups confectioners' sugar*

1. Heat the oven to 350°F. Lightly coat a 6-cup Bundt pan with vegetable oil cooking spray; dust with some flour and shake out the excess.

2. In a small skillet or saucepan over low heat, heat the butter, swirling the skillet until it begins to brown, about 1 minute. Pour the browned butter into a bowl, add the buttermilk, and set aside.

3. Sift the 1¹/₂ cups flour, baking powder, baking soda, and salt into a bowl; set aside. Grate 2 teaspoons lemon zest (just the yellow part) from the lemons and then squeeze enough juice to make ¹/₂ cup; set the zest and juice aside.

(continued)

4. In another bowl, beat the eggs, sugar, and oil until they become thick and pale, about 3 to 5 minutes. Blend in the vanilla, lemon zest, and 1 tablespoon of the lemon juice; set aside the remaining juice.

5. With a rubber spatula, fold about one-fourth of the dry ingredients and then one-third of the liquid ingredients into the beaten eggs, folding just until blended. Repeat adding ingredients alternately. Spoon the batter into the prepared pan and bake for 30 to 35 minutes or until a toothpick inserted into the cake comes out clean. Let cool on a wire rack for 5 minutes before removing from the pan.

6. Meanwhile, whisk together 1 cup of the confectioners' sugar and the reserved lemon juice to make a syrup. While the cake is still warm, poke holes all over it with a wooden skewer. Spoon the lemon syrup over the cake. Just before serving, dust with the reserved confectioners' sugar.

Nutrient analysis per serving: 205 calories, 3 grams protein, 40 grams carbohydrate, 4 grams fat, 1.5 grams saturated fat, 0 milligrams cholesterol, 0 grams fiber, 247 milligrams sodium.

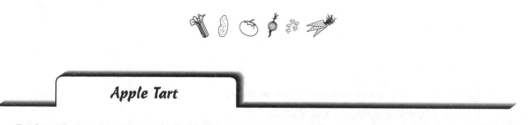

Apple Tart

Rather than a two-crust apple pie, which is typical of most apple pie recipes, this one has one and a half crusts. Use your own recipe for a single crust pie or start with a ready-made pie crust as we do here.

Preparation time: 20 minutes

Cooking time: 45 minutes

Yield: 8 servings

1 refrigerated rolled ready-made pie crust (not a preshaped frozen shell)

1 lemon

1$^{1}/_{2}$ pounds tart cooking apples, such as Rome, Empire, or Granny Smith, peeled and thinly sliced (about 4 medium to large)

$^{1}/_{2}$ cup raisins

$^{1}/_{3}$ cup sugar

1 tablespoon butter

2 tablespoons all-purpose flour

1 large egg white

1. Heat the oven to 400°F. Lightly coat a large baking sheet with vegetable oil cooking spray.

2. Unfold the pie crust on a lightly floured work surface. Using a lightly floured rolling pin, roll it out into a 15-inch circle. Transfer it to the baking sheet.

(continued)

3. Grate ¹/₂ teaspoon lemon zest (just the yellow part) from the lemon and then squeeze 1 tablespoon of juice. Toss the peel and juice with the apples and raisins.

4. Set aside 1 teaspoon of the sugar. In a small bowl, combine the butter, flour, and remaining sugar with the tines of a fork until it resembles oatmeal and then add it to the apples.

5. Place the apples in the center of the pie crust. Beat the egg white with 1 tablespoon water and brush it over the pasty and exposed apples; sprinkle the tart with the reserved teaspoon of sugar.

6. Bake for 30 minutes or until the crust is golden. Place a sheet of aluminum foil loosely on the top of the pie and bake for about 15 minutes longer or until the apples are very tender when tested with a fork. Let the pie cool for about 15 minutes in the pan and then run a metal spatula under it and remove it to a serving plate.

Nutrient analysis per serving: 200 calories, 3 grams protein, 27 grams carbohydrate, 9 grams fat, 2.5 grams saturated fat, 5 milligrams cholesterol, 1 gram fiber, 146 milligrams sodium.

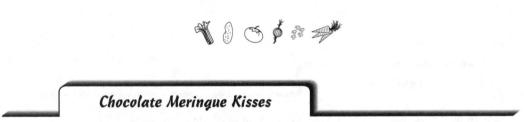

Chocolate Meringue Kisses

Chocolate is one food that's tough to pass up. And there's no need to if you know this recipe's secret: Instead of using lots of chocolate, which contains lots of fat, use some cocoa, which is virtually fat-free and therefore lower in calories. You still get the chocolate flavor that you crave, and because the cookies are crisp and fudgy at the same time, you don't have to compromise on chewing satisfaction, either.

Preparation time: 10 minutes

Cooking time: 20 minutes

Yield: About 3¹/₂ dozen cookies

3 large egg whites

¹/₂ teaspoon instant coffee powder or granules

4 tablespoons unsweetened cocoa powder

1 ounce unsweetened chocolate, chopped

¹/₄ cup sifted confectioners' sugar

1¹/₂ tablespoons cornstarch

1 teaspoon ground cinnamon

³/₄ cup granulated sugar

1 teaspoon vanilla extract

(continued)

1. Set the racks in the center and upper positions of the oven and heat the oven to 325°F.

2. Line two baking sheets with aluminum foil.

3. In a grease-free, non-plastic mixing bowl, combine the egg whites and coffee powder; let stand for 5 minutes.

4. Pulverize the cocoa powder and chocolate in a food processor for about 30 seconds or until the chocolate is ground to a fine powder. Pour into a bowl and stir in the confectioners' sugar, cornstarch, and cinnamon until evenly incorporated. Set aside.

5. With an electric mixer on medium speed, beat the egg whites and coffee until frothy. Increase the speed to high and beat until soft peaks form. Gradually add the granulated sugar, about 2 tablespoons at a time, until all the sugar is incorporated. Add the vanilla. Beat until stiff and glossy. Gently fold in the chocolate and cocoa until evenly incorporated but not overmixed.

6. Drop the batter by rounded teaspoonfuls on the prepared baking sheets, spacing the kisses about 1^1/$_2$ inches apart. (Alternatively, spoon the batter into a pastry bag fitted with a ^{1}/$_2$-inch-diameter open-star tip and pipe the kisses about 1 inch in diameter.)

7. Bake for 14 to 18 minutes, switching the baking sheets halfway through; the cookies should be almost firm to the touch. (Bake all the cookies at once; the batter does not hold.) For chewy cookies, underbake slightly; for crispy, drier ones, overbake slightly.

8. Remove the sheets to wire racks and let cool for a minute or two. Then slide the aluminum foil from the baking sheets to a flat surface and let the cookies stand until completely cool. Carefully peel the cookies off the foil. Store in an airtight container for up to 4 days. Freeze for longer storage.

Nutrient analysis per cookie: *25 calories, 0.5 grams protein, 5 grams carbohydrate, 0 grams fat, 0 grams saturated fat, 0 milligrams cholesterol, 0 grams fiber, 4 milligrams sodium.*

Chocolate Cheesecake

Did you know that the number-one most ordered dessert in restaurants is cheesecake? And for good reason. Few foods deliver the richness and creaminess that cheesecake can. This one, while being calorie and fat reduced, offers an added bonus: chocolate. What could be better?

Preparation time: *20 minutes*

Cooking time: *60 minutes*

Chilling time: *8 hours*

Yield: *16 servings*

Crust

4 ounces chocolate wafers (about 18 wafers)

1 cup graham cracker crumbs

2 tablespoons unsweetened cocoa powder

2 tablespoons sugar

3 tablespoons vegetable oil

3 tablespoons water

Filling

2 ounces unsweetened chocolate

2 tablespoons instant coffee powder

2 16-ounce containers nonfat cottage cheese (4 cups)

1 8-ounce package low-fat cream cheese at room temperature

1 cup low-fat sour cream

1 cup granulated sugar

1 large egg

2 large egg whites

$3/4$ cup unsweetened cocoa powder

2 tablespoons cornstarch

1 teaspoon vanilla extract

$1/8$ teaspoon salt

1. Heat the oven to 325° F. Coat a 9-inch springform pan with vegetable oil cooking spray.

2. **Make the crust:** Place the chocolate wafers, graham cracker crumbs, cocoa, and sugar in a food processor. Using an on/off motion, process to fine crumbs. Add the oil and water and process until the crumbs are moistened. Pour the crumbs into the springform pan and press them into the bottom and about $1^{1}/_{2}$ inches up the side of the pan. Set aside.

3. **Make the filling:** Melt the chocolate in the top of a double boiler over hot, not boiling, water or in a microwave at medium (50 percent) power. Let cool slightly.

(continued)

4. Dissolve the instant coffee in 1 tablespoon boiling water and set aside.

5. Place the cottage cheese in a strainer lined with a double thickness of cheesecloth. Gather up the cheesecloth and squeeze out the moisture.

6. Put the pressed cottage cheese in a food processor and blend until smooth. Add the cream cheese, sour cream, sugar, egg, egg whites, cocoa, cornstarch, vanilla, salt, melted chocolate, and dissolved coffee and process until smooth. Pour the mixture into the crust-lined pan.

7. Bake for about 1 hour or until firm around the edge but still shiny and slightly soft in the center. Remove from the oven.

8. Run a knife around the inside of the pan to loosen the edge. Let cool in the pan on a rack. Cover and refrigerate until well chilled, for at least 8 hours or up to 2 days.

9. When ready to serve, remove the side of the springform pan. To facilitate cutting, dip a sharp knife in hot water and wipe dry before cutting each slice.

Nutrient analysis per serving: 260 calories, 12 grams protein, 31 grams carbohydrate, 11 grams fat, 6 grams saturated fat, 25 milligrams cholesterol, 2 grams fiber, 326 milligrams sodium.

For picture-perfect slices of cheesecake, use a long piece of dental floss instead of a knife. Cut the cake first in half, then in quarters, then in eighths, and then in sixteenths.

Sane snacking

Don't try to white-knuckle the times between meals without a nosh. No need. Studies show that people who eat frequently have better success at reaching their weight-loss goals.

The perfect snack is a mini-meal. It should be based on carbohydrate for fast energy but also include a tiny bit of fat for staying power and a wee bit of protein so that the carbs can be used for energy and not be shunted off for muscle repair. You can improve even a healthy snack such as an apple by adding a small piece of low-fat cheese or a thin schmear of peanut butter to it.

Here are some great snacks to try:

- **Whole-grain cereal and low-fat milk:** Buy single-serving packages of cereal to make portion control a no-brainer.

- **Low-fat yogurt with fresh fruit:** Fat-free yogurt doesn't have the same staying power that yogurt with a little fat does. If you prefer the nonfat kind, sprinkle in a scant handful of chopped nuts or granola to add some fat and fiber.

- **Peanut butter on whole-wheat crackers:** Relying on peanut butter as a good source of protein is not a calorie-wise move, but eating it in snack-size amounts does make sense. You can use the low-fat variety of peanut butter if you like, but there are no calorie savings over the regular kind. Better still, use natural peanut butter and pour off the oil that accumulates on the top — you're pouring off some of its calories. If the peanut butter is too dry, add a dab of jelly.

- **Pita bread stuffed with lettuce, tomato, cucumber, and shredded low-fat cheese:** Buy whole-wheat, mini pitas for extra fiber and automatic portion control.

- **A small baked potato topped with low-fat cottage cheese:** Small-curd cottage cheese, whirled in a blender, has a creamy texture. Cottage cheese with added calcium, vegetables, or chives is even better nutritionally and flavor-wise.

- **A hard-cooked egg with salsa:** A handful of baked tortilla chips for a little crunch would be tasty, too.

- **A single-serving-size can of tuna mixed with sweet pickle relish and a little low-fat mayo:** Spread it on crackers, toast, rice cakes, celery, or apple wedges.

- **A baked apple with nuts:** Core it, and then fill the cavity with a tablespoon of nuts, a little brown sugar, and a sprinkle of ground cinnamon. Cover it with plastic wrap and nuke it until soft. Eat it with low-fat vanilla yogurt. Bananas are yummy flavored and heated this way, too.

- **Frozen fruit and dairy dips:** Freeze grapes until crunchy and then dip them into low-fat sour cream. Or try frozen peach slices with low-fat ricotta cheese and raisins.

- **A soft microwave pretzel:** Eat it Manhattan sidewalk–style with a bit of mustard and a handful of peanuts.

Appendix A

Weight Management Resources

* *

*I*n this appendix, you can find books, Web sites, and organizations that can help you in your search for more information about weight management.

Books

With *so* many books about diet and nutrition out there, telling what's legit and what's not is sometimes hard. Here are a few of our all-time favorites:

- ✔ *The American Dietetic Association's Complete Food & Nutrition Guide,* by Roberta Larson Duyff. Chronimed Publishing, 1998.

- ✔ *The American Dietetic Association's Guide to Women's Nutrition for Healthy Living,* by Susan Calvert Finn, Ph.D., R.D., with Jane Grant Tougas. Perigee Books, 1997.

- ✔ *The Diet-Free Solution,* by Laurel Mellin, M.A., R.D. Regan Books, 1997.

- ✔ *Helping Your Child Lose Weight the Healthy Way,* by Judith Levine, M.S., R.D., and Linda Bine. Birch Lane Press, 1996.

- ✔ *How to Get Your Kid to Eat . . . But Not Too Much,* by Ellyn Satter, R.D. Bull Publishing Co., 1987.

- ✔ *Intuitive Eating,* by Evelyn Tribole, M.S., R.D., and Elyse Resch, M.S., R.D. St. Martin's Paperbacks, 1995.

- ✔ *Nutrition For Dummies,* by Carol Ann Rinzler. IDG Books Worldwide, Inc., 1997.

- ✔ *The Supermarket Guide,* by Mary Abbott Hess, M.S., R.D. Chronimed Publishing, 1997.

Newsletters

Newsletters are a great way to keep up on the latest nutrition information. They frequently include articles about healthy eating and weight loss, among other topics of interest.

Consumer Reports on Health

P. O. Box 52148
Boulder, CO 80322
800-234-2188

Environmental Nutrition

P. O. Box 420235
Palm Coast, FL 32142
800-829-5384

Tufts University Health & Nutrition Letter

P. O. Box 57857
Boulder, CO 80322
800-274-7581

healthletter.tufts.edu

University of California at Berkeley Wellness Letter

Health Letter Associates
P. O. Box 420235
Palm Coast, FL 32142
800-829-9080

Web Sites

You can find a ton of information out in cyberspace about nutrition and health, but view it with a wary eye. As with books, it can be difficult to tell whether the information a Web site provides is from a knowledgeable, sound source or simply from someone who *thinks* they know about nutrition. The sites listed in this section provide balanced, accurate information about diet, nutrition, and health. For ways to evaluate sites not listed here, see Chapter 20.

Calorie Control Council

This site can help you reduce your fat and calorie intake, figure out what weight is healthy for you, and attain and maintain that weight. It also provides information about low-calorie, reduced-fat foods and beverages and the ingredients they contain.

```
www.caloriecontrol.org
```

Children's Nutrition Research Center (CNRC)

The CNRC is one of six United States Department of Agriculture's human nutrition research centers for the nutrient needs of healthy children and pregnant and nursing women.

```
www.bcm.tmc.edu/cnrc/
```

Fat City

Fat City is a diet and weight-loss fraud watchdog group with Canadian ties.

```
www.healthwatch.org/Dietfraud/fatcity.html
```

Food and Drug Administration

This government site tells you more than you'd ever want to know about food and drugs, including information about dietary supplements, additives, food labeling, and kids' and women's health.

```
www.fda.gov
```

Food Guide Pyramid

The official site of the USDA's Food Guide Pyramid, which recommends numbers of servings from the five food groups. You can also find information about what makes a serving.

www.nal.usda.gov:8001/py/pmap.htm

Healthy Weight Network

Healthy Weight Network provides research and practical information about weight and eating issues, including how to identify fraudulent claims and programs. This site gives information about seminars that can help reduce your fear of eating, and also offers access to a Healthy Weight Journal.

www.healthyweightnetwork.com

LEARN Program

Developed by psychologist Kelly D. Brownell, Ph.D., the LEARN program incorporates lessons on lifestyles, exercise, attitudes, relationships, and nutrition.

www.learneducation.com

Nutrition and Your Health: Dietary Guidelines for Americans

Here, you can view the USDA's Dietary Guidelines for Healthy Americans, published in 1995. The guidelines involve seven intertwining principles of healthy eating.

www.nal.usda.gov/fnic/dga/dguide95.html

Shape Up America!

This site gives information about safe weight management and physical fitness, including a free Body Mass Index calculator. You can also visit the Cyberkitchen and enter your height, weight, age, and activity level to determine an appropriate daily calorie intake for yourself.

www.shapeup.org

Tufts University Nutrition Navigator

This online rating and review guide to Internet nutrition information is designed to help you find accurate, useful nutrition information that you can trust. A great resource for helping determine whether sites are legitimate — and it provides links only to those sites it approves.

```
www.navigator.tufts.edu
```

Weight Control Information Network

This national information service of the National Institute of Diabetes and Digestive and Kidney Diseases (NIDDK) of the National Institutes of Health (NIH) provides science-based information on obesity, weight control, and nutrition in an easy-to-read fact sheet format.

```
www.niddk.nih.gov/health/nutriti/pubs/wtloss/wtloss.htm
```

Organizations

The following organizations provide information about a variety of health topics, ranging from exercise to nutrition to the special needs of children.

Children

American Academy of Pediatrics
141 Northwest Point Boulevard
P. O. Box 747
Elk Grove Village, IL 60009
800-433-9016

```
www.aap.org
```

American Dietetic Association (ADA)
National Center for Nutrition and Dietetics
216 West Jackson Boulevard
Chicago, IL 60606
800-366-1655

```
www.eatright.org
```

Eating disorders

When it comes to eating disorders, being informed is always a good idea. This section lists some organizations that can help.

Anorexia Nervosa and Related Eating Disorders (ANRED)

P.O. Box 5102
Eugene, OR 97405
541-344-1144

www.anred.com

This nonprofit organization provides information about anorexia nervosa, bulimia nervosa, binge eating disorder, and weight disorders.

National Association of Anorexia Nervosa and Associated Disorders (ANAD)

Box 7
Highland Park, IL 60035
847-831-3438

www.aureate.com

ANAD offers free eating disorder information and prevention services, hotline counseling, support groups, and referrals to health care professionals.

Overeaters Anonymous (OA)

P. O. Box 44020
Rio Rancho, NM 87174-4020
505-891-2664

www.overeatersanonymous.org

OA is an international self-help group for anorexics, bulimics, and compulsive overeaters. The office answers calls, distributes meeting lists, gives general information about the program, and sells literature.

Exercise

American College of Sports Medicine (ACSM)

P. O. Box 1440
Indianapolis, IN 46206-1440
317-637-9200

www.acsm.org/sportsmed

American Council on Exercise (ACE)
5820 Overlain Dr., Suite 102
San Diego, CA 92121-3787
800-825-3636

www.acefitness.org/index.html

President's Council on Physical Fitness and Sports
701 Pennsylvania Avenue, NW
Suite 250
Washington, DC 20004
202-272-3421

Nutrition

American Dietetic Association (ADA)
National Center for Nutrition and Dietetics
216 West Jackson Boulevard
Chicago, IL 60606
800-366-1655

www.eatright.org

Surgical centers for obesity

American Society of Bariatric Physicians (ASBP)
5600 South Quebec Street
Suite 109-A
Englewood, CO 80111
303-779-2526

American Society for Bariatric Surgeons (ASBS)
6717 NW 11th Place
Suite C
Gainesville, FL 32605
352-331-4900

www.asbs.org

Recipes

Healthy eating *can* be delicious! Just check out these Web sites that offer
recipes — perfect whether you're looking for a quick work-night meal or
planning a more extravagant dinner party.

FATFREE: The Low Fat Vegetarian Archive

Even if you're not a vegetarian, you can appreciate the interesting veggie-based recipes for soups, casseroles, desserts, appetizers, and more — more than 2,500 in all. Many — but not all — recipes are fat-free.

```
www.fatfree.com
```

Mayo Clinic's Virtual Cookbook

This site features more than 200 recipes, each analyzed and taste-tested by staff dietitians at the Mayo Clinic. You can submit recipes for makeovers and view the "before" and "after" versions of favorite desserts, main dishes, breads, and appetizers. All recipes include calorie, fat, and sodium counts.

```
www.mayo.ivi.com/mayo/recipe/htm/maintoc.htm
```

Appendix B
The Nutrients in Food

• •

*T*he chart on the following pages is an adaptation of the USDA Nutrient Database prepared by the Human Nutrition Information Service. It lists the nutrient values for specific, real-life servings of hundreds of different foods and beverages. Each entry on the chart is identified with an NDB (Nutrition Data Base) number and gives you a snap-shot of a specific food serving ("raw apple with skin") that shows how much the serving weighs (in grams) and lists the amount of

- ✔ Water (as a percentage of the serving's weight)
- ✔ Food energy (calories)
- ✔ Protein
- ✔ Carbohydrates
- ✔ Dietary fiber
- ✔ Calcium
- ✔ Phosphorus
- ✔ Iron
- ✔ Sodium
- ✔ Potassium
- ✔ Magnesium
- ✔ Zinc
- ✔ Copper
- ✔ Vitamin A
- ✔ Thiamin (vitamin B$_1$)
- ✔ Riboflavin (vitamin B$_2$)
- ✔ Niacin
- ✔ Vitamin B$_6$
- ✔ Folate
- ✔ Vitamin B$_{12}$
- ✔ Vitamin C
- ✔ Fat
- ✔ Saturated, monounsaturated, and polyunsaturated fat
- ✔ Cholesterol

The Foods on This Chart

The actual Human Nutrition Information Service chart has more than 5,000 entries, including baby food and fast food. The *Dieting For Dummies* chart is considerably shorter, of course. To access the *big* chart, go to the search page for the USDA Nutrient Database at www.nal.usda.gov/fnic/foodcomp

What you find here are absolutely basic foods — for example, a raw apple with skin rather than a baked apple or apple pie. Why the distinction? Because it's relatively easy to figure out how many calories and what nutrients you get from a plain raw apple, but when you bake the apple or put it into a pie, you begin to add ingredients in amounts that may vary from one dish to another.

For fresh foods (that raw apple again), the values in this chart apply to the part of the food you actually eat — corn without the cob, meat without bones, the apple without pits and core. The values for cooked foods, such as vegetables or toast, do not include extra ingredients, such as butter or salt.

Sometimes you find two sets of values for the same portion of cooked meat or poultry — one for a simple combination of fat and lean parts, a second for lean meat (meat from which the fat has been removed before or after cooking) or poultry without skin.

For the most part, there are no brand-name foods on this list. The recipes used to determine the nutrient values of breads or pastas or jellies and jams are based on standard recipes. The bread or pasta or jelly or jam that you buy may not conform precisely to these recipes. But not to worry: Food labels tell you everything you need to know about foods. Think of them as your government's gift to healthy eating!

Eating by the Numbers

The *Dieting For Dummies* chart and the Human Nutrition Information Service database listings can give you the real facts about what's in the food on your plate. After you know why you need the various nutrients — protein, fat, carbs, vitamins, and minerals — the charts give you the information you need to make healthy food choices that also satisfy your palate.

NDB #	Description & Serving	Grams	Water	Calories	Protein	Carbohydrates	Fiber	Calcium	Phosphorus	Iron	Sodium	Potassium	Magnesium
		gm	gm	kcal	gm	gm	gm	mg	mg	mg	mg	mg	mg

Beans (legumes) and bean products

NDB #	Description & Serving	Grams	Water	Calories	Protein	Carbohydrates	Fiber	Calcium	Phosphorus	Iron	Sodium	Potassium	Magnesium
16015	Black beans, cooked, boiled, wo/salt 1 cup	172	113.07	227.04	15.24	40.78	14.96	46.44	240.8	3.61	1.72	610.6	120.4
16053	Broadbeans (fava beans), cooked, boiled, wo/salt 1 cup	170	121.62	187	12.92	33.41	9.18	61.2	212.5	2.55	8.5	455.6	73.1
16058	Chickpeas (garbanzo beans, bengal gram), seeds, canned 1 cup	240	167.26	285.6	11.88	54.29	10.56	76.8	216	3.24	717.6	412.8	69.6
16025	Great northern beans, cooked, boiled, wo/salt 1 cup	177	122.13	208.86	14.74	37.33	12.39	120.36	292.05	3.77	3.54	692.07	88.5
16028	Kidney beans, all types, cooked, boiled, wo/salt 1 cup	177	118.48	224.79	15.35	40.37	11.33	49.56	251.34	5.2	3.54	713.31	79.65
16070	Lentils, cooked, boiled, wo/salt 1 cup	198	137.89	229.68	17.86	39.88	15.64	37.62	356.4	6.59	3.96	730.62	71.28
16072	Lima beans, lrg, cooked, boiled, wo/salt 1 cup	188	131.21	216.2	14.66	39.27	13.16	31.96	208.68	4.49	3.76	955.04	80.84
16038	Navy beans, cooked, boiled, wo/salt 1 cup	182	114.99	258.44	15.83	47.88	11.65	127.4	285.74	4.51	1.82	669.76	107.38
16086	Peas, split, cooked, boiled, wo/salt 1 cup	196	136.2	231.28	16.35	41.38	16.27	27.44	194.04	2.53	3.92	709.52	70.56
16090	Peanuts, all types, dry-roasted, w/salt 1 oz	28.35	0.44	165.85	6.71	6.1	2.27	15.31	101.49	0.64	230.49	186.54	49.9
16097	Peanut butter, chunk style, w/salt 2 tablespoons	32	0.36	188.48	7.7	6.91	2.11	13.12	101.44	0.61	155.52	239.04	50.88
16098	Peanut butter, smooth style, w/salt 2 tablespoons	32	0.39	189.76	8.07	6.17	1.89	12.16	118.08	0.59	149.44	214.08	50.88
16109	Soybeans, cooked, boiled, wo/salt 1 cup	172	107.59	297.56	28.62	17.06	10.32	175.44	421.4	8.84	1.72	885.8	147.92
16120	Soy milk, fluid 1 cup	245	228.51	80.85	6.74	4.43	3.19	9.8	120.05	1.42	29.4	345.45	46.55
16123	Soy sauce made from soy & wheat (shoyu) 1 tablespoon	16	11.37	8.48	0.83	1.36	0.13	2.72	17.6	0.32	914.4	28.8	5.44
16124	Soy sauce made from soy (tamari) 1 tablespoon	18	11.88	10.8	1.89	1	0.14	3.6	23.4	0.43	1005.48	38.16	7.2
16114	Tempeh 1 cup	166	91.22	330.34	31.46	28.27	0	154.38	341.96	3.75	9.96	609.22	116.2
16127	Tofu, raw, regular 1 cup (1/2" cubes)	248	209.68	188.48	20.04	4.66	2.98	260.4	240.56	13.29	17.36	300.08	255.44
16046	White beans, small, cooked, boiled, wo/salt 1 cup	179	113.2	254.18	16.06	46.2	18.62	130.67	302.51	5.08	3.58	828.77	121.72

Beverages

Alcohol beverages

NDB #	Description & Serving	Grams	Water	Calories	Protein	Carbohydrates	Fiber	Calcium	Phosphorus	Iron	Sodium	Potassium	Magnesium
14037	Alcoholic bev, distilled, all (gin, rum, vodka, whiskey) 80 proof 1 fl oz	27.8	18.51	64.22	0	0	0	0	1.11	0.01	0.28	0.56	0
14550	Alcoholic bev (gin, rum, vodka, whiskey) 86 proof 1 fl oz	27.8	17.76	69.5	0	0.03	0	0	1.11	0.01	0.28	0.56	0
14533	Alcoholic bev, distilled, all 100 proof 1 fl oz	27.8	15.99	82.01	0	0	0	0	1.11	0.01	0.28	0.56	0

NDB #	Zinc	Copper	Vitamin A	Thiamin	Riboflavin	Niacin	Vitamin B6	Folate	Vitamin B12	Vitamin C	Fat	Fat: Saturated	Fat: Monounsaturated	Fat: Polyunsaturated	Cholesterol
	mg	mg	IU	mg	mg	mg	mg	mcg	mcg	mg	gm	gm	gm	gm	mg
Beans (legumes) and bean products															
16015	1.93	0.36	10.32	0.42	0.1	0.87	0.12	255.94	0	0	0.93	0.24	0.08	0.4	0
16053	1.72	0.44	25.5	0.16	0.15	1.21	0.12	176.97	0	0.51	0.68	0.11	0.13	0.28	0
16058	2.54	0.42	57.6	0.07	0.08	0.33	1.14	160.32	0	9.12	2.74	0.28	0.62	1.22	0
16025	1.56	0.44	1.77	0.28	0.1	1.21	0.21	180.89	0	2.3	0.8	0.25	0.04	0.33	0
16028	1.89	0.43	0	0.28	0.1	1.02	0.21	229.39	0	2.12	0.89	0.13	0.07	0.49	0
16070	2.51	0.5	15.84	0.33	0.14	2.1	0.35	357.98	0	2.97	0.75	0.1	0.13	0.35	0
16072	1.79	0.44	0	0.3	0.1	0.79	0.3	156.23	0	0	0.71	0.17	0.06	0.32	0
16038	1.93	0.54	3.64	0.37	0.11	0.97	0.3	254.62	0	1.64	1.04	0.27	0.09	0.45	0
16086	1.96	0.35	13.72	0.37	0.11	1.74	0.09	127.2	0	0.78	0.76	0.11	0.16	0.32	0
16090	0.94	0.19	0	0.12	0.03	3.83	0.07	41.19	0	0	14.08	1.95	6.99	4.45	0
16097	0.89	0.16	0	0.04	0.04	4.38	0.14	29.44	0	0	15.98	3.07	7.54	4.53	0
16098	0.93	0.04	0	0.03	0.03	4.29	0.15	23.68	0	0	16.33	3.31	7.77	4.41	0
16109	1.98	0.7	15.48	0.27	0.49	0.69	0.4	92.54	0	2.92	15.43	2.23	3.41	8.71	0
16120	0.56	0.29	78.4	0.39	0.17	0.36	0.1	3.68	0	0	4.68	0.52	0.8	2.04	0
16123	0.06	0.02	0	0.01	0.02	0.54	0.03	2.48	0	0	0.01	0	0	0.01	0
16124	0.08	0.02	0	0.01	0.03	0.71	0.04	3.28	0	0	0.02	0	0	0.01	0
16114	3	1.11	1138.76	0.22	0.18	7.69	0.5	86.32	1.66	0	12.75	1.84	2.81	7.19	0
16127	1.98	0.48	210.8	0.2	0.13	0.48	0.12	37.2	0	0.25	11.85	1.71	2.62	6.69	0
16046	1.95	0.27	0	0.42	0.11	0.49	0.23	245.05	0	0	1.15	0.3	0.1	0.49	0
Beverages															
Alcohol beverages															
14037	0.01	0.01	0	0	0	0	0	0	0	0	0	0	0	0	0
14550	0.01	0.01	0	0	0	0	0	0	0	0	0	0	0	0	0
14533	0.01	0.01	0	0	0	0	0	0	0	0	0	0	0	0	0

NDB #	Description & Serving	Grams	Water	Calories	Protein	Carbohydrates	Fiber	Calcium	Phosphorus	Iron	Sodium	Potassium	Magnesium
			gm	kcal	gm	gm	gm	mg	mg	mg	mg	mg	mg
14003	Beer, reg 1 can (12 fl oz)	356	328.59	145.96	1.07	13.17	0.71	17.8	42.72	0.11	17.8	89	21.36
14006	Beer, light 1 can (12 fl oz)	354	337.01	99.12	0.71	4.6	0	17.7	42.48	0.14	10.62	63.72	17.7
14096	Wine, red 1 wine glass (3.5 fl oz)	103	91.16	74.16	0.21	1.75	0	8.24	14.42	0.44	5.15	115.36	13.39
14104	Wine, rosé 1 wine glass (3.5 fl oz)	103	91.57	73.13	0.21	1.44	0	8.24	15.45	0.39	5.15	101.97	10.3
14106	Wine, white 1 wine glass (3.5 fl oz)	103	92.29	70.04	0.1	0.82	0	9.27	14.42	0.33	5.15	82.4	10.3
Carbonated beverages													
14121	Club soda 1 can (16 fl oz)	474	473.53	0	0	0	0	23.7	0	0.05	99.54	9.48	4.74
14400	Cola 1 can (16 fl oz)	492	439.85	201.72	0	51.17	0	14.76	59.04	0.15	19.68	4.92	4.92
14416	Cola, low-cal, w/aspartame 1 can (16 fl oz)	474	473.05	4.74	0.47	0.47	0	18.96	42.66	0.14	28.44	0	4.74
14166	Cola, low-cal, or pepper-types, w/saccharin 1 can (16 fl oz)	474	473.05	0	0	0.47	0	18.96	52.14	0.19	75.84	9.48	4.74
14136	Ginger ale 1 can (16 fl oz)	488	445.06	165.92	0	42.46	0	14.64	0	0.88	34.16	4.88	4.88
14155	Tonic water 1 bottle (11 fl oz)	336	306.1	114.24	0	29.57	0	3.36	0	0.03	13.44	0	0
Coffee and tea													
14209	Coffee, brewed, prep w/tap water 1 cup (8 fl oz)	237	235.34	4.74	0.24	0.95	0	4.74	2.37	0.12	4.74	127.98	11.85
14215	Coffee, instant, reg, prep w/water 6 fl oz	179	177.21	3.58	0.18	0.72	0	5.37	5.37	0.09	5.37	64.44	7.16
14219	Coffee, instant, decaffeinated, powder, prep w/water 1 cup (6 fl oz)	179	177.21	3.58	0.18	0.72	0	5.37	5.37	0.07	5.37	62.65	7.16
14237	Coffee sub, cereal grain bev, prep w/water 1 cup (8 fl oz)	240	236.88	12	0.24	2.4	0	7.2	16.8	0.14	9.6	57.6	9.6
14355	Tea, brewed, prep w/tap water 1 cup (8 fl oz)	237	236.29	2.37	0	0.71	0	0	2.37	0.05	7.11	87.69	7.11
14381	Tea, herb, other than chamomile, brewed 1 cup (8 fl oz)	178	177.47	1.78	0	0.36	0	3.56	0	0.14	1.78	16.02	1.78
14545	Tea, herb, chamomile, brewed 1 cup (8 fl oz)	237	236.29	2.37	0	0.47	0	4.74	0	0.19	2.37	21.33	2.37
Dairy products													
Butter													
01145	Butter, wo/salt 1 tablespoon	14.2	2.55	101.81	0.12	0.01	0	3.34	3.24	0.02	1.56	3.69	0.28
Cheese													
01004	Blue 1 oz	28.35	12.02	100.09	6.07	0.66	0	149.57	109.83	0.09	395.57	72.66	6.5
01007	Camembert 1 oz	28.35	14.69	84.93	5.61	0.13	0	109.89	98.26	0.09	238.62	52.90	5.66

NDB #	Zinc	Copper	Vitamin A	Thiamin	Riboflavin	Niacin	Vitamin B6	Folate	Vitamin B12	Vitamin C	Fat	Fat: Saturated	Fat: Monounsaturated	Fat: Polyunsaturated	Cholesterol
	mg	mg	IU	mg	mg	mg	mg	mcg	mcg	mg	gm	gm	gm	gm	mg
14003															
	0.07	0.03	0	0.02	0.09	1.61	0.18	21.36	0.07	0	0	0	0	0	0
14006															
	0.11	0.08	0	0.03	0.11	1.39	0.12	14.51	0.04	0	0	0	0	0	0
14096															
	0.09	0.02	0	0.01	0.03	0.08	0.04	2.06	0.01	0	0	0	0	0	0
14104															
	0.06	0.05	0	0	0.02	0.08	0.02	1.13	0.01	0	0	0	0	0	0
14106															
	0.07	0.02	0	0	0.01	0.07	0.01	0.21	0	0	0	0	0	0	0
Carbonated beverages															
14121															
	0.47	0.03	0	0	0	0	0	0	0	0	0	0	0	0	0
14400															
	0.05	0.05	0	0	0	0	0	0	0	0	0	0	0	0	0
14416															
	0.38	0.05	0	0.02	0.11	0	0	0	0	0	0	0	0	0	0
14166															
	0.24	0.12	0	0	0	0	0	0	0	0	0	0	0	0	0
14136															
	0.24	0.09	0	0	0	0	0	0	0	0	0	0	0	0	0
14155															
	0.34	0.02	0	0	0	0	0	0	0	0	0	0	0	0	0
Coffee and tea															
14209															
	0.05	0.02	0	0	0	0.53	0	0.24	0	0	0	0	0	0	0
14215															
	0.05	0.01	0	0	0	0.51	0	0	0	0	0	0	0	0	0
14219															
	0.05	0.01	0	0	0.03	0.5	0	0	0	0	0	0	0	0	0
14237															
	0.07	0.02	0	0.02	0	0.52	0.03	0.72	0	0	0	0.02	0.01	0.05	0
14355															
	0.05	0.02	0	0	0.03	0	0	12.32	0	0	0	0	0	0.01	0
14381															
	0.07	0.03	0	0.02	0.01	0	0	1.07	0	0	0	0	0	0.01	0
14545															
	0.09	0.04	47.4	0.02	0.01	0	0	1.42	0	0	0	0	0	0.01	0
Dairy products															
Butter															
01145															
	0.01	0	434.24	0	0	0.01	0	0.4	0.02	0	11.52	7.17	3.33	0.43	31.08
Cheese															
01004															
	0.75	0.01	204.4	0.01	0.11	0.29	0.05	10.32	0.35	0	8.15	5.29	2.21	0.23	21.32
01007															
	0.68	0.01	261.67	0.01	0.14	0.18	0.06	17.63	0.37	0	6.89	4.33	1.99	0.21	20.41

NDB #	Description & Serving	Grams	Water	Calories	Protein	Carbohydrates	Fiber	Calcium	Phosphorus	Iron	Sodium	Potassium	Magnesium
			gm	kcal	gm	gm	gm	mg	mg	mg	mg	mg	mg
01009	Cheddar 1 oz	28.35	10.42	114.13	7.1	0.36	0	204.49	145.18	0.19	175.91	27.90	7.88
01011	Colby 1 oz	28.35	10.83	111.60	6.74	0.73	0	194.08	129.42	0.22	171.29	35.86	7.32
01012	Cottage cheese, creamed, lrg curd 1 cup (not packed, large curd)	210	165.82	217.03	26.23	5.63	0	126	276.78	0.29	850.08	177.03	11.05
01014	Cottage cheese, uncreamed, dry, lrg or sml curd 1 cup (not packed)	145	115.67	122.66	25.04	2.68	0	45.97	150.8	0.33	18.56	46.98	5.71
01015	Cottage cheese, 2% fat 1 cup (not packed)	226	179.24	202.68	31.05	8.2	0	154.81	340.13	0.36	917.56	217.41	13.56
01016	Cottage cheese, 1% fat 1 cup (not packed)	226	186.4	163.62	28	6.15	0	137.63	302.39	0.32	917.56	193.23	12.07
01017	Cream cheese 1 tablespoon	14.5	7.79	50.61	1.09	0.39	0	11.59	15.14	0.17	42.85	17.31	0.93
01018	Edam 1 oz	28.35	11.78	101.1	7.08	0.41	0	207.24	151.84	0.12	273.58	53.21	8.44
01019	Feta 1 oz	28.35	15.65	74.72	4.03	1.16	0	139.62	95.6	0.18	316.41	17.52	5.45
01157	Goat cheese, semisoft type 1 oz	28.35	12.9	103.19	6.12	0.72	0	84.48	106.31	0.46	146	44.79	8.22
01022	Gouda 1 oz	28.35	11.75	101.01	7.07	0.63	0	198.39	154.88	0.07	232.27	34.16	8.22
01023	Gruyere 1 oz	28.35	9.41	117.07	8.45	0.10	0	286.62	171.60	0.05	95.26	22.96	10.18
01024	Limburger 1 oz	28.35	13.73	92.71	5.68	0.14	0	140.81	111.42	0.04	226.8	36.29	5.95
01025	Monterey 1 oz	28.35	11.63	105.84	6.94	0.19	0	211.60	125.87	0.20	152.04	22.88	7.66
01026	Mozzarella, whole milk 1 oz	28.35	15.35	79.77	5.51	0.63	0	146.57	105.09	0.05	105.77	19.02	5.27
01028	Mozzarella, part skim milk 1 oz	28.35	15.25	72.08	6.88	0.79	0	183.06	131.26	0.06	132.11	23.73	6.58
01030	Muenster 1 oz	28.35	11.84	104.43	6.64	0.32	0	203.36	132.59	0.12	177.95	38.10	7.75
01031	Neufchatel 1 oz	28.35	17.64	73.67	2.82	0.83	0	21.35	38.64	0.08	113.23	32.35	2.15
01032	Parmesan, grated 1 tablespoon	5	0.88	22.79	2.08	0.19	0	68.79	40.36	0.05	93.08	5.36	2.54
01034	Port de salut 1 oz	28.35	12.89	99.69	6.74	0.16	0	184.22	102.06	0.12	151.39	38.5	6.9
01035	Provolone 1 oz	28.35	11.61	99.65	7.25	0.61	0	214.3	140.64	0.15	248.2	39.21	7.82
01036	Ricotta, whole milk 1/2 cup	124	88.91	215.68	13.96	3.77	0	256.68	196.04	0.47	104.28	129.7	14.01

NDB #	Zinc	Copper	Vitamin A	Thiamin	Riboflavin	Niacin	Vitamin B6	Folate	Vitamin B12	Vitamin C	Fat	Fat: Saturated	Fat: Monounsaturated	Fat: Polyunsaturated	Cholesterol
	mg	mg	IU	mg	mg	mg	mg	mcg	mcg	mg	gm	gm	gm	gm	mg
01009	0.88	0.01	300.23	0.01	0.12	0.02	0.02	5.16	0.23	0	9.40	5.98	2.66	0.27	29.74
01011	0.87	0.01	293.14	0	0.11	0.03	0.02	5.16	0.23	0	9.10	5.73	2.63	0.27	26.90
01012	0.78	0.06	342.3	0.04	0.34	0.26	0.14	25.62	1.31	0	9.47	5.99	2.7	0.29	31.29
01014	0.68	0.04	43.5	0.04	0.21	0.22	0.12	21.40	1.2	0	0.61	0.4	0.16	0.02	9.72
01015	0.95	0.06	158.2	0.05	0.42	0.33	0.17	29.61	1.61	0	4.36	2.76	1.24	0.13	18.98
01016	0.86	0.06	83.62	0.05	0.37	0.29	0.15	28.02	1.43	0	2.31	1.46	0.66	0.07	9.94
01017	0.08	0	206.92	0	0.03	0.01	0.01	1.91	0.06	0	5.06	3.19	1.43	0.18	15.91
01018	1.06	0.01	259.69	0.01	0.11	0.02	0.02	4.59	0.44	0	7.88	4.98	2.3	0.19	25.29
01019	0.82	0.01	126.72	0.04	0.24	0.28	0.12	9.07	0.48	0	6.03	4.24	1.31	0.17	25.23
01157	0.19	0.16	378.19	0.02	0.19	0.33	0.02	0.57	0.06	0	8.46	5.85	1.93	0.2	22.4
01022	1.11	0.01	182.57	0.01	0.09	0.02	0.02	5.93	0.44	0	7.78	4.99	2.2	0.19	32.32
01023	1.11	0.01	345.59	0.02	0.08	0.03	0.02	2.95	0.45	0	9.17	5.36	2.85	0.49	31.19
01024	0.6	0.01	363.16	0.02	0.14	0.04	0.02	16.3	0.29	0	7.73	4.75	2.44	0.14	25.52
01025	0.85	0.01	269.33	0	0.11	0.03	0.02	5.16	0.23	0	8.58	5.14	2.48	0.26	25.23
01026	0.63	0.01	224.53	0	0.07	0.02	0.02	1.98	0.19	0	6.12	3.73	1.86	0.22	22.23
01028	0.78	0.01	165.56	0.01	0.09	0.03	0.02	2.49	0.23	0	4.51	2.87	1.28	0.13	16.39
01030	0.8	0.01	317.52	0	0.09	0.03	0.02	3.43	0.42	0	8.52	5.42	2.48	0.19	27.10
01031	0.15	0	321.49	0	0.06	0.04	0.01	3.2	0.07	0	6.64	4.19	1.92	0.18	21.57
01032	0.16	0	35.05	0	0.02	0.02	0.01	0.4	0.07	0	1.5	0.95	0.44	0.03	3.94
01034	0.74	0.01	377.91	0	0.07	0.02	0	5.16	0.43	0	8	4.73	2.65	0.21	34.87
01035	0.92	0.01	231.05	0.01	0.09	0.04	0.02	2.95	0.41	0	7.55	4.84	2.1	0.22	19.53
01036	1.44	0.03	607.6	0.02	0.24	0.13	0.05	15.13	0.42	0	16.1	10.29	4.5	0.48	62.74

NDB #	Description & Serving	Grams	Water	Calories	Protein	Carbohydrates	Fiber	Calcium	Phosphorus	Iron	Sodium	Potassium	Magnesium
			gm	kcal	gm	gm	gm	mg	mg	mg	mg	mg	mg
01037	Ricotta, part skim milk 1/2 cup	246	92.27	171.19	14.12	6.37	0	337.28	226.42	0.55	154.63	155	18.32
01038	Romano 1 oz	28.35	8.76	109.61	9.02	1.03	0	301.59	215.46	0.22	340.2	24.47	11.6
01039	Roquefort 1 oz	28.35	11.16	104.62	6.11	0.57	0	187.62	111.16	0.16	512.85	25.71	8.37
01040	Swiss 1 cup, diced	132	49.12	496.01	37.53	4.46	0	1268.39	798.07	0.22	343.2	146.12	47.4
Eggs													
01123	Egg, whole, raw, fresh 1 extra large	58	43.69	86.42	7.24	0.71	0	28.42	103.24	0.84	73.08	70.18	5.8
01124	Egg, white, raw, fresh 1 large egg white	33.4	29.33	16.7	3.51	0.34	0	2	4.34	0.01	54.78	47.76	3.67
01125	Egg, yolk, raw, fresh 1 large egg yolk	16.6	8.1	59.43	2.78	0.3	0	22.74	81.01	0.59	7.14	15.6	1.49
Milk and cream													
Milk													
01077	Milk, whole, 3.3% fat 1 cup	244	214.7	149.92	8.03	11.37	0	291.34	227.9	0.12	119.56	369.66	32.79
01079	Milk, low-fat, 2% fat, w/vit A 1 cup	244	217.67	121.2	8.13	11.71	0	296.7	232.04	0.12	121.76	376.74	33.35
01082	Milk, low-fat, 1% fat, w/vit A 1 cup	244	219.8	102.15	8.03	11.66	0	300.12	234.73	0.12	123.22	380.88	33.72
01085	Milk, fat-free (skim), w/vit A 1 cup	245	222.46	85.53	8.35	11.88	0	302.33	247.21	0.1	126.18	405.72	27.83
01088	Milk, bttrmlk, cultured, from fat-free (skim) milk 1 cup	245	220.82	98.99	8.11	11.74	0	285.18	218.54	0.12	257.01	370.69	26.83
01154	Milk, dry, fat-free (skim), non-fat solids, reg, w/vit A 1 cup	120	3.79	434.8	43.39	62.38	0	1508.28	1161.84	0.38	642.36	2152.92	132
01090	Milk, dry, whole 1 cup	128	3.16	634.69	33.69	49.18	0	1167.87	992.64	0.6	475.26	1702.27	108.17
01095	Milk, canned, cond, sweetened 1 cup	306	83.11	981.58	24.2	166.46	0	867.51	775.1	0.58	388.62	1136.48	78.49
01153	Milk, canned, evap, whole, w/vit A 1 fl oz	31.5	23.32	42.33	2.15	3.16	0	82.15	63.79	0.06	33.33	95.48	7.62
01097	Milk, canned, evap, fat-free (skim) 1 cup	256	203.26	199.48	19.33	29.06	0	741.12	498.94	0.74	294.4	848.64	69.12
01106	Milk, goat 1 cup	244	212.35	167.9	8.69	10.86	0	325.74	270.11	0.12	121.51	498.74	34.09
Cream													
01049	Cream, half and half 1 tablespoon	15	12.09	19.55	0.44	0.65	0	15.74	14.28	0.01	6.11	19.44	1.53
01052	Cream, light whipping 1 cup, fluid (yields 2 cups whipped)	239	151.77	698.88	5.19	7.07	0	165.87	146.03	0.07	81.98	231.35	17.28

NDB #	Zinc	Copper	Vitamin A	Thiamin	Riboflavin	Niacin	Vitamin B6	Folate	Vitamin B12	Vitamin C	Fat	Fat: Saturated	Fat: Monounsaturated	Fat: Polyunsaturated	Cholesterol
	mg	mg	IU	mg	mg	mg	mg	mcg	mcg	mg	gm	gm	gm	gm	mg
01037	1.66	0.04	535.68	0.03	0.23	0.10	0.03	16.24	0.36	0	9.81	6.11	2.87	0.32	38.19
01038	0.73	0.01	161.88	0.01	0.1	0.02	0.02	1.93	0.32	0	7.64	4.85	2.22	0.17	29.48
01039	0.59	0.01	296.82	0.01	0.17	0.21	0.04	13.89	0.18	0	8.69	5.46	2.4	0.37	25.52
01040	5.15	0.04	1115.4	0.03	0.48	0.12	0.11	8.45	2.21	0	36.23	23.47	9.6	1.28	121.04
Eggs															
01123	0.64	0.01	368.3	0.04	0.29	0.04	0.08	27.26	0.58	0	5.81	1.8	2.21	0.79	246.5
01124	0	0	0	0	0.15	0.03	0	1	0.07	0	0	0	0	0	0
01125	0.52	0	322.87	0.03	0.11	0	0.07	24.24	0.52	0	5.12	1.59	1.95	0.7	212.65
Milk and cream															
Milk															
01077	0.93	0.02	307.44	0.09	0.4	0.2	0.1	12.2	0.87	2.29	8.15	5.07	2.35	0.3	33.18
01079	0.95	0.02	500.2	0.1	0.4	0.21	0.1	12.44	0.89	2.32	4.68	2.92	1.35	0.17	18.3
01082	0.95	0.02	500.2	0.1	0.41	0.21	0.1	12.44	0.9	2.37	2.59	1.61	0.75	0.1	9.76
01085	0.98	0.03	499.8	0.09	0.34	0.22	0.1	12.74	0.93	2.4	0.44	0.29	0.12	0.02	4.41
01088	1.03	0.03	80.85	0.08	0.38	0.14	0.08	12.25	0.54	2.4	2.16	1.34	0.62	0.08	8.58
01154	4.9	0.05	2637.6	0.5	1.86	1.14	0.43	60	4.84	8.11	0.92	0.6	0.24	0.04	23.52
01090	4.28	0.1	1180.16	0.36	1.54	0.83	0.39	47.36	4.16	11.06	34.19	21.43	10.14	0.85	124.29
01095	2.88	0.05	1003.68	0.28	1.27	0.64	0.16	34.27	1.36	7.96	26.62	16.79	7.43	1.03	103.73
01153	0.24	0.01	125.06	0.01	0.1	0.06	0.02	2.49	0.05	0.59	2.38	1.45	0.74	0.08	9.26
01097	2.3	0.04	1003.52	0.12	0.79	0.45	0.14	22.02	0.61	3.17	0.51	0.31	0.16	0.02	9.22
01106	0.73	0.11	451.4	0.12	0.34	0.68	0.11	1.46	0.16	3.15	10.1	6.51	2.71	0.36	27.82
Cream															
01049	0.08	0	65.1	0.01	0.02	0.01	0.01	0.38	0.05	0.13	1.73	1.07	0.5	0.06	5.54
01052	0.6	0.02	2693.53	0.06	0.3	0.1	0.07	8.84	0.47	1.46	73.87	46.22	21.73	2.11	265.29

NDB #	Description & Serving	Grams	Water	Calories	Protein	Carbohydrates	Fiber	Calcium	Phosphorus	Iron	Sodium	Potassium	Magnesium
		gm	gm	kcal	gm	gm	gm	mg	mg	mg	mg	mg	mg
01053	Cream, heavy whipping 1 cup, fluid (yields 2 cups whipped)	238	137.35	820.58	4.88	6.64	0	153.75	148.51	0.07	89.49	179.45	16.73
01053	Cream, heavy whipping 1 tablespoon	15	10.28	36.56	0.37	0.52	0	13.53	10.59	0.01	5.55	17.18	1.26
01056	Cream, sour, cultured 1 cup	230	163.19	492.79	7.27	9.82	0	267.72	195.27	0.14	122.59	331.2	25.83
01056	Cream, sour, cultured 1 tablespoon	12	8.51	25.71	0.38	0.51	0	13.97	10.19	0.01	6.4	17.28	1.35
01074	Cream, sour, imitation, cultured 1 cup	230	163.65	479.46	5.52	15.25	0	5.75	102.35	0.9	234.6	369.15	14.67
Ice cream, ice milk													
19270	Ice cream, chocolate 1/2 cup (4 fl oz)	66	36.76	142.56	2.51	18.61	0.79	71.94	70.62	0.61	50.16	164.34	19.14
19271	Ice cream, strawberry 1/2 cup (4 fl oz)	66	39.6	126.72	2.11	18.22	0.2	79.2	66	0.14	39.6	124.08	9.24
19095	Ice cream, vanilla 1/2 cup (4 fl oz)	66	40.26	132.66	2.31	15.58	0	84.48	69.3	0.06	52.8	131.34	9.24
19088	Ice milk, vanilla 1/2 cup (4 fl oz)	66	45.01	91.74	2.51	14.98	0	91.74	71.94	0.07	56.1	139.26	9.9
Yogurt													
01116	Yogurt, plain, whole milk 1 cup (8 fl oz)	245	215.36	150.48	8.5	11.42	0	295.72	232.51	0.12	113.68	378.77	28.37
01117	Yogurt, plain, low-fat 1 cup (8 fl oz)	245	208.42	155.05	12.86	17.25	0	447.37	351.58	0.2	171.99	572.81	42.75
01118	Yogurt, plain, fat-free (skim) milk 1 cup (8 fl oz)	245	208.81	136.64	14.04	18.82	0	487.8	383.43	0.22	187.43	624.51	46.8
Fats and oils													
Fats													
04542	Chicken fat 1 tablespoon	12.8	0.03	115.25	0	0	0	0	0	0	0	0	0
04002	Lard 1 tablespoon	12.8	0	115.46	0	0	0	0.01	0	0	0	0	0
04071	Margarine, reg, hard, corn (hydrogenated) 1 teaspoon	4.7	0.74	33.78	0.04	0.04	0	1.41	1.08	0	44.34	1.99	0.12
04092	Margarine, soft, corn (hydrogenated & reg) 1 teaspoon	4.7	0.76	33.67	0.04	0.02	0	1.25	0.95	0	50.7	1.77	0.11
04585	Margarine blend, 60% corn oil & 40% butter 1 tablespoon	14.2	2.24	101.96	0.12	0.09	0	3.98	3.27	0.01	127.37	5.11	0.28
Oils													
04582	Canola oil 1 tablespoon	14	0	123.76	0	0	0	0	0	0	0	0	0
04518	Corn, salad or cooking oil 1 tablespoon	13.6	0	120.22	0	0	0	0	0	0	0	0	0
04053	Olive, salad or cooking oil 1 tablespoon	13.5	0	119.34	0	0	0	0.02	0.16	0.05	0.01	0	0

NDB #	Zinc	Copper	Vitamin A	Thiamin	Riboflavin	Niacin	Vitamin B6	Folate	Vitamin B12	Vitamin C	Fat	Fat: Saturated	Fat: Monounsaturated	Fat: Polyunsaturated	Cholesterol
	mg	mg	IU	mg	mg	mg	mg	mcg	mcg	mg	gm	gm	gm	gm	mg
01053	0.55	0.01	3498.6	0.05	0.26	0.09	0.06	8.81	0.43	1.38	88.06	54.82	25.43	3.27	326.3
01053	0.04	0	141.3	0	0.02	0.01	0	0.35	0.03	0.11	3.75	2.33	1.08	0.14	13.13
01056	0.62	0.04	1817	0.08	0.34	0.15	0.04	24.84	0.69	1.98	48.21	30.01	13.92	1.79	102.12
01056	0.03	0	94.8	0	0.02	0.01	0	1.3	0.04	0.1	2.52	1.57	0.73	0.09	5.33
01074	2.71	0.13	0	0	0	0	0	0	0	0	44.9	40.92	1.35	0.13	0
Ice cream, ice milk															
19270	0.38	0.09	274.56	0.03	0.13	0.15	0.04	10.56	0.19	0.46	7.26	4.49	2.12	0.27	22.44
19271	0.22	0.02	211.2	0.03	0.17	0.11	0.03	7.92	0.2	5.08	5.54	3.43	0	0	19.14
19095	0.46	0.02	269.94	0.03	0.16	0.08	0.03	3.3	0.26	0.4	7.26	4.48	2.09	0.27	29.04
19088	0.29	0.01	108.9	0.04	0.17	0.06	0.04	3.96	0.44	0.53	2.84	1.74	0.81	0.11	9.24
Yogurt															
01116	1.45	0.02	301.35	0.07	0.35	0.18	0.08	18.13	0.91	1.3	7.96	5.14	2.19	0.23	31.12
01117	2.18	0.03	161.7	0.11	0.52	0.28	0.12	27.44	1.38	1.96	3.8	2.45	1.04	0.11	14.95
01118	2.38	0.04	17.15	0.12	0.57	0.3	0.13	29.89	1.5	2.13	0.44	0.28	0.12	0.01	4.41
Fats and oils															
Fats															
04542	0	0	0	0	0	0	0	0	0	0	12.77	3.81	5.72	2.68	10.88
04002	0.01	0	0	0	0	0	0	0	0	0	12.8	5.02	5.77	1.43	12.16
04071	0	0	167.84	0	0	0	0	0.06	0	0.01	3.78	0.62	2.15	0.85	0
04092	0	0	167.84	0	0	0	0	0.05	0	0.01	3.78	0.66	1.49	1.47	0
04585	0	0	507.08	0	0	0	0	0.28	0.01	0.01	11.46	4.04	4.65	2.26	12.5
Oils															
04582	0	0	0	0	0	0	0	0	0	0	14	0.99	8.25	4.14	0
04518	0	0	0	0	0	0	0	0	0	0	13.6	1.73	3.29	7.98	0
04053	0.01	0	0	0	0	0	0	0	0	0	13.5	1.82	9.95	1.13	0

NDB #	Description & Serving	Grams	Water	Calories	Protein	Carbohydrates	Fiber	Calcium	Phosphorus	Iron	Sodium	Potassium	Magnesium
		gm	gm	kcal	gm	gm	gm	mg	mg	mg	mg	mg	mg
04042	Peanut, salad or cooking oil 1 tablespoon	13.5	0	119.34	0	0	0	0.01	0	0	0.01	0	0.01
04058	Sesame, salad or cooking oil 1 tablespoon	13.6	0	120.22	0	0	0	0	0	0	0	0	0
04044	Soybean, salad or cooking oil (hydrogenated) 1 tablespoon	13.6	0	120.22	0	0	0	0.01	0.03	0	0	0	0
Fruits and fruit juices													
09003	Apples, raw, with skin 1 cup, quartered or chopped	125	104.91	73.75	0.24	19.06	3.38	8.75	8.75	0.23	0	143.75	6.25
09011	Apples, dried, sulfured, uncooked 1 cup	86	27.31	208.98	0.8	56.67	7.48	12.04	32.68	1.2	74.82	387	13.76
09400	Apple juice, canned or bottled, unsweetened, w/ vit C 1 cup	248	218.07	116.56	0.15	28.97	0.25	17.36	17.36	0.92	7.44	295.12	7.44
09021	Apricots, raw 1 cup, halves	155	133.84	74.4	2.17	17.24	3.72	21.7	29.45	0.84	1.55	458.8	12.4
09024	Apricots, canned, juice pk, w/skin, solids & liquids 1 cup, halves	244	211.35	117.12	1.54	30.11	3.9	29.28	48.8	0.73	9.76	402.6	24.4
09032	Apricots, dried, sulfured, uncooked 1 half fruit	3.5	1.09	8.33	0.13	2.16	0.32	1.58	4.1	0.16	0.35	48.23	1.65
09403	Apricot nectar, canned, w/ vit C 1 cup	251	213.02	140.56	0.93	36.12	1.51	17.57	22.59	0.95	7.53	286.14	12.55
09038	Avocados, raw, California 1 fruit, without skin and seeds	173	125.53	306.21	3.65	11.95	8.48	19.03	72.66	2.04	20.76	1096.82	70.93
09039	Avocados, raw, Florida 1 fruit, without skin and seeds	304	242.38	340.48	4.83	27.09	16.11	33.44	118.56	1.61	15.2	1483.52	103.36
09040	Bananas, raw 1 cup, sliced	150	111.39	138	1.55	35.15	3.6	9	30	0.47	1.5	594	43.5
09042	Blackberries, raw 1 cup	144	123.32	74.88	1.04	18.37	7.63	46.08	30.24	0.82	0	282.24	28.8
09050	Blueberries, raw 1 pint, as purchased, yields	402	340.13	225.12	2.69	56.8	10.85	24.12	40.2	0.68	24.12	357.78	20.1
09063	Cherries, sour, red, raw 1 cup with pits	103	0	0	0	0	0	0	0	0	0	0	0
09070	Cherries, sweet, raw 1 cup, with pits	117	94.49	84.24	1.4	19.36	2.69	17.55	22.23	0.46	0	262.08	12.87
09087	Cranberries, raw 1 cup, whole	95	82.21	46.55	0.37	12.05	3.99	6.65	8.55	0.19	0.95	67.45	4.75
09083	Currants, European black, raw 1 cup	112	91.8	70.56	1.57	17.23	0	61.6	66.08	1.72	2.24	360.64	26.88
09085	Currants, zante, dried 1 cup	144	27.66	407.52	5.88	106.68	9.79	123.84	180	4.69	11.52	1284.48	59.04
09087	Dates, domestic, natural & dry 1 cup, pitted, chopped	178	40.05	489.5	3.51	130.85	13.35	56.96	71.2	2.05	5.34	1160.56	62.3
09088	Elderberries, raw 1 cup	145	115.71	105.85	0.96	26.68	10.15	55.1	56.55	2.32	8.7	406	7.25
09089	Figs, raw 1 medium (2-1/4" dia)	50	39.55	37	0.38	9.59	1.65	17.5	7	0.19	0.5	116	8.5

NDB #	Zinc	Copper	Vitamin A	Thiamin	Riboflavin	Niacin	Vitamin B6	Folate	Vitamin B12	Vitamin C	Fat	Fat: Saturated	Fat: Monounsaturated	Fat: Polyunsaturated	Cholesterol
	mg	mg	IU	mg	mg	mg	mg	mcg	mcg	mg	gm	gm	gm	gm	mg
04042	0	0	0	0	0	0	0	0	0	0	13.5	2.28	6.24	4.32	0
04058	0	0	0	0	0	0	0	0	0	0	13.6	1.93	5.4	5.67	0
04044	0	0	0	0	0	0	0	0	0	0	13.6	1.96	3.17	7.87	0
Fruits and fruit juices															
09003	0.05	0.05	66.25	0.02	0.02	0.1	0.06	3.5	0	7.13	0.45	0.07	0.02	0.13	0
09011	0.17	0.16	0	0	0.14	0.8	0.11	0	0	3.35	0.28	0.04	0.01	0.08	0
09400	0.07	0.05	2.48	0.05	0.04	0	0.07	0.25	0	103.17	0.27	0.05	0.01	0.08	0
09021	0.4	0.14	4048.6	0.05	0.06	0.93	0.08	13.33	0	15.5	0.6	0.04	0.26	0.12	0
09024	0.27	0.13	4126.04	0.04	0.05	0.84	0.13	4.15	0	11.96	0.1	0.01	0.04	0.02	0
09032	0.03	0.02	253.4	0	0.01	0.1	0.01	0.36	0	0.08	0.02	0	0.01	0	0
09403	0.23	0.18	3303.10	0.02	0.04	0.05	0.06	3.20	0	136.54	0.23	0.02	0.1	0.04	0
09038	0.73	0.46	1058.76	0.19	0.21	3.32	0.48	113.32	0	13.67	29.98	4.48	19.4	3.53	0
09039	1.28	0.76	1860.48	0.33	0.37	5.84	0.85	162.03	0	24.02	26.96	5.34	14.8	4.5	0
09040	0.24	0.16	121.5	0.07	0.15	0.81	0.87	28.65	0	13.65	0.72	0.28	0.06	0.13	0
09042	0.39	0.2	237.6	0.04	0.06	0.58	0.08	48.96	0	30.24	0.56	0.02	0.05	0.32	0
09050	0.44	0.25	402	0.19	0.2	1.44	0.14	25.73	0	52.26	1.53	0.13	0.22	0.67	0
09063	0	0	0	0	0	0	0	0	0	0	0	0	0	0	0
09070	0.07	0.11	250.38	0.06	0.07	0.47	0.04	4.91	0	8.19	1.12	0.25	0.31	0.34	0
09087	0.12	0.06	43.70	0.03	0.02	0.10	0.06	1.62	0	12.83	0.19	0.02	0.03	0.08	0
09083	0.3	0.1	257.6	0.06	0.06	0.34	0.07	0	0	202.72	0.46	0.04	0.06	0.2	0
09085	0.95	0.67	105.12	0.23	0.2	2.33	0.43	14.69	0	6.77	0.39	0.04	0.07	0.26	0
09087	0.52	0.51	89	0.16	0.18	3.92	0.34	22.43	0	0	0.8	0.34	0.27	0.06	0
09088	0.16	0.09	870	0.1	0.09	0.73	0.33	8.7	0	52.2	0.73	0.03	0.12	0.36	0
09089	0.08	0.04	71	0.03	0.03	0.2	0.06	3	0	1	0.15	0.03	0.03	0.07	0

NDB #	Description & Serving	Grams	Water	Calories	Protein	Carbohydrates	Fiber	Calcium	Phosphorus	Iron	Sodium	Potassium	Magnesium
			gm	kcal	gm	gm	gm	mg	mg	mg	mg	mg	mg
09094	Figs, dried, uncooked 1 fig	19	5.4	48.45	0.58	12.42	1.77	27.36	12.92	0.42	2.09	135.28	11.21
09109	Gooseberries, canned, light syrup pk, solids & liquids 1 cup	252	201.85	183.96	1.64	47.25	6.05	40.32	17.64	0.83	5.04	194.04	15.12
09111	Grapefruit, raw, pink & red & white, all areas 1 cup sections with juice	230	209.05	73.6	1.45	18.58	2.53	27.6	18.4	0.21	0	319.7	18.4
09123	Grapefruit juice, canned, unsweetened 1 cup	247	222.55	93.86	1.28	22.13	0.25	17.29	27.17	0.49	2.47	377.91	24.7
09131	Grapes, American type (slip skin), raw 1 cup	92	74.8	57.96	0.58	15.78	0.92	12.88	9.2	0.27	1.84	175.72	4.6
09132	Grapes, European type (adherent skin), raw 1 cup, seedless	160	128.9	113.6	1.06	28.43	1.6	17.6	20.8	0.42	3.2	296	9.6
09135	Grape juice, canned or bottled, unsweetened, wo/vit C 1 cup	253	212.82	154.33	1.42	37.85	0.25	22.77	27.83	0.61	7.59	333.96	25.3
09139	Guavas, common, raw 1 cup, strawberry	244	210.08	124.44	2	28.99	13.18	48.8	61	0.76	7.32	692.96	24.4
09148	Kiwi fruit, (Chinese gooseberries), fresh, raw 1 large fruit, without skin	91	75.58	55.51	0.9	13.54	3.09	23.66	36.4	0.37	4.55	302.12	27.3
09149	Kumquats, raw 1 fruit, without refuse	19	15.52	11.97	0.17	3.12	1.25	8.36	3.61	0.07	1.14	37.05	2.47
09152	Lemon juice, raw 1 fl oz	30.5	27.67	7.63	0.12	2.63	0.12	2.14	1.83	0.01	0.31	37.82	1.83
09160	Lime juice, raw 1 fl oz	30.8	27.78	8.32	0.14	2.78	0.12	2.77	2.16	0.01	0.31	33.57	1.85
09176	Mangos, raw 1 fruit, without refuse	207	169.14	134.55	1.06	35.19	3.73	20.7	22.77	0.27	4.14	322.92	18.63
09181	Melons, cantaloupe, raw 1 cup, balls	177	158.91	61.95	1.56	14.8	1.42	19.47	30.09	0.37	15.93	546.93	19.47
09184	Melons, honeydew, raw 1 cup, diced (approx 20 pieces per cup)	170	152.42	59.5	0.78	15.61	1.02	10.2	17	0.12	17	460.7	11.9
09191	Nectarines, raw 1 fruit (2-1/2" dia)	136	117.34	66.64	1.28	16.02	2.18	6.8	21.76	0.2	0	288.32	10.88
09201	Oranges, raw, California, Valencias 1 fruit (2-5/8" dia, sphere)	121	104.47	59.29	1.26	14.39	3.03	48.4	20.57	0.11	0	216.59	12.1
09202	Oranges, raw, California, navels 1 fruit (2-7/8" dia)	140	121.53	64.4	1.44	16.28	3.36	56	26.6	0.17	1.4	249.2	14
09203	Oranges, raw, Florida 1 fruit (2-5/8" dia, sphere)	141	122.87	64.86	0.99	16.27	3.38	60.63	16.92	0.13	0	238.29	14.1
09206	Orange juice, raw 1 cup	248	218.98	111.6	1.74	25.79	0.5	27.28	42.16	0.5	2.48	496	27.28
09218	Tangerines (mandarin oranges), raw 1 large (2-1/2" dia)	98	85.85	43.12	0.62	10.97	2.25	13.72	9.8	0.1	0.98	153.86	11.76

NDB #	Zinc	Copper	Vitamin A	Thiamin	Riboflavin	Niacin	Vitamin B6	Folate	Vitamin B12	Vitamin C	Fat	Fat: Saturated	Fat: Monounsaturated	Fat: Polyunsaturated	Cholesterol
	mg	mg	IU	mg	mg	mg	mg	mcg	mcg	mg	gm	gm	gm	gm	mg
09094	0.1	0.06	25.27	0.01	0.02	0.13	0.04	1.43	0	0.15	0.22	0.04	0.05	0.11	0
09109	0.28	0.55	347.76	0.05	0.13	0.39	0.03	8.06	0	25.2	0.5	0.03	0.05	0.28	0
09111	0.16	0.11	285.2	0.08	0.05	0.58	0.1	23.46	0	79.12	0.23	0.03	0.03	0.06	0
09123	0.22	0.09	17.29	0.1	0.05	0.57	0.05	25.69	0	72.12	0.25	0.03	0.03	0.06	0
09131	0.04	0.04	92	0.08	0.05	0.28	0.1	3.59	0	3.68	0.32	0.1	0.01	0.09	0
09132	0.08	0.14	116.8	0.15	0.09	0.48	0.18	6.24	0	17.28	0.93	0.3	0.04	0.27	0
09135	0.13	0.07	20.24	0.07	0.09	0.66	0.16	6.58	0	0.25	0.2	0.06	0.01	0.06	0
09139	0.56	0.25	1932.48	0.12	0.12	2.93	0.35	34.16	0	447.74	1.46	0.42	0.13	0.62	0
09148	0.15	0.14	159.25	0.02	0.05	0.46	0.08	34.58	0	89.18	0.4	0.03	0.04	0.22	0
09149	0.02	0.02	57.38	0.02	0.02	0.1	0.01	3.04	0	7.11	0.02	0	0	0	0
09152	0.02	0.01	6.1	0.01	0	0.03	0.02	3.93	0	14.03	0	0	0	0	0
09160	0.02	0.01	3.08	0.01	0	0.03	0.01	2.53	0	9.02	0.03	0	0	0.01	0
09176	0.08	0.23	8060.58	0.12	0.12	1.21	0.28	28.98	0	57.34	0.56	0.14	0.21	0.11	0
09181	0.28	0.07	5706.48	0.06	0.04	1.02	0.2	30.09	0	74.69	0.5	0.13	0.01	0.19	0
09184	0.12	0.07	68	0.13	0.03	1.02	0.1	10.2	0	42.16	0.17	0.04	0	0.07	0
09191	0.12	0.1	1000.96	0.02	0.06	1.35	0.03	5.03	0	7.34	0.63	0.07	0.24	0.31	0
09201	0.07	0.04	278.3	0.11	0.05	0.33	0.08	46.71	0	58.69	0.36	0.04	0.07	0.07	0
09202	0.08	0.08	256.2	0.12	0.06	0.41	0.1	47.18	0	80.22	0.13	0.02	0.02	0.03	0
09203	0.11	0.05	282	0.14	0.06	0.56	0.07	24.39	0	63.45	0.3	0.04	0.05	0.06	0
09206	0.12	0.11	496	0.22	0.07	0.99	0.1	75.14	0	124	0.5	0.06	0.09	0.1	0
09218	0.24	0.03	901.6	0.1	0.02	0.16	0.07	19.99	0	30.18	0.19	0.02	0.03	0.04	0

NDB #	Description & Serving	Grams	Water	Calories	Protein	Carbohydrates	Fiber	Calcium	Phosphorus	Iron	Sodium	Potassium	Magnesium
		gm	gm	kcal	gm	gm	gm	mg	mg	mg	mg	mg	mg
09219	Tangerines (mandarin oranges), canned, juice pk 1 cup	249	222.88	92.13	1.54	23.83	1.74	27.39	24.9	0.67	12.45	331.17	27.39
09226	Papayas, raw 1 cup, cubes	140	124.36	54.6	0.85	13.73	2.52	33.6	7	0.14	4.2	359.8	14
09229	Papaya nectar, canned 1 cup	250	212.55	142.5	0.43	36.28	1.5	25	0	0.85	12.5	77.5	7.5
09231	Passion-fruit (granadilla), purple, raw 1 fruit, without refuse	18	13.13	17.46	0.4	4.21	1.87	2.16	12.24	0.29	5.04	62.64	5.22
09236	Peaches, raw 1 large (2-3/4" dia) (approx 2 1/2 per lb)	157	137.63	67.51	1.1	17.43	3.14	7.85	18.84	0.17	0	309.29	10.99
09246	Peaches, dried, sulfured, uncooked 1 half	13	4.13	31.07	0.47	7.97	1.07	3.64	15.47	0.53	0.91	129.48	5.46
09251	Peach nectar, canned, wo/vit C 1 cup	249	213.24	134.46	0.67	34.66	1.49	12.45	14.94	0.47	17.43	99.6	9.96
09252	Pears, raw 1 medium (approx 2 1/2 per lb)	166	139.12	97.94	0.65	25.08	3.98	18.26	18.26	0.42	0	207.5	9.96
09259	Pears, dried, sulfured, uncooked 1 half with liquid	76	20.28	199.12	1.42	52.97	5.7	25.84	44.84	1.6	4.56	405.08	25.08
09265	Persimmons, native, raw 1 fruit, without refuse	25	16.1	31.75	0.2	8.38	0	6.75	6.5	0.63	0.25	77.5	0
09266	Pineapple, raw 1 cup, diced	155	134.08	75.95	0.6	19.2	1.86	10.85	10.85	0.57	1.55	175.15	21.7
09273	Pineapple juice, canned, unsweetened, wo/vit C 1 cup	250	213.83	140	0.8	34.45	0.5	42.5	20	0.65	2.5	335	32.5
09278	Plantains, cooked 1 cup, slices	154	103.64	178.64	1.22	47.97	3.54	3.08	43.12	0.89	7.7	716.1	49.28
09279	Plums, raw 1 fruit (2-1/8" dia)	66	56.23	36.3	0.52	8.59	0.99	2.64	6.6	0.07	0	113.52	4.62
09286	Pomegranates, raw 1 pomegranate (3-3/8" dia)	154	124.69	104.72	1.46	26.44	0.92	4.62	12.32	0.46	4.62	398.86	4.62
09287	Prickly pears, raw 1 fruit	103	90.18	42.23	0.75	9.86	3.71	57.68	24.72	0.31	5.15	226.6	87.55
09291	Prunes, dried, uncooked 1 prune	8.4	2.72	20.08	0.22	5.27	0.6	4.28	6.64	0.21	0.34	62.58	3.78
09294	Prune juice, canned 1 cup	256	207.97	181.76	1.56	44.67	2.56	30.72	64	3.02	10.24	706.56	35.84
09296	Quinces, raw 1 fruit, without refuse	92	77.1	52.44	0.37	14.08	1.75	10.12	15.64	0.64	3.68	181.24	7.36
09298	Raisins, seedless 1 cup, packed	165	25.44	495	5.31	130.56	6.6	80.85	160.05	3.43	19.8	1239.15	54.45
09302	Raspberries, raw 1 cup	123	106.48	60.27	1.12	14.23	8.36	27.06	14.76	0.7	0	186.96	22.14
09309	Rhubarb, frozen, uncooked 1 cup, diced	137	128.11	28.77	0.75	6.99	2.47	265.78	16.44	0.4	2.74	147.96	24.66
09316	Strawberries, raw 1 cup, halves	152	139.19	45.6	0.93	10.67	3.5	21.28	28.88	0.58	1.52	252.32	15.2

NDB #	Zinc	Copper	Vitamin A	Thiamin	Riboflavin	Niacin	Vitamin B6	Folate	Vitamin B12	Vitamin C	Fat	Fat: Saturated	Fat: Monounsaturated	Fat: Polyunsaturated	Cholesterol
	mg	mg	IU	mg	mg	mg	mg	mcg	mcg	mg	gm	gm	gm	gm	mg
09219	1.27	0.08	2121.48	0.2	0.07	1.11	0.1	11.45	0	85.16	0.07	0.01	0.01	0.01	0
09226	0.1	0.02	397.6	0.04	0.04	0.47	0.03	53.2	0	86.52	0.2	0.06	0.05	0.04	0
09229	0.38	0.03	277.5	0.02	0.01	0.38	0.02	5.25	0	7.5	0.38	0.12	0.1	0.09	0
09231	0.02	0.02	126	0	0.02	0.27	0.02	2.52	0	5.4	0.13	0.01	0.02	0.07	0
09236	0.22	0.11	839.95	0.03	0.06	1.55	0.03	5.34	0	10.36	0.14	0.02	0.05	0.07	0
09246	0.07	0.05	281.19	0	0.03	0.57	0.01	0.04	0	0.62	0.1	0.01	0.04	0.05	0
09251	0.2	0.17	642.42	0.01	0.03	0.72	0.02	3.49	0	13.2	0.05	0	0.02	0.03	0
09252	0.2	0.18	33.2	0.03	0.07	0.17	0.03	12.12	0	6.64	0.66	0.04	0.14	0.16	0
09259	0.3	0.28	2.28	0.01	0.11	1.04	0.05	0	0	5.32	0.48	0.03	0.1	0.11	0
09265	0	0	0	0	0	0	0	0	0	16.5	0.1	0	0	0	0
09266	0.12	0.17	35.65	0.14	0.06	0.65	0.13	16.43	0	23.87	0.67	0.05	0.07	0.23	0
09273	0.28	0.23	12.5	0.14	0.06	0.64	0.24	57.75	0	26.75	0.2	0.01	0.02	0.07	0
09278	0.2	0.1	1399.86	0.07	0.08	1.16	0.37	40.04	0	16.79	0.28	0.11	0.02	0.05	0
09279	0.07	0.03	213.18	0.03	0.06	0.33	0.05	1.45	0	6.27	0.41	0.03	0.27	0.09	0
09286	0.18	0.11	0	0.05	0.05	0.46	0.16	9.24	0	9.39	0.46	0.06	0.07	0.1	0
09287	0.12	0.08	52.53	0.01	0.06	0.47	0.06	6.18	0	14.42	0.53	0.07	0.08	0.22	0
09291	0.04	0.04	166.91	0.01	0.01	0.16	0.02	0.31	0	0.28	0.04	0	0.03	0.01	0
09294	0.54	0.17	7.68	0.04	0.18	2.01	0.56	1.02	0	10.5	0.08	0.01	0.05	0.02	0
09296	0.04	0.12	36.8	0.02	0.03	0.18	0.04	2.76	0	13.8	0.09	0.01	0.03	0.05	0
09298	0.45	0.51	13.2	0.26	0.15	1.35	0.41	5.45	0	5.45	0.76	0.25	0.03	0.22	0
09302	0.57	0.09	159.9	0.04	0.11	1.11	0.07	31.98	0	30.75	0.68	0.02	0.07	0.38	0
09309	0.14	0.03	146.59	0.04	0.04	0.28	0.03	11.23	0	6.58	0.15	0.04	0.03	0.07	0
09316	0.2	0.07	41.04	0.03	0.1	0.35	0.09	26.9	0	86.18	0.56	0.03	0.08	0.28	0

NDB #	Description & Serving	Grams	Water	Calories	Protein	Carbohydrates	Fiber	Calcium	Phosphorus	Iron	Sodium	Potassium	Magnesium
		gm	*gm*	*kcal*	*gm*	*gm*	*gm*	*mg*	*mg*	*mg*	*mg*	*mg*	*mg*
09326	**Watermelon, raw** 1 cup, balls	154	140.93	49.28	0.95	11.06	0.77	12.32	13.86	0.26	3.08	178.64	16.94

Grain products

Breads

NDB #	Description & Serving	Grams	Water	Calories	Protein	Carbohydrates	Fiber	Calcium	Phosphorus	Iron	Sodium	Potassium	Magnesium
18001	**Bagels, plain, enriched, w/calcium propionate (incl onion, poppy, sesame)** 1 bagel (3" dia)	57	18.58	156.75	5.99	30.44	1.31	42.18	54.72	2.03	304.38	57.57	16.53
18007	**Bagels, oat bran** 1 bagel (3" dia)	57	18.75	145.35	6.1	30.38	2.05	6.84	94.05	1.76	288.99	116.28	32.49
18079	**Bread crumbs, dry, grated, plain** 1 cup	108	6.7	426.6	13.5	78.3	2.59	245.16	158.76	6.61	930.96	238.68	49.68
18080	**Breadsticks, plain** 1 small stick (approx 4-1/4" long)	5	0.31	20.6	0.6	3.42	0.15	1.1	6.05	0.21	32.85	6.2	1.6
18347	**Dinner rolls, wheat** 1 roll (1 oz)	28.35	10.49	77.4	2.44	13.04	1.07	49.9	33.45	1.01	96.39	37.71	11.91
18258	**English muffins, plain, enriched, w/calcium propionate (incl sourdough)** 1 muffin	57	24	133.95	4.39	26.22	1.54	99.18	75.81	1.43	264.48	74.67	11.97
18266	**English muffins, whole-wheat** 1 muffin	66	30.16	133.98	5.81	26.66	4.42	174.9	186.12	1.62	420.42	138.6	46.86
18349	**French rolls** 1 roll	38	13.22	105.26	3.27	19.08	1.22	34.58	31.92	1.03	231.42	43.32	7.6
18029	**French or Vienna bread (incl sourdough)** 1 large slice (5" x 2-1/2" x 1")	35	12.01	95.9	3.08	18.17	1.05	26.25	36.75	0.89	213.15	39.55	9.45
18350	**Hamburger or hotdog, plain rolls** 1 roll	43	14.62	122.98	3.66	21.63	1.16	59.77	37.84	1.36	240.8	60.63	8.6
18353	**Hard (incl kaiser) rolls** 1 roll (3-1/2" dia)	57	17.67	167.01	5.64	30.04	1.31	54.15	57	1.87	310.08	61.56	15.39
18033	**Italian bread** 1 large slice (4-1/2" x 3-1/4" x 3/4")	30	10.71	81.3	2.64	15	0.81	23.4	30.9	0.88	175.2	33	8.1
18035	**Mixed-grain (incl whole-grain, 7-grain) bread** 1 large slice	32	12.06	80	3.2	14.85	2.05	29.12	56.32	1.11	155.84	65.28	16.96
18041	**Pita, white, enriched bread** 1 large pita (6-1/2" dia)	60	19.26	165	5.46	33.42	1.32	51.6	58.2	1.57	321.6	72	15.6
18042	**Pita, whole-wheat bread** 1 large pita (6-1/2" dia)	64	19.58	170.24	6.27	35.2	4.74	9.6	115.2	1.85	340.48	108.8	44.16
18044	**Pumpernickel bread** 1 regular slice	26	9.85	65	2.26	12.35	1.69	17.68	46.28	0.75	174.46	54.08	14.04
18047	**Raisin, enriched bread** 1 large slice	32	10.75	87.68	2.53	16.74	1.38	21.12	34.88	0.93	124.8	72.64	8.32
18060	**Rye bread** 1 slice	32	11.94	82.88	2.72	15.46	1.86	23.36	40	0.91	211.2	53.12	12.8
18064	**Wheat (incl wheat berry) bread** 1 slice	25	9.28	65	2.28	11.8	1.08	26.25	37.5	0.83	132.5	50.25	11.5
18069	**White bread, commercially prep (incl soft bread crumbs)** 1 cup, crumbs	45	16.52	120.15	3.69	22.28	1.04	48.6	42.3	1.36	242.1	53.55	10.8
18360	**Taco shells, baked** 1 large (6-1/2" dia)	21	1.26	98.28	1.51	13.1	1.58	33.6	52.08	0.53	77.07	37.59	22.05

NDB #	Zinc	Copper	Vitamin A	Thiamin	Riboflavin	Niacin	Vitamin B6	Folate	Vitamin B12	Vitamin C	Fat	Fat. Saturated	Fat. Monounsaturated	Fat. Polyunsaturated	Cholesterol
	mg	mg	IU	mg	mg	mg	mg	mcg	mcg	mg	gm	gm	gm	gm	mg
09326	0.11	0.05	563.64	0.12	0.03	0.31	0.22	3.39	0	14.78	0.66	0.07	0.16	0.22	0

Grain products

Breads

NDB #	Zinc	Copper	Vitamin A	Thiamin	Riboflavin	Niacin	Vitamin B6	Folate	Vitamin B12	Vitamin C	Fat	Fat. Saturated	Fat. Monounsaturated	Fat. Polyunsaturated	Cholesterol
18001	0.5	0.09	0	0.31	0.18	2.6	0.03	12.54	0	0	0.91	0.13	0.07	0.4	0
18007	1.19	0.07	2.28	0.19	0.19	1.69	0.12	26.22	0	0.11	0.68	0.11	0.14	0.28	0
18079	1.32	0.18	1.08	0.83	0.47	7.4	0.11	27	0.02	0	5.83	1.36	2.26	1.68	0
18080	0.04	0.01	0	0.03	0.03	0.26	0	1.5	0	0	0.48	0.07	0.19	0.18	0
18347	0.29	0.04	0	0.12	0.08	1.15	0.02	4.25	0	0	1.79	0.43	0.92	0.3	0
18258	0.4	0.07	0	0.25	0.16	2.21	0.02	21.09	0.02	0.06	1.03	0.15	0.17	0.51	0
18266	1.06	0.14	0	0.2	0.09	2.25	0.11	32.34	0	0	1.39	0.22	0.34	0.55	0
18349	0.29	0.07	1.52	0.2	0.11	1.65	0.02	12.54	0	0	1.63	0.37	0.75	0.32	0
18029	0.3	0.07	0	0.18	0.12	1.66	0.02	10.85	0	0	1.05	0.22	0.43	0.24	0
18350	0.27	0.05	0	0.21	0.13	1.69	0.02	11.61	0.01	0	2.19	0.51	1.07	0.39	0
18353	0.54	0.09	0	0.27	0.19	2.42	0.03	8.55	0	0	2.45	0.35	0.65	0.98	0
18033	0.26	0.06	0	0.14	0.09	1.31	0.01	9	0	0	1.05	0.26	0.24	0.42	0
18035	0.41	0.08	0	0.13	0.11	1.4	0.11	15.36	0.02	0.1	1.22	0.26	0.49	0.3	0
18041	0.5	0.1	0	0.36	0.2	2.78	0.02	14.4	0	0	0.72	0.1	0.06	0.32	0
18042	0.97	0.18	0	0.22	0.05	1.82	0.15	22.4	0	0	1.66	0.26	0.22	0.68	0
18044	0.38	0.07	0	0.09	0.08	0.8	0.03	8.84	0	0	0.81	0.11	0.24	0.32	0
18047	0.23	0.06	0.64	0.11	0.13	1.11	0.02	10.88	0	0.16	1.41	0.35	0.73	0.22	0
18060	0.36	0.06	1.28	0.14	0.11	1.22	0.02	16.32	0	0.06	1.06	0.2	0.42	0.26	0
18064	0.26	0.05	0	0.1	0.07	1.03	0.02	10.25	0	0	1.03	0.22	0.43	0.23	0
18069	0.28	0.06	0	0.21	0.15	1.79	0.03	15.3	0.01	0	1.62	0.36	0.73	0.33	0.45
18360	0.29	0.03	73.5	0.05	0.01	0.28	0.08	1.26	0	0	4.75	0.7	1.99	1.81	0

NDB #	Description & Serving	Grams	Water	Calories	Protein	Carbohydrates	Fiber	Calcium	Phosphorus	Iron	Sodium	Potassium	Magnesium
			gm	kcal	gm	gm	gm	mg	mg	mg	mg	mg	mg
18363	Tortillas, ready-to-bake or -fry, corn 1 medium tortilla (approx 6" dia) 26		11.47	57.72	1.48	12.12	1.35	45.5	81.64	0.36	41.86	40.04	16.9
18364	Tortillas, ready-to-bake or -fry, flour 1 medium tortilla (approx 6" dia) 32		8.58	104	2.78	17.79	1.06	40	39.68	1.06	152.96	41.92	8.32
Crackers													
18214	Cheese, regular 1 cup, bite size	62	1.92	311.86	6.26	36.08	1.49	93.62	135.16	2.96	616.9	89.9	22.32
18215	Cheese, sandwich-type w/peanut butter filling 1 sandwich	7	0.27	33.74	0.88	3.99	0.2	5.53	22.68	0.2	69.44	17.15	4.06
18216	Crispbread, rye 1 crispbread or cracker	10	0.61	36.6	0.79	8.22	1.65	3.1	26.9	0.24	26.4	31.9	7.8
18217	Matzoh, plain 1 matzoh	28.35	1.22	111.98	2.84	23.73	0.85	3.69	25.23	0.9	0.57	31.75	7.09
18220	Melba toast, plain 1 cup, pieces	30	1.53	117	3.63	22.98	1.89	27.9	58.8	1.11	248.7	60.6	17.7
18226	Rye, wafers, plain 1 cracker (4-1/2" x 2-1/2" x 1/8")	11	0.55	36.74	1.06	8.84	2.52	4.4	36.74	0.65	87.34	54.45	13.31
18228	Saltines (incl oyster, soda, soup) 1 cup, oyster crackers	45	1.85	195.3	4.14	32.18	1.35	53.55	47.25	2.43	585.9	57.6	12.15
18232	Wheat, regular 1 euphrates	4	0.12	18.92	0.34	2.6	0.18	1.96	8.8	0.18	31.8	7.32	2.48
Flours and meals													
20011	Buckwheat flour, whole-groat 1 cup	120	13.38	402	15.14	84.71	12	49.2	404.4	4.87	13.2	692.4	301.2
20322	Cornmeal, degermed, enriched, white 1 cup	138	15.99	505.08	11.7	107.2	10.21	6.9	115.92	5.7	4.14	223.56	55.2
20022	Cornmeal, degermed, enriched, yellow 1 cup	138	15.99	505.08	11.7	107.2	10.21	6.9	115.92	5.7	4.14	223.56	55.2
20320	Cornmeal, whole-grain, white 1 cup	122	12.52	441.64	9.91	93.81	8.91	7.32	294.02	4.21	42.7	350.14	154.94
20020	Cornmeal, whole-grain, yellow 1 cup	122	12.52	441.64	9.91	93.81	8.91	7.32	294.02	4.21	42.7	350.14	154.94
18236	Cracker meal 1 cup	115	8.74	440.45	10.7	93.04	2.94	26.45	119.6	5.34	32.2	132.25	27.6
20090	Rice flour, brown 1 cup	158	18.91	573.54	11.42	120.84	7.27	17.38	532.46	3.13	12.64	456.62	176.96
20061	Rice flour, white 1 cup	158	18.79	578.28	9.4	126.61	3.79	15.8	154.84	0.55	0	120.08	55.3
20063	Rye flour, dark 1 cup	128	14.17	414.72	17.96	87.99	28.93	71.68	808.96	8.26	1.28	934.4	317.44
20064	Rye flour, medium 1 cup	102	10.05	361.08	9.58	79.04	14.89	24.48	211.14	2.16	3.06	346.8	76.5
20065	Rye flour, light 1 cup	102	8.96	374.34	8.56	81.83	14.89	21.42	197.88	1.84	2.04	237.66	71.4
20076	Wheat flour, durum 1 cup	192	21	650.88	26.27	136.57	0	65.28	975.36	6.76	3.84	827.52	276.48
20080	Wheat flour, whole-grain 1 cup	120	12.32	406.8	16.44	87.08	14.64	40.8	415.2	4.66	6	486	165.6

NDB #	Zinc	Copper	Vitamin A	Thiamin	Riboflavin	Niacin	Vitamin B6	Folate	Vitamin B12	Vitamin C	Fat	Fat: Saturated	Fat: Monounsaturated	Fat: Polyunsaturated	Cholesterol
	mg	mg	IU	mg	mg	mg	mg	mcg	mcg	mg	gm	gm	gm	gm	mg
18363	0.24	0.04	62.92	0.03	0.02	0.39	0.06	3.9	0	0	0.65	0.09	0.17	0.29	0
18364	0.23	0.09	0	0.17	0.09	1.14	0.02	3.84	0	0	2.27	0.35	0.92	0.89	0
Crackers															
18214	0.7	0.13	100.44	0.35	0.27	2.9	0.34	15.5	0.29	0	15.69	5.81	5.58	3	8.06
18215	0.08	0.02	22.33	0.03	0.02	0.46	0.1	1.75	0	0	1.62	0.36	0.85	0.31	0.35
18216	0.24	0.03	0	0.02	0.01	0.1	0.02	2.2	0	0	0.13	0.01	0.02	0.06	0
18217	0.19	0.02	0	0.11	0.08	1.1	0.03	3.97	0	0	0.4	0.06	0.04	0.17	0
18220	0.6	0.09	0	0.12	0.08	1.23	0.03	7.8	0	0	0.96	0.13	0.23	0.38	0
18226	0.31	0.05	2.53	0.05	0.03	0.17	0.03	4.95	0	0.01	0.1	0.01	0.02	0.04	0
18228	0.35	0.09	0	0.25	0.21	2.36	0.02	13.95	0	0	5.31	0.95	2.91	0.83	0
18232	0.06	0.01	0	0.02	0.01	0.2	0.01	0.72	0	0	0.82	0.15	0.47	0.12	0
Flours and meals															
20011	3.74	0.62	0	0.5	0.23	7.38	0.7	64.8	0	0	3.72	0.81	1.14	1.14	0
20322	0.99	0.11	0	0.99	0.56	6.95	0.35	66.24	0	0	2.28	0.31	0.57	0.98	0
20022	0.99	0.11	569.94	0.99	0.56	6.95	0.35	66.24	0	0	2.28	0.31	0.57	0.98	0
20320	2.22	0.24	0	0.47	0.25	4.43	0.37	30.99	0	0	4.38	0.62	1.16	2	0
20020	2.22	0.24	572.18	0.47	0.25	4.43	0.37	30.99	0	0	4.38	0.62	1.16	2	0
18236	0.79	0.26	0	0.8	0.54	6.56	0.04	25.3	0	0	1.96	0.31	0.17	0.83	0
20090	3.87	0.36	0	0.7	0.13	10.02	1.16	25.28	0	0	4.39	0.88	1.59	1.57	0
20061	1.26	0.21	0	0.22	0.03	4.09	0.69	6.32	0	0	2.24	0.61	0.7	0.6	0
20063	7.19	0.96	0	0.4	0.32	5.47	0.57	76.8	0	0	3.44	0.4	0.42	1.54	0
20064	2.03	0.29	0	0.29	0.12	1.76	0.27	19.38	0	0	1.81	0.2	0.21	0.78	0
20065	1.79	0.26	0	0.34	0.09	0.82	0.24	22.44	0	0	1.39	0.15	0.16	0.58	0
20076	7.99	1.06	0	0.8	0.23	12.94	0.8	83.14	0	0	4.74	0.87	0.66	1.88	0
20080	3.52	0.46	0	0.54	0.26	7.64	0.41	52.8	0	0	2.24	0.39	0.28	0.93	0

NDB #	Description & Serving	Grams	Water	Calories	Protein	Carbohydrates	Fiber	Calcium	Phosphorus	Iron	Sodium	Potassium	Magnesium
			gm	kcal	gm	gm	gm	mg	mg	mg	mg	mg	mg
20081	Wheat flour, white, all-purpose, enriched, bleached 1 cup	125	14.9	455	12.91	95.39	3.38	18.75	135	5.8	2.5	133.75	27.5
20581	Wheat flour, white, all-purpose, enriched, unbleached 1 cup	125	14.9	455	12.91	95.39	3.38	18.75	135	5.8	2.5	133.75	27.5

Grains and cereals

NDB #	Description & Serving	Grams	Water	Calories	Protein	Carbohydrates	Fiber	Calcium	Phosphorus	Iron	Sodium	Potassium	Magnesium
20006	Barley, pearled, cooked 1 cup	157	108.02	193.11	3.55	44.31	5.97	17.27	84.78	2.09	4.71	146.01	34.54
20010	Buckwheat groats, roasted, cooked 1 cup	168	127.06	154.56	5.68	33.5	4.54	11.76	117.6	1.34	6.72	147.84	85.68
20013	Bulghur, cooked 1 cup	182	141.52	151.06	5.61	33.82	8.19	18.2	72.8	1.75	9.1	123.76	58.24
08161	Corn grits, white, reg & quick, enriched, cooked w/water, w/salt 1 cup	242	206.43	145.2	3.39	31.46	0.48	0	29.04	1.55	539.66	53.24	9.68
08164	Corn grits, yellow, reg & quick, enriched, cooked w/water, wo/salt (corn) 1 cup	242	206.43	145.2	3.39	31.46	0.48	0	29.04	1.55	0	53.24	9.68
20029	Couscous, cooked 1 cup, cooked	157	113.93	175.84	5.95	36.46	2.2	12.56	34.54	0.6	7.85	91.06	12.56
08174	Farina, unenriched, cooked w/water, wo/salt (wheat) 1 cup	233	204.81	116.5	3.26	24.7	3.26	4.66	27.96	0.05	0	30.29	4.66
20030	Hominy, canned, white 1 cup	165	136.17	118.8	2.44	23.53	4.13	16.5	57.75	1.02	346.5	14.85	26.4
20330	Hominy, canned, yellow 1 cup	160	132.05	115.2	2.37	22.82	4	16	56	0.99	336	14.4	25.6
20032	Millet, cooked 1 cup	240	171.38	285.6	8.42	56.81	3.12	7.2	240	1.51	4.8	148.8	105.6
20034	Oat bran, cooked 1 cup	219	183.96	87.6	7.03	25.05	5.69	21.9	260.61	1.93	2.19	201.48	87.6
08121	Oats, reg & quick & instant, wo/fortification, cooked w/water, wo/salt (oats) 1 cup	234	199.6	145.08	6.08	25.27	3.98	18.72	177.84	1.59	2.34	131.04	56.16
08123	Oats, instant, fortified, plain, prep w/water (oats) 1 cup, cooked	234	200.07	138.06	5.85	23.87	3.98	215.28	175.5	8.33	376.74	131.04	56.16
20037	Rice, brown, long-grain, cooked 1 cup	195	142.53	216.45	5.03	44.77	3.51	19.5	161.85	0.82	9.75	83.85	83.85
20041	Rice, brown, medium-grain, cooked 1 cup	195	142.27	218.4	4.52	45.84	3.51	19.5	150.15	1.03	1.95	154.05	85.8
20345	Rice, white, long-grain, reg, cooked, enriched, w/salt 1 cup	158	108.14	205.4	4.25	44.51	0.63	15.8	67.94	1.9	603.56	55.3	18.96
20055	Rice, white, glutinous, cooked 1 cup, cooked	174	133.34	168.78	3.51	36.7	1.74	3.48	13.92	0.24	8.7	17.4	8.7
20066	Semolina, enriched 1 cup	167	21.16	601.2	21.18	121.63	6.51	28.39	227.12	7.28	1.67	310.62	78.49
08084	Wheat germ, toasted, plain 1 cup	113	6.33	431.66	32.88	56.05	14.58	50.85	1294.98	10.27	4.52	1070.11	361.6
08145	Whole wheat hot natural cereal, cooked w/water, wo/salt (wheat) 1 cup	242	202.31	150.04	4.84	33.15	3.87	16.94	166.98	1.5	0	171.82	53.24
20089	Wild rice, cooked 1 cup	164	121.25	165.64	6.54	35	2.95	4.92	134.48	0.98	4.92	165.64	52.48

NDB #	Zinc	Copper	Vitamin A	Thiamin	Riboflavin	Niacin	Vitamin B6	Folate	Vitamin B12	Vitamin C	Fat	Fat, Saturated	Fat, Monounsaturated	Fat, Polyunsaturated	Cholesterol
	mg	mg	IU	mg	mg	mg	mg	mcg	mcg	mg	gm	gm	gm	gm	mg
20081	0.88	0.18	0	0.98	0.62	7.38	0.06	32.5	0	0	1.23	0.19	0.11	0.52	0
20581	0.88	0.18	0	0.98	0.62	7.38	0.06	32.5	0	0	1.23	0.19	0.11	0.52	0

Grains and cereals

NDB #	Zinc	Copper	Vitamin A	Thiamin	Riboflavin	Niacin	Vitamin B6	Folate	Vitamin B12	Vitamin C	Fat	Fat, Saturated	Fat, Monounsaturated	Fat, Polyunsaturated	Cholesterol
20006	1.29	0.16	10.99	0.13	0.1	3.24	0.18	25.12	0	0	0.69	0.15	0.09	0.34	0
20010	1.02	0.25	0	0.07	0.07	1.58	0.13	23.52	0	0	1.04	0.23	0.32	0.32	0
20013	1.04	0.14	0	0.1	0.05	1.82	0.15	32.76	0	0	0.44	0.08	0.06	0.18	0
08161	0.17	0.03	0	0.24	0.15	1.96	0.06	2.42	0	0	0.48	0.07	0.12	0.19	0
08164	0.17	0.03	145.2	0.24	0.15	1.96	0.06	2.42	0	0	0.48	0.07	0.12	0.19	0
20029	1.37	0.22	0	0.33	0.14	5.19	0.27	79.2	0	0	0.84	0.15	0.12	0.34	0
08174	0.16	0.03	0	0.02	0.02	0.23	0.02	4.66	0	0	0.23	0.02	0.02	0.07	0
20030	1.73	0.05	0	0	0.01	0.05	0.01	1.65	0	0	1.45	0.2	0.38	0.66	0
20330	1.68	0.05	176	0	0.01	0.05	0.01	1.6	0	0	1.41	0.2	0.37	0.64	0
20032	2.18	0.39	0	0.25	0.2	3.19	0.26	45.6	0	0	2.4	0.41	0.44	1.22	0
20034	1.16	0.14	0	0.35	0.07	0.32	0.05	13.14	0	0	1.88	0.36	0.64	0.74	0
08121	1.15	0.13	37.44	0.26	0.05	0.3	0.05	9.36	0	0	2.34	0.42	0.75	0.87	0
08123	1.15	0.13	1996.02	0.7	0.37	7.23	0.98	198.9	0	0	2.34	0.42	0.75	0.87	0
20037	1.23	0.2	0	0.19	0.05	2.98	0.28	7.8	0	0	1.76	0.35	0.64	0.63	0
20041	1.21	0.16	0	0.2	0.02	2.59	0.29	7.8	0	0	1.62	0.32	0.59	0.58	0
20345	0.77	0.11	0	0.26	0.02	2.33	0.15	4.74	0	0	0.44	0.12	0.14	0.12	0
20055	0.71	0.09	0	0.03	0.02	0.5	0.05	1.74	0	0	0.33	0.07	0.12	0.12	0
20066	1.75	0.32	0	1.35	0.95	10	0.17	120.24	0	0	1.75	0.25	0.21	0.72	0
08084	18.84	0.7	0	1.89	0.93	6.32	1.11	397.76	0	6.78	12.09	2.07	1.7	7.48	0
08145	1.16	0.2	0	0.17	0.12	2.15	0.18	26.62	0	0	0.97	0.15	0.14	0.49	0
20089	2.2	0.2	0	0.09	0.14	2.11	0.22	42.64	0	0	0.56	0.08	0.08	0.35	0

NDB #	Description & Serving	Grams	Water	Calories	Protein	Carbohydrates	Fiber	Calcium	Phosphorus	Iron	Sodium	Potassium	Magnesium
			gm	kcal	gm	gm	gm	mg	mg	mg	mg	mg	mg
Pasta													
20100	Macaroni, cooked, enriched 1 cup elbow shaped	140	92.39	197.4	6.68	39.68	1.82	9.8	75.6	1.96	1.4	43.4	25.2
20108	Macaroni, whole-wheat, cooked 1 cup elbow shaped	140	94.01	173.6	7.46	37.16	3.92	21	124.6	1.48	4.2	61.6	42
20110	Noodles, egg, cooked, enriched 1 cup	160	109.92	212.8	7.6	39.74	1.76	19.2	110.4	2.54	11.2	44.8	30.4
20112	Noodles, egg, spinach, cooked, enriched 1 cup	160	109.63	211.2	8.06	38.8	3.68	30.4	91.2	1.74	19.2	59.2	38.4
20113	Noodles, Chinese, chow mein 1 cup	45	0.33	237.15	3.77	25.89	1.76	9	72.45	2.13	197.55	54	23.4
20115	Noodles, Japanese, soba, cooked 1 cup	114	83.23	112.86	5.77	24.44	0	4.56	28.5	0.55	68.4	39.9	10.26
20121	Spaghetti, cooked, enriched, wo/ salt 1 cup	140	92.39	197.4	6.68	39.68	2.38	9.8	75.6	1.96	1.4	43.4	25.2
20127	Spaghetti, spinach, cooked 1 cup	140	95.4	182	6.41	36.61	0	42	151.2	1.46	19.6	81.2	86.8
20125	Spaghetti, whole-wheat, cooked 1 cup	140	94.01	173.6	7.46	37.16	6.3	21	124.6	1.48	4.2	61.6	42
Condiments													
11935	Catsup 1 tablespoon	15	9.99	15.6	0.23	4.09	0.2	2.85	5.85	0.11	177.9	72.15	3.3
11215	Garlic, raw 1 teaspoon	2.8	1.64	4.17	0.18	0.93	0.06	5.07	4.28	0.05	0.48	11.23	0.7
11937	Pickles, cucumber, dill 1 cup (about 23 slices)	155	142.09	27.9	0.96	6.4	1.86	13.95	32.55	0.82	1987.1	179.8	17.05
11940	Pickles, cucumber, sweet 1 cup, sliced	170	110.94	198.9	0.63	54.08	1.87	6.8	20.4	1	1596.3	54.4	6.8
11941	Pickle, cucumber, sour 1 large (4" long)	135	127.01	14.85	0.45	3.04	1.62	0	18.9	0.54	1630.8	31.05	5.4
11945	Pickle relish, sweet 1 tablespoon	15	9.31	19.5	0.06	5.26	0.17	0.45	2.1	0.13	121.65	3.75	0.75
11943	Pimento, canned 1 tablespoon	12	11.17	2.76	0.13	0.61	0.23	0.72	2.04	0.2	1.68	18.96	0.72
02047	Salt, table 1 tablespoon	18	0.04	0	0	0	0	4.32	0	0.06	6976.44	1.44	0.18
Meat													
Beef													
13369	Brisket, flat half, lean & fat, 0" fat, braised 3 oz	85	49.08	182.75	25.91	0	0	4.25	210.8	2.34	52.7	245.65	20.4
13034	Chuck, arm pot roast, lean & fat, 1/4" fat, braised 3 oz	85	40.79	282.2	23.32	0	0	8.5	187	2.64	51	209.1	16.15

NDB #	Zinc	Copper	Vitamin A	Thiamin	Riboflavin	Niacin	Vitamin B6	Folate	Vitamin B12	Vitamin C	Fat	Fat: Saturated	Fat: Monounsaturated	Fat: Polyunsaturated	Cholesterol
	mg	mg	IU	mg	mg	mg	mg	mcg	mcg	mg	gm	gm	gm	gm	mg
Pasta															
20100	0.74	0.14	0	0.29	0.14	2.34	0.05	9.8	0	0	0.94	0.13	0.11	0.38	0
20108	1.13	0.23	0	0.15	0.06	0.99	0.11	7	0	0	0.76	0.14	0.11	0.3	0
20110	0.99	0.14	32	0.3	0.13	2.38	0.06	11.2	0.14	0	2.35	0.5	0.69	0.65	52.8
20112	1.01	0.13	164.8	0.39	0.2	2.36	0.18	33.6	0.22	0	2.51	0.58	0.79	0.56	52.8
20113	0.63	0.08	38.25	0.26	0.19	2.68	0.05	9.9	0	0	13.84	1.97	3.46	7.8	0
20115	0.14	0.01	0	0.11	0.03	0.58	0.05	7.98	0	0	0.11	0.02	0.03	0.04	0
20121	0.74	0.14	0	0.29	0.14	2.34	0.05	9.8	0	0	0.94	0.13	0.11	0.38	0
20127	1.51	0.29	212.8	0.14	0.14	2.14	0.13	16.8	0	0	0.88	0.13	0.1	0.36	0
20125	1.13	0.23	0	0.15	0.06	0.99	0.11	7	0	0	0.76	0.14	0.11	0.3	0
Condiments															
11935	0.03	0.03	152.4	0.01	0.01	0.21	0.03	2.25	0	2.27	0.05	0.01	0.01	0.02	0
11215	0.03	0.01	0	0.01	0	0.02	0.03	0.09	0	0.87	0.01	0	0	0.01	0
11937	0.22	0.12	509.95	0.02	0.04	0.09	0.02	1.55	0	2.95	0.29	0.07	0	0.12	0
11940	0.14	0.18	214.2	0.02	0.05	0.3	0.03	1.7	0	2.04	0.44	0.11	0.01	0.18	0
11941	0.03	0.11	195.75	0	0.01	0	0.01	0.96	0	1.35	0.27	0.07	0	0.11	0
11945	0.02	0.01	23.25	0	0	0.03	0	0.15	0	0.15	0.07	0.01	0.03	0.02	0
11943	0.02	0.01	318.6	0	0.01	0.07	0.03	0.72	0	10.19	0.04	0.01	0	0.02	0
02047	0.02	0.01	0	0	0	0	0	0	0	0	0	0	0	0	0
Meat															
Beef															
13369	5.19	0.1	0	0.06	0.18	3.18	0.26	6.8	2.19	0	8	2.85	3.53	0.31	80.75
13034	5.81	0.11	0	0.06	0.2	2.7	0.24	7.65	2.51	0	20.24	7.97	8.68	0.77	84.15

NDB #	Description & Serving	Grams	Water	Calories	Protein	Carbohydrates	Fiber	Calcium	Phosphorus	Iron	Sodium	Potassium	Magnesium
			gm	kcal	gm	gm	gm	mg	mg	mg	mg	mg	mg
13073	Rib, whole (ribs 6-12), lean & fat, 1/4" fat, roasted 3 oz	85	40.37	304.3	19.13	0	0	9.35	148.75	1.99	53.55	255.85	17
13148	Shortribs, lean & fat, choice, braised 3 oz	85	30.36	400.35	18.33	0	0	10.2	137.7	1.96	42.5	190.4	12.75
13160	Bottom round, lean & fat, 1/4" fat, all grades, braised 3 oz	85	44.32	233.75	24.36	0	0	5.1	208.25	2.65	42.5	239.7	18.7
13176	Eye of round, lean & fat, 1/4" fat, roasted 3 oz	85	50.52	194.65	22.77	0	0	5.1	176.8	1.56	50.15	307.7	20.4
13184	Eye of round, lean, 1/4" fat, roasted 3 oz	85	55.25	142.8	24.64	0	0	4.25	192.1	1.66	52.7	335.75	22.95
13238	Tenderloin, lean & fat, 1/4" fat, broiled 3 oz	85	45.08	247.35	21.47	0	0	6.8	178.5	2.68	50.15	312.8	22.1
13299	Ground, extra lean, broiled, well done 85	85	45.79	225.25	24.29	0	0	7.65	161.5	2.35	69.7	313.65	21.25
13306	Ground, lean, broiled, well done 85	85	44.93	238	23.97	0	0	10.2	154.7	2.08	75.65	296.65	20.4
13313	Ground, regular, broiled, well done 85	85	44.2	248.2	23.12	0	0	10.2	162.35	2.33	79.05	277.95	18.7
13322	Heart, simmered 3 oz	85	54.47	148.75	24.47	0.36	0	5.1	212.5	6.38	53.55	198.05	21.25
13324	Kidneys, simmered 3 oz	85	58.51	122.4	21.66	0.82	0	14.45	260.1	6.21	113.9	152.15	15.3
13327	Liver, pan-fried 3 oz	85	47.33	184.45	22.71	6.67	0	9.35	391.85	5.34	90.1	309.4	19.55
13340	Tongue, simmered 3 oz	85	47.64	240.55	18.79	0.28	0	5.95	120.7	2.88	51	153	14.45
13347	Corned beef, brisket 3 oz	85	50.82	213.35	15.44	0.4	0	6.8	106.25	1.58	963.9	123.25	10.2
Lamb													
17014	Domestic, leg, whole (shk & sirl), lean, 1/4" fat, choice, roasted 3 oz	85	54.31	162.35	24.06	0	0	6.8	175.1	1.8	57.8	287.3	22.1
17025	Domestic, loin, lean & fat, 1/4" fat, choice, roasted 3 oz	85	44.63	262.65	19.17	0	0	15.3	153	1.8	54.4	209.1	19.55
17060	Domestic, cubed for stew (leg & shoulder), lean, 1/4" fat, braised 3 oz	85	47.8	189.55	28.64	0	0	12.75	174.25	2.38	59.5	221	23.8
17073	New Zealand, imp, frz, leg, whole (shk & sirl), lean & fat, roasted 3 oz	85	49.19	209.1	21.09	0	0	8.5	185.3	1.79	36.55	141.95	17
17075	New Zealand, imp, frz, leg, whole (shk & sirl), lean, roasted 3 oz	85	54.33	153.85	23.53	0	0	5.95	198.9	1.9	38.25	155.55	17.85
Veal													
17103	Leg, lean, roasted 3 oz	85	56.96	127.5	23.86	0	0	5.1	200.6	0.77	57.8	334.05	23.8
17109	Loin, lean, roasted 3 oz	85	54.9	148.75	22.37	0	0	17.85	188.7	0.72	81.6	289	22.1
17115	Rib, lean, roasted 3 oz	85	54.94	150.45	21.9	0	0	10.2	175.95	0.82	82.45	264.35	20.4
17143	Ground, broiled 3 oz	85	56.75	146.2	20.72	0	0	14.45	184.45	0.84	70.55	286.45	20.4

NDB #	Zinc	Copper	Vitamin A	Thiamin	Riboflavin	Niacin	Vitamin B6	Folate	Vitamin B12	Vitamin C	Fat	Fat: Saturated	Fat: Monounsaturated	Fat: Polyunsaturated	Cholesterol
	mg	mg	IU	mg	mg	mg	mg	mcg	mcg	mg	gm	gm	gm	gm	mg
13073	4.55	0.07	0	0.06	0.14	2.9	0.2	5.95	2.16	0	24.66	9.95	10.6	0.88	71.4
13148	4.15	0.08	0	0.04	0.13	2.08	0.19	4.25	2.23	0	35.68	15.13	16.05	1.3	79.9
13160	4.17	0.1	0	0.06	0.2	3.17	0.28	8.5	2	0	14.37	5.41	6.25	0.54	81.6
13176	3.69	0.08	0	0.07	0.14	2.97	0.3	5.95	1.79	0	10.84	4.23	4.66	0.39	61.2
13184	4.03	0.09	0	0.08	0.14	3.19	0.32	5.95	1.84	0	4.17	1.51	1.77	0.14	58.65
13238	4.15	0.13	0	0.09	0.22	2.99	0.33	5.1	2.05	0	17.22	6.76	7.06	0.65	73.1
13299	5.47	0.07	0	0.06	0.27	4.97	0.27	9.35	2.18	0	13.43	5.28	5.88	0.5	84.15
13306	5.27	0.07	0	0.05	0.2	5.07	0.26	9.35	2.31	0	14.99	5.89	6.56	0.56	85.85
13313	4.94	0.08	0	0.03	0.18	5.5	0.26	8.50	2.79	0	16.54	6.50	7.24	0.62	85.85
13322	2.66	0.63	0	0.12	1.31	3.46	0.18	1.7	12.16	1.28	4.78	1.43	1.06	1.16	164.05
13324	3.59	0.58	1054.85	0.16	3.45	5.12	0.44	83.3	43.61	0.68	2.92	0.93	0.63	0.63	328.95
13327	4.63	3.8	30689.25	0.18	3.52	12.27	1.22	187	95.03	19.55	6.8	2.27	1.38	1.45	409.7
13340	4.08	0.19	0	0.03	0.3	1.83	0.14	4.25	5.02	0.43	17.63	7.59	8.05	0.66	90.95
13347	3.89	0.13	0	0.02	0.14	2.58	0.2	5.1	1.39	0	16.13	5.39	7.84	0.57	83.3
Lamb															
17014	4.2	0.1	0	0.09	0.25	5.39	0.14	19.55	2.24	0	6.58	2.35	2.88	0.43	75.65
17025	2.9	0.1	0	0.09	0.2	6.04	0.09	16.15	1.88	0	20.05	8.7	8.23	1.59	80.75
17060	5.59	0.12	0	0.06	0.2	5.06	0.1	17.85	2.32	0	7.48	2.68	3.01	0.69	91.8
17073	3.04	0.09	0	0.1	0.38	6.45	0.11	0.85	2.21	0	13.23	6.47	5.11	0.64	85.85
17075	3.43	0.09	0	0.1	0.43	6.38	0.12	0	2.24	0	5.96	2.59	2.34	0.35	85
Veal															
17103	2.62	0.11	0	0.05	0.28	8.57	0.26	13.6	1	0	2.88	1.04	1.01	0.25	87.55
17109	2.75	0.1	0	0.05	0.26	8.04	0.31	13.6	1.11	0	5.9	2.19	2.12	0.48	90.1
17115	3.82	0.09	0	0.05	0.25	6.38	0.23	11.9	1.34	0	6.32	1.77	2.26	0.57	97.75
17143	3.29	0.09	0	0.06	0.23	6.83	0.33	9.35	1.08	0	6.43	2.58	2.41	0.47	87.55

NDB #	Description & Serving	Grams	Water	Calories	Protein	Carbohydrates	Fiber	Calcium	Phosphorus	Iron	Sodium	Potassium	Magnesium
		gm	gm	kcal	gm	gm	gm	mg	mg	mg	mg	mg	mg
Pork													
10011	Fresh, (ham), whole, lean, roasted 3 oz	85	51.56	179.35	25	0	0	5.95	238.85	0.95	54.4	317.05	21.25
10019	Fresh, (ham), shank half, lean, roasted 3 oz	85	51.37	182.75	23.98	0	0	5.95	236.3	0.94	54.4	306	21.25
10027	Fresh, loin, whole, lean, roasted 3 oz	85	51.87	177.65	24.33	0	0	15.3	211.65	0.93	49.3	361.25	23.8
10042	Fresh, center loin (chops), bone-in, lean, broiled 3 oz	85	51.98	171.7	25.66	0	0	26.35	204.85	0.72	51	318.75	22.95
10050	Fresh, center rib (chops), bone-in, lean, broiled 3 oz	85	48.41	186.15	26.15	0	0	26.35	208.25	0.7	55.25	357	23.8
10059	Fresh, sirloin (roasts), bone-in, lean, roasted 3 oz	85	51.46	183.6	24.49	0	0	17	193.8	0.95	53.55	311.1	21.25
10079	Fresh, shoulder, arm picnic, lean, roasted 3 oz	85	51.23	193.8	22.68	0	0	7.65	209.95	1.21	68	298.35	17
10089	Fresh, spareribs, lean & fat, braised 3 oz	85	34.36	337.45	24.7	0	0	39.95	221.85	1.57	79.05	272	20.4
10124	Cured, bacon, broiled, pan-fried or roasted 3 medium slices packed 20/lb raw, after cooking	19	2.46	109.44	5.79	0.11	0	2.28	63.84	0.31	303.24	92.34	4.56
10131	Cured, Canadian-style bacon, grilled 2 slices (6 per 6-oz pkg.)	46.5	28.69	86.03	11.27	0.63	0	4.65	137.64	0.38	718.89	181.35	9.77
10132	Cured, feet, pickled 1 lb	453.6	311.26	920.81	61.33	0.09	0	145.15	154.22	2.81	4186.73	1065.96	18.14
10134	Cured, ham, boneless, extra lean (approx 5% fat), roasted 3 oz	85	57.52	123.25	17.79	1.28	0	6.8	166.6	1.26	1022.55	243.95	11.9
10136	Cured, ham, boneless, reg (approx 11% fat), roasted 3 oz	85	54.86	151.3	19.23	0	0	6.8	238.85	1.14	1275	347.65	18.7
10153	Cured, ham, whole, lean, roasted 3 oz	85	55.91	133.45	21.29	0	0	5.95	192.95	0.8	1127.95	268.6	18.7
10169	Cured, shoulder, arm picnic, lean, roasted 3 oz	85	54.28	144.5	21.2	0	0	9.35	206.55	0.92	1046.35	248.2	13.6
Poultry: Chicken (broilers or fryers)													
05030	Light meat, meat & skin, fried, batter 1/2 chicken, bone removed	188	94.43	520.76	44.27	17.86	0	37.6	315.84	2.37	539.56	347.8	41.36
05031	Light meat, meat & skin, fried, flour 1/2 chicken, bone removed	130	71.06	319.8	39.59	2.37	0.13	20.8	276.9	1.57	100.1	310.7	35.1
05032	Light meat, meat & skin, roasted 1/2 chicken, bone removed	132	79.87	293.04	38.31	0	0	19.8	264	1.5	99	299.64	33
05033	Light meat, meat & skin, stewed 1/2 chicken, bone removed	150	97.7	301.5	39.21	0	0	19.5	219	1.47	94.5	250.5	30
05035	Dark meat, meat & skin, fried, batter 1/2 chicken, bone removed	278	135.72	828.44	60.74	26.08	0	58.38	403.1	4	820.1	514.3	55.6
05037	Dark meat, meat & skin, roasted 1/2 chicken, bone removed	167	97.91	422.51	43.37	0	0	25.05	280.56	2.27	145.29	367.4	36.74
05038	Dark meat, meat & skin, stewed 1/2 chicken, bone removed	184	115.9	428.72	43.24	0	0	25.76	244.72	2.41	128.8	305.44	33.12

NDB #	Zinc	Copper	Vitamin A	Thiamin	Riboflavin	Niacin	Vitamin B6	Folate	Vitamin B12	Vitamin C	Fat	Fat: Saturated	Fat: Monounsaturated	Fat: Polyunsaturated	Cholesterol
	mg	mg	IU	mg	mg	mg	mg	mcg	mcg	mg	gm	gm	gm	gm	mg
Pork															
10011	2.77	0.09	7.65	0.59	0.3	4.19	0.38	10.2	0.61	0.34	8.02	2.81	3.78	0.72	79.9
10019	2.93	0.09	6.8	0.54	0.29	4.15	0.39	5.1	0.6	0.34	8.93	3.09	4.27	0.77	78.2
10027	2.15	0.05	6.8	0.86	0.28	5.01	0.47	5.95	0.62	0.51	8.19	2.98	3.67	0.65	68.85
10042	2.02	0.04	6.8	0.98	0.26	4.71	0.4	5.1	0.63	0.34	6.86	2.51	3.09	0.49	69.7
10050	2.02	0.06	5.1	0.95	0.28	5.24	0.4	2.55	0.65	0.26	8.28	2.94	3.78	0.53	68.85
10059	2.18	0.07	5.95	0.68	0.28	4.72	0.36	5.1	0.66	0.26	8.75	3.08	3.84	0.74	73.1
10079	3.46	0.11	5.95	0.49	0.3	3.67	0.35	4.25	0.66	0.26	10.73	3.66	5.08	1.02	80.75
10089	3.91	0.12	8.5	0.35	0.32	4.65	0.3	3.4	0.92	0	25.76	9.45	11.46	2.32	102.85
10124	0.62	0.03	0	0.13	0.05	1.39	0.05	0.95	0.33	0	9.36	3.31	4.5	1.1	16.15
10131	0.79	0.03	0	0.38	0.09	3.22	0.21	1.86	0.36	0	3.92	1.32	1.88	0.38	26.97
10132	5.62	0.23	0	0.03	0.19	1.66	1.72	18.14	2.81	0	73.21	25.27	34.34	7.94	417.31
10134	2.45	0.07	0	0.64	0.17	3.42	0.34	2.55	0.55	0	4.7	1.54	2.23	0.46	45.05
10136	2.1	0.12	0	0.62	0.28	5.23	0.26	2.55	0.6	0	7.67	2.65	3.77	1.2	50.15
10153	2.18	0.07	0	0.58	0.22	4.27	0.4	3.4	0.6	0	4.68	1.56	2.15	0.54	46.75
10169	2.5	0.11	0	0.62	0.19	4.08	0.31	3.4	0.94	0	5.98	2.01	2.75	0.69	40.8
Poultry: Chicken (broilers or fryers)															
05030	1.99	0.11	148.52	0.21	0.28	17.21	0.73	11.28	0.53	0	29.03	7.75	11.98	6.77	157.92
05031	1.64	0.08	88.4	0.1	0.17	15.65	0.7	5.2	0.43	0	15.72	4.32	6.24	3.5	113.1
05032	1.62	0.07	145.2	0.08	0.16	14.7	0.69	3.96	0.42	0	14.32	4.03	5.62	3.05	110.88
05033	1.71	0.07	144	0.06	0.17	10.4	0.41	4.5	0.3	0	14.96	4.2	5.88	3.18	111
05035	5.78	0.22	286.34	0.33	0.61	15.59	0.7	25.02	0.75	0	51.82	13.76	21.07	12.32	247.42
05037	4.16	0.13	335.67	0.11	0.35	10.62	0.52	11.69	0.48	0	26.35	7.3	10.34	5.83	151.97
05038	4.16	0.13	342.24	0.09	0.33	8.3	0.31	11.04	0.37	0	26.97	7.47	10.58	5.96	150.88

NDB #	Description & Serving	Grams	Water	Calories	Protein	Carbohydrates	Fiber	Calcium	Phosphorus	Iron	Sodium	Potassium	Magnesium
			gm	kcal	gm	gm	gm	mg	mg	mg	mg	mg	mg
05040	**Light meat, meat only, fried** 1 cup	140	84.2	268.8	45.95	0.59	0	22.4	323.4	1.6	113.4	368.2	40.6
05041	**Light meat, meat only, roasted** 1 cup, chopped or diced	140	90.66	242.2	43.27	0	0	21	302.4	1.48	107.8	345.8	37.8
05042	**Light meat, meat only, stewed** 1 cup, chopped or diced	140	95.23	222.6	40.43	0	0	18.2	222.6	1.3	91	252	30.8
05044	**Dark meat, meat only, fried** 1 cup	140	77.98	334.6	40.59	3.63	0	25.2	261.8	2.09	135.8	354.2	35
05045	**Dark meat, meat only, roasted** 1 cup, chopped or diced	140	88.28	287	38.32	0	0	21	250.6	1.86	130.2	336	32.2
05046	**Dark meat, meat only, stewed** 1 cup, chopped or diced	140	92.16	268.8	36.36	0	0	19.6	200.2	1.9	103.6	253.4	28
05028	**Chicken, liver, all classes, simmered** 1 cup, chopped or diced	140	95.63	219.8	34.1	1.23	0	19.6	436.8	11.86	71.4	196	29.4
05310	**Cornish game hens, meat only, roasted** 1/2 bird	110	79.09	147.4	25.63	0	0	14.3	163.9	0.85	69.3	275	20.9
	Poultry: Duck												
05140	**Duck, domesticated, meat & skin, roasted** 1 cup, chopped or diced	140	72.58	471.8	26.59	0	0	15.4	218.4	3.78	82.6	285.6	22.4
05142	**Duck, domesticated, meat only, roasted** 1 cup, chopped or diced	140	89.91	281.4	32.87	0	0	16.8	284.2	3.78	91	352.8	28
	Poultry: Goose												
05147	**Goose, domesticated, meat & skin, roasted** 1 cup, chopped or diced	140	72.73	427	35.22	0	0	18.2	378	3.96	98	460.6	30.8
05149	**Goose, domesticated, meat only, roasted** 1/2 goose	591	338.23	1406.58	171.21	0	0	82.74	1826.19	16.96	449.16	2293.08	147.75
	Poultry: Turkey												
05192	**Turkey, breast, meat & skin, roasted** 1/2 breast, bone removed	864	546.22	1632.96	248.05	0	0	181.44	1814.4	12.1	544.32	2488.32	233.28
05194	**Turkey, leg, meat & skin, roasted** 1 leg, bone removed	546	334.1	1135.68	152.17	0	0	174.72	1086.54	12.56	420.42	1528.8	125.58
05186	**Turkey, all classes, light meat, cooked, roasted** 1 cup, chopped or diced	140	92.78	219.8	41.86	0	0	26.6	306.6	1.89	89.6	427	39.2
05188	**Turkey, all classes, dark meat, cooked, roasted** 1 cup, chopped or diced	140	88.33	261.8	39.1	0	0	44.8	285.6	3.26	110.6	406	33.6
	Luncheon meat												
07007	**Bologna, beef** 1 slice (4" dia x 1/8" thick)	23	12.72	71.76	2.81	0.18	0	2.76	20.24	0.38	225.63	36.11	2.76
07011	**Bologna, turkey** 2 slices	56.7	36.9	112.83	7.78	0.55	0	47.63	74.28	0.87	497.83	112.83	7.94
07017	**Chicken roll, light meat** 2 slices	56.7	38.9	90.15	11.07	1.39	0	24.38	89.02	0.55	331.13	129.28	10.77
07022	**Frankfurter, beef** 1 frankfurter (5 in long x 3/4 in dia, 10 per pound)	45	24.62	141.75	5.4	0.81	0	9	39.15	0.64	461.7	74.7	1.35
07024	**Frankfurter, chicken** 1 frankfurter	45	25.89	115.65	5.82	3.06	0	42.75	48.15	0.9	616.5	37.8	4.5

NDB #	Zinc	Copper	Vitamin A	Thiamin	Riboflavin	Niacin	Vitamin B6	Folate	Vitamin B12	Vitamin C	Fat	Fat: Saturated	Fat: Monounsaturated	Fat: Polyunsaturated	Cholesterol
	mg	mg	IU	mg	mg	mg	mg	mcg	mcg	mg	gm	gm	gm	gm	mg
05040	1.78	0.08	42	0.1	0.18	18.71	0.88	5.6	0.5	0	7.76	2.13	2.76	1.76	126
05041	1.72	0.07	40.6	0.09	0.16	17.39	0.84	5.6	0.48	0	6.31	1.78	2.16	1.37	119
05042	1.67	0.06	37.8	0.06	0.16	10.91	0.46	4.2	0.32	0	5.59	1.57	1.89	1.22	107.8
05044	4.07	0.12	110.6	0.13	0.35	9.9	0.52	12.6	0.46	0	16.27	4.37	6.05	3.88	134.4
05045	3.92	0.11	100.8	0.1	0.32	9.17	0.5	11.2	0.45	0	13.62	3.72	4.98	3.16	130.2
05046	3.72	0.11	96.6	0.08	0.28	6.63	0.29	9.8	0.31	0	12.57	3.43	4.56	2.93	123.2
05028	6.08	0.52	22925	0.21	2.45	6.23	0.81	1078	27.15	22.12	7.63	2.58	1.88	1.26	883.4
05310	1.68	0.06	71.5	0.08	0.25	6.9	0.39	2.2	0.33	0.66	4.26	1.09	1.36	1.03	116.6
Poultry: Duck															
05140	2.6	0.32	294	0.24	0.38	6.76	0.25	8.4	0.42	0	39.69	13.54	18.06	5.11	117.6
05142	3.64	0.32	107.8	0.36	0.66	7.14	0.35	14	0.56	0	15.68	5.84	5.18	2	124.6
Poultry: Goose															
05147	3.67	0.37	98	0.11	0.45	5.84	0.52	2.8	0.57	0	30.69	9.62	14.35	3.53	127.4
05149	18.73	1.63	236.4	0.54	2.3	24.12	2.78	70.92	2.9	0	74.88	26.95	25.65	9.1	567.36
Poultry: Turkey															
05192	17.54	0.41	0	0.49	1.13	54.99	4.15	51.84	3.11	0	64.02	18.14	21.17	15.55	639.36
05194	23.31	0.84	0	0.33	1.32	19.44	1.8	49.14	1.97	0	53.62	16.71	15.67	14.85	464.1
05186	2.86	0.06	0	0.08	0.18	9.57	0.76	8.4	0.52	0	4.51	1.44	0.78	1.2	96.6
05188	6.24	0.22	0	0.09	0.35	5.11	0.5	12.6	0.52	0	10.11	3.39	2.29	3.02	119
Luncheon meat															
07007	0.5	0.01	0	0.01	0.03	0.55	0.03	1.15	0.33	0	6.56	2.78	3.17	0.25	13.34
07011	0.99	0.02	0	0.03	0.09	2	0.12	3.97	0.15	0	8.62	2.87	2.72	2.43	56.13
07017	0.41	0.02	46.49	0.04	0.07	3	0.12	1.13	0.09	0	4.18	1.15	1.68	0.91	28.35
07022	0.98	0.03	0	0.02	0.05	1.09	0.05	1.8	0.69	0	12.83	5.42	6.13	0.62	27.45
07024	0.47	0.02	58.5	0.03	0.05	1.39	0.14	1.8	0.11	0	8.77	2.49	3.82	1.82	45.45

NDB #	Description & Serving	Grams	Water	Calories	Protein	Carbohydrates	Fiber	Calcium	Phosphorus	Iron	Sodium	Potassium	Magnesium
			gm	kcal	gm	gm	gm	mg	mg	mg	mg	mg	mg
07025	**Frankfurter, turkey** 1 frankfurter	45	28.35	101.7	6.43	0.67	0	47.7	60.3	0.83	641.7	80.55	6.3
07028	**Ham, sliced, extra lean (approx 5% fat)** 1 slice (6-1/4" x 4" x 1/16")	28.35	19.99	37.14	5.49	0.27	0	1.98	61.8	0.22	405.12	99.23	4.82
07029	**Ham, sliced, reg (approx 11% fat)** 1 slice (6-1/4" x 4" x 1/16")	28.35	18.33	51.6	4.98	0.88	0	1.98	70.02	0.28	373.37	94.12	5.39
07069	**Salami, beef & pork** 1 slice (4" dia x 1/8" thick) (10 per 8 oz package)	23	13.89	57.5	3.2	0.52	0	2.99	26.45	0.61	244.95	45.54	3.45
07070	**Salami, cooked, turkey** 2 slices	56.7	37.34	111.13	9.28	0.31	0	11.34	60.1	0.91	569.27	138.35	8.51
07071	**Salami, dry or hard, pork** 1 slice (3-1/8" dia x 1/16" thick)	10	3.62	40.7	2.26	0.16	0	1.3	22.9	0.13	226	37.8	2.2
07079	**Turkey breast meat** 1 slice (3-1/2" square; 8 per 6 oz package)	21	15.09	23.1	4.73	0	0	1.47	48.09	0.08	300.51	58.38	4.2
07081	**Turkey roll, light meat** 2 slices	56.7	40.57	83.35	10.6	0.3	0	22.68	103.76	0.73	277.26	142.32	9.07
07082	**Turkey roll, light & dark meat** 2 slices	56.7	39.78	84.48	10.29	1.21	0	18.14	95.26	0.77	332.26	153.09	10.21
Nuts, seeds, and related products													
12061	**Almonds, dried, unblanched** 1 cup, sliced, unblanched	95	4.2	559.55	18.95	19.38	10.36	252.7	494	3.48	10.45	695.4	281.2
12063	**Almonds, dry roasted, unblanched, wo/salt** 1 cup whole kernels	138	4.14	810.06	22.54	33.35	18.91	389.16	756.24	5.24	15.18	1062.6	419.52
12065	**Almonds, oil roasted, unblanched, wo/salt** 1 cup whole kernels	157	4.84	970.26	32.01	24.93	17.58	367.38	858.79	6.01	15.7	1072.31	477.28
12078	**Brazil nuts, dried, unblanched** 1 cup, shelled (32 kernels)	140	4.68	918.4	20.08	17.92	7.56	246.4	840	4.76	2.8	840	315
12085	**Cashew nuts, dry roasted, wo/salt** 1 cup, halves and whole	137	2.33	786.38	20.97	44.79	4.11	61.65	671.3	8.22	21.92	774.05	356.2
12086	**Cashew nuts, oil roasted, wo/salt** 1 cup, halves and whole	130	5.08	748.8	21	37.08	4.94	53.3	553.8	5.33	22.1	689	331.5
12096	**Chestnuts, Chinese, roasted** 1 oz	28.35	11.4	67.76	1.27	14.84	0	5.39	28.92	0.43	1.13	135.23	25.52
12104	**Coconut meat, raw** 1 cup, shredded	80	37.59	283.2	2.66	12.18	7.2	11.2	90.4	1.94	16	284.8	25.6
12108	**Coconut meat, dried (desiccated), not sweetened** 1 oz	28.35	0.85	187.11	1.95	6.92	4.62	7.37	58.4	0.94	10.49	153.94	25.52
12115	**Coconut cream, raw (liquid expressed from grated meat)** 1 tablespoon	15	8.09	49.5	0.54	1	0.33	1.65	18.3	0.34	0.6	48.75	4.2
12121	**Filberts or hazelnuts, dried, blanched** 1 oz	28.35	0.54	190.51	3.61	4.53	1.81	55.28	91.57	0.96	0.85	130.98	83.92
12122	**Filberts or hazelnuts, dry roasted, unblanched, wo/salt** 1 oz	28.35	0.54	187.68	2.84	5.07	2.04	55.28	91.57	0.96	0.85	130.98	83.92
12123	**Filberts or hazelnuts, oil roasted, unblanched, wo/salt** 1 oz	28.35	0.34	187.11	4.04	5.43	1.81	55.57	92.42	0.97	0.85	131.83	84.48

NDB #	Zinc	Copper	Vitamin A	Thiamin	Riboflavin	Niacin	Vitamin B6	Folate	Vitamin B12	Vitamin C	Fat	Fat: Saturated	Fat: Monounsaturated	Fat: Polyunsaturated	Cholesterol
	mg	mg	IU	mg	mg	mg	mg	mcg	mcg	mg	gm	gm	gm	gm	mg
07025															
	1.4	0.05	0	0.02	0.08	1.86	0.1	3.6	0.13	0	7.97	2.65	2.51	2.25	48.15
07028															
	0.55	0.02	0	0.26	0.06	1.37	0.13	1.13	0.21	0	1.41	0.46	0.67	0.14	13.32
07029															
	0.61	0.03	0	0.24	0.07	1.49	0.1	0.85	0.24	0	3	0.96	1.4	0.34	16.16
07069															
	0.49	0.05	0	0.05	0.09	0.82	0.05	0.46	0.84	0	4.63	1.86	2.11	0.46	14.95
07070															
	1.03	0.03	0	0.04	0.1	2	0.14	2.27	0.12	0	7.82	2.28	2.58	2	46.49
07071															
	0.42	0.02	0	0.09	0.03	0.56	0.06	0.2	0.28	0	3.37	1.19	1.6	0.37	7.9
07079															
	0.24	0.01	0	0.01	0.02	1.75	0.08	0.84	0.42	0	0.33	0.1	0.09	0.06	8.61
07081															
	0.88	0.02	0	0.05	0.13	3.97	0.18	2.27	0.14	0	4.09	1.15	1.42	0.99	24.38
07082															
	1.13	0.04	0	0.05	0.16	2.72	0.15	2.84	0.13	0	3.96	1.16	1.3	1.01	31.19

Nuts, seeds, and related products

NDB #	Zinc	Copper	Vitamin A	Thiamin	Riboflavin	Niacin	Vitamin B6	Folate	Vitamin B12	Vitamin C	Fat	Fat: Saturated	Fat: Monounsaturated	Fat: Polyunsaturated	Cholesterol
12061															
	2.77	0.89	0	0.2	0.74	3.19	0.11	55.77	0	0.57	49.6	4.7	32.21	10.41	0
12063															
	6.76	1.69	0	0.18	0.83	3.89	0.1	88.04	0	0.97	71.21	6.75	46.24	14.94	0
12065															
	7.69	1.92	0	0.2	1.55	5.5	0.13	100.17	0	1.1	90.54	8.58	58.79	19	0
12078															
	6.43	2.48	0	1.4	0.17	2.27	0.35	5.6	0	0.98	92.71	22.62	32.22	33.78	0
12085															
	7.67	3.04	0	0.27	0.27	1.92	0.35	94.8	0	0	63.5	12.66	37.42	10.74	0
12086															
	6.18	2.82	0	0.55	0.23	2.34	0.33	88.01	0	0	62.67	12.38	36.94	10.6	0
12096															
	0.17	0.07	39.12	0.03	0.03	0.16	0.08	13.15	0	7	0.22	0.03	0.11	0.06	0
12104															
	0.88	0.35	0	0.05	0.02	0.43	0.04	21.12	0	2.64	26.79	23.76	1.14	0.29	0
12108															
	0.57	0.23	0	0.02	0.03	0.17	0.09	2.55	0	0.43	18.29	16.22	0.78	0.2	0
12115															
	0.14	0.06	0	0	0	0.13	0.01	3.45	0	0.42	5.2	4.61	0.22	0.06	0
12121															
	0.71	0.44	19.56	0.15	0.03	0.33	0.18	21.12	0	0.28	19.08	1.4	14.95	1.83	0
12122															
	0.71	0.44	19.56	0.06	0.06	0.79	0.18	21.12	0	0.28	18.8	1.38	14.73	1.8	0
12123															
	0.71	0.45	19.85	0.06	0.06	0.79	0.18	21.29	0	0.28	18.03	1.33	14.13	1.73	0

NDB #	Description & Serving	Grams	Water	Calories	Protein	Carbohydrates	Fiber	Calcium	Phosphorus	Iron	Sodium	Potassium	Magnesium
		gm	gm	kcal	gm	gm	gm	mg	mg	mg	mg	mg	mg
12131	Macadamia nuts, dried 1 oz (11 whole kernels)	28.35	0.82	199.02	2.35	3.89	2.64	19.85	38.56	0.68	1.42	104.33	32.89
12133	Macadamia nuts, oil roasted, wo/salt 1 cup, whole or halves	134	2.24	962.12	9.73	17.29	12.46	60.3	268	2.41	9.38	440.86	156.78
09193	Olives, ripe, canned (small-extra lrg) 1 large	4.4	3.52	5.06	0.04	0.28	0.14	3.87	0.13	0.15	38.37	0.35	0.18
09194	Olives, ripe, canned (jumbo-super colossal) 1 jumbo	8.3	7	6.72	0.08	0.47	0.21	7.8	0.25	0.28	74.53	0.75	0.33
12143	Pecans, dry roasted, wo/salt 1 oz	28.35	0.31	186.83	2.26	6.33	2.64	9.92	86.18	0.62	0.28	104.9	37.71
12144	Pecans, oil roasted, wo/salt 1 oz (15 halves)	28.35	1.19	194.2	1.97	4.55	1.9	9.64	83.35	0.6	0.28	101.78	36.57
12152	Pistachio nuts, dry roasted, wo/salt 1 cup	128	2.68	775.68	19.11	35.24	13.82	89.6	609.28	4.06	7.68	1241.6	166.4
02033	Poppy seed 1 teaspoon	2.8	0.19	14.93	0.51	0.66	0.28	40.56	23.76	0.26	0.59	19.59	9.28
12166	Sesame butter, tahini, from roasted & toasted kernels (most common type) 1 tablespoon	15	0.46	89.25	2.55	3.18	1.4	63.9	109.8	1.34	17.25	62.1	14.25
12537	Sunflower seed kernels, dry roasted, w/salt 1 cup	128	1.54	744.96	24.74	30.81	11.52	89.6	1478.4	4.86	998.4	1088	165.12
12023	Sesame seeds, whole, dried 1 tablespoon	9	0.42	51.57	1.6	2.11	1.06	87.75	56.61	1.31	0.99	42.12	31.59
12036	Sunflower seed kernels, dried 1 cup, with hulls, edible yield	46	2.47	262.2	10.48	8.63	4.83	53.36	324.3	3.11	1.38	316.94	162.84
12154	Walnuts, black, dried 1 cup, chopped	125	5.45	758.75	30.44	15.13	6.25	72.5	580	3.84	1.25	655	252.5

Seafood

Fish

NDB #	Description & Serving	Grams	Water	Calories	Protein	Carbohydrates	Fiber	Calcium	Phosphorus	Iron	Sodium	Potassium	Magnesium
15187	Bass, freshwater, mxd sp, cooked, dry heat 3 oz	85	58.47	124.1	20.55	0	0	87.55	217.6	1.62	76.5	387.6	32.3
15188	Bass, striped, cooked, dry heat 3 oz	85	62.36	105.4	19.32	0	0	16.15	215.9	0.92	74.8	278.8	43.35
15189	Bluefish, cooked, dry heat 3 oz	85	53.24	135.15	21.84	0	0	7.65	247.35	0.53	65.45	405.45	35.7
15009	Carp, cooked, dry heat 3 oz	85	59.19	137.7	19.43	0	0	44.2	451.35	1.35	53.55	362.95	32.3
15235	Catfish, channel, farmed, cooked, dry heat 3 oz	85	60.84	129.2	15.91	0	0	7.65	208.25	0.7	68	272.85	22.1
15012	Caviar, black & red, granular 1 tablespoon	16	7.6	40.32	3.94	0.64	0	44	56.96	1.9	240	28.96	48
15016	Cod, Atlantic, cooked, dry heat 3 oz	85	64.53	89.25	19.41	0	0	11.9	117.3	0.42	66.3	207.4	35.7
15192	Cod, Pacific, cooked, dry heat 3 oz	85	64.6	89.25	19.51	0	0	7.65	189.55	0.28	77.35	439.45	26.35
15229	Cuttlefish, mixed species, cooked, moist heat 3 oz	85	51.95	134.3	27.61	1.39	0	153	493	9.21	632.4	541.45	51
15194	Dolphinfish, cooked, dry heat 3 oz	85	60.54	92.65	20.16	0	0	16.15	155.55	1.23	96.05	453.05	32.3

NDB #	Zinc	Copper	Vitamin A	Thiamin	Riboflavin	Niacin	Vitamin B6	Folate	Vitamin B12	Vitamin C	Fat	Fat: Saturated	Fat: Monounsaturated	Fat: Polyunsaturated	Cholesterol
	mg	mg	IU	mg	mg	mg	mg	mcg	mcg	mg	gm	gm	gm	gm	mg
12131	0.48	0.08	0	0.1	0.03	0.61	0.06	4.45	0	0	20.9	3.13	16.49	0.36	0
12133	1.47	0.4	12.06	0.29	0.15	2.71	0.27	21.31	0	0	102.54	15.35	80.91	1.77	0
09193	0.01	0.01	17.73	0	0	0	0	0	0	0.04	0.47	0.06	0.35	0.04	0
09194	0.02	0.02	28.72	0	0	0	0	0	0	0.12	0.57	0.08	0.42	0.05	0
12143	1.61	0.35	37.71	0.09	0.03	0.26	0.06	11.54	0	0.57	18.31	1.47	11.42	4.53	0
12144	1.56	0.34	36.57	0.09	0.03	0.25	0.05	11.17	0	0.57	20.19	1.62	12.58	5	0
12152	1.74	1.55	304.64	0.54	0.31	1.8	0.33	75.65	0	9.34	67.61	8.56	45.64	10.22	0
02033	0.29	0.05	0	0.02	0	0.03	0.01	1.62	0	0.08	1.25	0.14	0.18	0.86	0
12166	0.69	0.24	10.05	0.18	0.07	0.82	0.02	14.66	0	0	8.06	1.13	3.05	3.53	0
12537	6.77	2.34	0	0.14	0.31	9.01	1.03	303.87	0	1.79	63.74	6.68	12.17	42.09	0
12023	0.7	0.37	0.81	0.07	0.02	0.41	0.07	8.7	0	0	4.47	0.63	1.69	1.96	0
12036	2.33	0.81	23	1.05	0.12	2.07	0.35	104.6	0	0.64	22.8	2.39	4.35	15.06	0
12154	4.28	1.28	370	0.27	0.14	0.86	0.69	81.88	0	4	70.73	4.54	15.91	46.87	0

Seafood
Fish

NDB #	Zinc	Copper	Vitamin A	Thiamin	Riboflavin	Niacin	Vitamin B6	Folate	Vitamin B12	Vitamin C	Fat	Fat: Saturated	Fat: Monounsaturated	Fat: Polyunsaturated	Cholesterol
15187	0.71	0.1	97.75	0.07	0.08	1.29	0.12	14.45	1.96	1.79	4.02	0.85	1.56	1.16	73.95
15188	0.43	0.03	88.4	0.1	0.03	2.17	0.29	8.5	3.75	0	2.54	0.55	0.72	0.85	87.55
15189	0.88	0.06	390.15	0.06	0.08	6.16	0.39	1.7	5.29	0	4.62	1	1.95	1.15	64.6
15009	1.62	0.06	27.2	0.12	0.06	1.79	0.19	14.71	1.25	1.36	6.09	1.18	2.54	1.56	71.4
15235	0.89	0.1	42.5	0.36	0.06	2.14	0.14	5.95	2.38	0.68	6.82	1.52	3.53	1.18	54.4
15012	0.15	0.02	298.88	0.03	0.1	0.02	0.05	8	3.2	0	2.86	0.65	0.74	1.18	94.08
15016	0.49	0.03	39.1	0.07	0.07	2.14	0.24	6.89	0.89	0.85	0.73	0.14	0.11	0.25	46.75
15192	0.43	0.03	27.2	0.02	0.04	2.11	0.39	6.8	0.88	2.55	0.69	0.09	0.09	0.27	39.95
15229	2.94	0.85	573.75	0.01	1.47	1.86	0.23	20.4	4.59	7.23	1.19	0.2	0.14	0.23	190.4
15194	0.5	0.05	176.8	0.02	0.07	6.31	0.39	5.1	0.59	0	0.77	0.2	0.13	0.18	79.9

NDB #	Description & Serving	Grams	Water	Calories	Protein	Carbohydrates	Fiber	Calcium	Phosphorus	Iron	Sodium	Potassium	Magnesium
			gm	kcal	gm	gm	gm	mg	mg	mg	mg	mg	mg
15195	Drum, freshwater, cooked, dry heat 3 oz	85	60.3	130.05	19.12	0	0	65.45	196.35	0.98	81.6	300.05	32.3
15026	Eel, mixed species, cooked, dry heat 1 oz, boneless	28.35	16.81	66.91	6.7	0	0	7.37	78.53	0.18	18.43	98.94	7.37
15029	Flatfish (flounder & sole species), cooked, dry heat 3 oz	85	62.19	99.45	20.54	0	0	15.3	245.65	0.29	89.25	292.4	49.3
15032	Grouper, mixed species, cooked, dry heat 3 oz	85	62.36	100.3	21.11	0	0	17.85	121.55	0.97	45.05	403.75	31.45
15034	Haddock, cooked, dry heat 3 oz	85	63.11	95.2	20.6	0	0	35.7	204.85	1.15	73.95	339.15	42.5
15035	Haddock, smoked 1 oz, boneless	28.35	20.26	32.89	7.15	0	0	13.89	71.16	0.4	216.31	117.65	15.31
15037	Halibut, Atlantic & Pacific, cooked, dry heat 3 oz	85	60.94	119	22.69	0	0	51	242.25	0.91	58.65	489.6	90.95
15041	Herring, Atlantic, pickled 1 oz, boneless	28.35	15.65	74.28	4.02	2.73	0	21.83	25.23	0.35	246.65	19.56	2.27
15042	Herring, Atlantic, kippered 1 oz, boneless	28.35	16.92	61.52	6.97	0	0	23.81	92.14	0.43	260.25	126.72	13.04
15047	Mackerel, Atlantic, cooked, dry heat 3 oz	85	45.28	222.7	20.27	0	0	12.75	236.3	1.33	70.55	340.85	82.45
15201	Mackerel, Pacific & jack, mixed species, cooked, dry heat 1 oz, boneless	28.35	17.5	56.98	7.29	0	0	8.22	45.36	0.42	31.19	147.7	10.21
15203	Monkfish, cooked, dry heat 3 oz	85	66.73	82.45	15.78	0	0	8.5	217.6	0.35	19.55	436.05	22.95
15056	Mullet, striped, cooked, dry heat 3 oz	85	59.94	127.5	21.09	0	0	26.35	207.4	1.2	60.35	389.3	28.05
15061	Perch, mixed species, cooked, dry heat 3 oz	85	62.26	99.45	21.13	0	0	86.7	218.45	0.99	67.15	292.4	32.3
15063	Pike, northern, cooked, dry heat 3 oz	85	62.02	96.05	20.99	0	0	62.05	239.7	0.6	41.65	281.35	34
15204	Pike, walleye, cooked, dry heat 3 oz	85	62.45	101.15	20.86	0	0	119.85	228.65	1.42	55.25	424.15	32.3
15205	Pollock, Atlantic, cooked, dry heat 3 oz	85	61.23	100.3	21.18	0	0	65.45	240.55	0.5	93.5	387.6	73.1
15067	Pollock, walleye, cooked, dry heat 3 oz	85	62.95	96.05	19.98	0	0	5.1	409.7	0.24	98.6	328.95	62.05
15069	Pompano, Florida, cooked, dry heat 3 oz	85	53.52	179.35	20.14	0	0	36.55	289.85	0.57	64.6	540.6	26.35
15207	Roe, mixed species, cooked, dry heat 1 oz	28.35	16.62	57.83	8.11	0.54	0	7.94	146	0.22	33.17	80.23	7.37
15232	Roughy, orange, cooked, dry heat 3 oz	85	58.74	75.65	16.02	0	0	32.3	217.6	0.2	68.85	327.25	32.3
15075	Sablefish, smoked 3 oz	85	51.12	218.45	15	0	0	42.5	188.7	1.44	626.45	400.35	62.9
15179	Salmon, chinook, smoked (lox), reg 3 oz	85	61.2	99.45	15.54	0	0	9.35	139.4	0.72	1700	148.75	15.3
15209	Salmon, Atlantic, wild, cooked, dry heat 3 oz	85	50.68	154.7	21.62	0	0	12.75	217.6	0.88	47.6	533.8	31.45

NDB #	Zinc	Copper	Vitamin A	Thiamin	Riboflavin	Niacin	Vitamin B6	Folate	Vitamin B12	Vitamin C	Fat	Fat: Saturated	Fat: Monounsaturated	Fat: Polyunsaturated	Cholesterol
	mg	mg	IU	mg	mg	mg	mg	mcg	mcg	mg	gm	gm	gm	gm	mg
15195	0.72	0.25	166.6	0.07	0.18	2.43	0.29	14.45	1.96	0.85	5.37	1.22	2.39	1.26	69.7
15026	0.59	0.01	1073.61	0.05	0.01	1.27	0.02	4.9	0.82	0.51	4.24	0.86	2.61	0.34	45.64
15029	0.54	0.02	32.3	0.07	0.1	1.85	0.2	7.82	2.13	0	1.3	0.31	0.2	0.55	57.8
15032	0.43	0.04	140.25	0.07	0.01	0.32	0.3	8.67	0.59	0	1.11	0.25	0.23	0.34	39.95
15034	0.41	0.03	53.55	0.03	0.04	3.94	0.29	11.31	1.18	0	0.79	0.14	0.13	0.26	62.9
15035	0.14	0.01	20.7	0.01	0.01	1.44	0.11	4.34	0.45	0	0.27	0.05	0.04	0.09	21.83
15037	0.45	0.03	152.15	0.06	0.08	6.05	0.34	11.73	1.16	0	2.5	0.35	0.82	0.8	34.85
15041	0.15	0.03	244.09	0.01	0.04	0.94	0.05	0.68	1.21	0	5.1	0.68	3.39	0.48	3.69
15042	0.39	0.04	36.29	0.04	0.09	1.25	0.12	3.88	5.3	0.28	3.51	0.79	1.45	0.83	23.25
15047	0.8	0.08	153	0.14	0.35	5.82	0.39	1.28	16.15	0.34	15.14	3.55	5.96	3.66	63.75
15201	0.24	0.03	13.32	0.04	0.15	3.02	0.11	0.57	1.2	0.6	2.87	0.82	0.96	0.71	17.01
15203	0.45	0.03	39.1	0.02	0.06	2.17	0.24	6.8	0.88	0.85	1.66	0	0	0	27.2
15056	0.75	0.12	119.85	0.09	0.09	5.36	0.42	8.33	0.21	1.02	4.13	1.22	1.17	0.78	53.55
15061	1.22	0.16	27.2	0.07	0.1	1.62	0.12	4.93	1.87	1.45	1	0.2	0.17	0.4	97.75
15063	0.73	0.06	68.85	0.06	0.07	2.38	0.11	14.71	1.96	3.23	0.75	0.13	0.17	0.22	42.5
15204	0.67	0.19	68.85	0.27	0.17	2.38	0.12	14.45	1.96	0	1.33	0.27	0.32	0.49	93.5
15205	0.51	0.05	34	0.05	0.19	3.39	0.28	2.55	3.13	0	1.07	0.14	0.12	0.53	77.35
15067	0.51	0.05	64.6	0.06	0.06	1.4	0.06	3.06	3.57	0	0.95	0.2	0.15	0.45	81.6
15069	0.59	0.07	102	0.58	0.13	3.23	0.2	14.71	1.02	0	10.32	3.82	2.82	1.24	54.4
15207	0.36	0.04	85.9	0.08	0.27	0.62	0.05	26.08	3.27	4.65	2.33	0.53	0.6	0.97	135.8
15232	0.82	0.15	68.85	0.1	0.16	3.11	0.29	6.8	1.96	0	0.77	0.02	0.52	0.01	22.1
15075	0.37	0.03	346.8	0.11	0.1	4.51	0.33	16.75	1.7	0	17.12	3.58	9.01	2.28	54.4
15179	0.26	0.2	74.8	0.02	0.09	4.01	0.24	1.62	2.77	0	3.67	0.79	1.72	0.85	19.55
15209	0.7	0.27	37.4	0.23	0.41	8.57	0.8	24.65	2.59	0	6.91	1.07	2.29	2.77	60.35

NDB #	Description & Serving	Grams	Water	Calories	Protein	Carbohydrates	Fiber	Calcium	Phosphorus	Iron	Sodium	Potassium	Magnesium
			gm	kcal	gm	gm	gm	mg	mg	mg	mg	mg	mg
15210	Salmon, chinook, cooked, dry heat 3 oz	85	55.76	196.35	21.86	0	0	23.8	315.35	0.77	51	429.25	103.7
15211	Salmon, chum, cooked, dry heat 3 oz	85	58.17	130.9	21.95	0	0	11.9	308.55	0.6	54.4	467.5	23.8
15212	Salmon, pink, cooked, dry heat 3 oz	85	59.23	126.65	21.73	0	0	14.45	250.75	0.84	73.1	351.9	28.05
15086	Salmon, sockeye, cooked, dry heat 3 oz	85	52.56	183.6	23.21	0	0	5.95	234.6	0.47	56.1	318.75	26.35
15088	Sardine, Atlantic, canned in oil, drained solids w/bone 1 oz	28.35	16.9	58.97	6.98	0	0	108.3	138.92	0.83	143.17	112.55	11.06
15092	Sea bass, mixed species, cooked, dry heat 3 oz	85	61.32	105.4	20.09	0	0	11.05	210.8	0.31	73.95	278.8	45.05
15215	Shad, American, cooked, dry heat 3 oz	85	50.34	214.2	18.45	0	0	51	296.65	1.05	55.25	418.2	32.3
15100	Smelt, rainbow, cooked, dry heat 3 oz	85	61.87	105.4	19.21	0	0	65.45	250.75	0.98	65.45	316.2	32.3
15102	Snapper, mixed species, cooked, dry heat 3 oz	85	59.8	108.8	22.36	0	0	34	170.85	0.2	48.45	443.7	31.45
15106	Sturgeon, mixed species, smoked 3 oz	85	53.13	147.05	26.52	0	0	14.45	238.85	0.79	628.15	322.15	39.95
15109	Surimi 3 oz	85	64.89	84.15	12.9	5.82	0	7.65	239.7	0.22	121.55	95.2	36.55
15111	Swordfish, cooked, dry heat 3 oz	85	58.44	131.75	21.58	0	0	5.1	286.45	0.88	97.75	313.65	28.9
15116	Trout, rainbow, wild, cooked, dry heat 3 oz	85	59.93	127.5	19.48	0	0	73.1	228.65	0.32	47.6	380.8	26.35
15118	Tuna, fresh, bluefin, cooked, dry heat 3 oz	85	50.23	156.4	25.42	0	0	8.5	277.1	1.11	42.5	274.55	54.4
15119	Tuna, light, canned in oil, drained solids 3 oz	85	50.85	168.3	24.76	0	0	11.05	264.35	1.18	300.9	175.95	26.35
15121	Tuna, light, canned in water, drained solids 3 oz	85	63.33	98.6	21.68	0	0	9.35	138.55	1.3	287.3	201.45	22.95
15124	Tuna, white, canned in oil, drained solids 3 oz	85	54.42	158.1	22.55	0	0	3.4	226.95	0.55	336.6	283.05	28.9
15126	Tuna, white, canned in water, drained solids 3 oz	85	62.21	108.8	20.08	0	0	11.9	184.45	0.83	320.45	201.45	28.05
15221	Tuna, yellowfin, fresh, cooked, dry heat 3 oz	85	53.39	118.15	25.47	0	0	17.85	208.25	0.8	39.95	483.65	54.4
15222	Turbot, European, cooked, dry heat 3 oz	85	59.88	103.7	17.49	0	0	19.55	140.25	0.39	163.2	259.25	55.25
15131	Whitefish, mixed species, smoked 1 oz, boneless	28.35	20.08	30.62	6.63	0	0	5.1	37.42	0.14	288.89	119.92	6.52
Shellfish													
15156	Abalone, mixed species, cooked, fried 3 oz	85	51.09	160.65	16.69	9.39	0	31.45	184.45	3.23	502.35	241.4	47.6
15159	Clam, mixed species, cooked, moist heat 20 small clams	190	120.92	281.2	48.55	9.75	0	174.8	642.2	53.12	212.8	1193.2	34.2

NDB #	Zinc	Copper	Vitamin A	Thiamin	Riboflavin	Niacin	Vitamin B6	Folate	Vitamin B12	Vitamin C	Fat	Fat: Saturated	Fat: Monounsaturated	Fat: Polyunsaturated	Cholesterol
	mg	mg	IU	mg	mg	mg	mg	mcg	mcg	mg	gm	gm	gm	gm	mg
15210	0.48	0.05	421.6	0.04	0.13	8.54	0.39	29.75	2.44	3.49	11.37	2.73	4.88	2.26	72.25
15211	0.51	0.06	96.9	0.08	0.19	7.25	0.39	4.25	2.94	0	4.11	0.92	1.68	0.98	80.75
15212	0.6	0.08	115.6	0.17	0.06	7.25	0.2	4.25	2.94	0	3.76	0.61	1.02	1.47	56.95
15086	0.43	0.06	177.65	0.18	0.15	5.67	0.19	4.25	4.93	0	9.32	1.63	4.5	2.05	73.95
15088	0.37	0.05	63.5	0.02	0.06	1.49	0.05	3.35	2.53	0	3.25	0.43	1.1	1.46	40.26
15092	0.44	0.02	181.05	0.11	0.13	1.62	0.39	4.93	0.26	0	2.18	0.56	0.46	0.81	45.05
15215	0.4	0.07	102	0.16	0.26	9.15	0.39	14.45	0.12	0	15	0	0	0	81.6
15100	1.8	0.15	49.3	0.01	0.12	1.5	0.14	3.91	3.37	0	2.64	0.49	0.7	0.96	76.5
15102	0.37	0.04	97.75	0.05	0	0.29	0.39	4.93	2.98	1.36	1.46	0.31	0.27	0.5	39.95
15106	0.48	0.04	793.05	0.08	0.08	9.44	0.23	17	2.47	0	3.74	0.88	2	0.37	68
15109	0.28	0.03	56.1	0.02	0.02	0.19	0.03	1.36	1.36	0	0.77	0.15	0.12	0.39	25.5
15111	1.25	0.14	116.45	0.04	0.1	10.02	0.32	1.96	1.72	0.94	4.37	1.2	1.68	1	42.5
15116	0.43	0.05	42.5	0.13	0.08	4.9	0.29	16.15	5.36	1.7	4.95	1.38	1.48	1.56	58.65
15118	0.65	0.09	2142	0.24	0.26	8.96	0.45	1.87	9.25	0	5.34	1.37	1.75	1.57	41.65
15119	0.77	0.06	66.3	0.03	0.1	10.54	0.09	4.51	1.87	0	6.98	1.3	2.51	2.45	15.3
15121	0.66	0.04	47.6	0.03	0.06	11.29	0.3	3.4	2.54	0	0.68	0.2	0.14	0.29	25.5
15124	0.40	0.11	68	0.01	0.07	9.94	0.37	3.91	1.87	0	6.87	1.4	2.11	2.87	26.35
15126	0.41	0.03	16.15	0.01	0.04	4.93	0.18	1.7	0.99	0	2.53	0.67	0.67	0.94	35.7
15221	0.57	0.07	57.8	0.43	0.05	10.15	0.88	1.7	0.51	0.85	1.04	0.26	0.17	0.31	49.3
15222	0.24	0.04	34	0.06	0.08	2.28	0.21	7.65	2.16	1.45	3.21	0	0	0	52.7
15131	0.14	0.09	53.87	0.01	0.03	0.68	0.11	2.07	0.92	0	0.26	0.06	0.08	0.08	9.36
Shellfish															
15156	0.81	0.19	4.25	0.19	0.11	1.62	0.13	4.59	0.59	1.53	5.76	1.4	2.33	1.42	79.9
15159	5.19	1.31	1083	0.29	0.81	6.37	0.21	54.72	187.89	41.99	3.71	0.36	0.33	1.05	127.3

NDB #	Description & Serving	Grams	Water	Calories	Protein	Carbohydrates	Fiber	Calcium	Phosphorus	Iron	Sodium	Potassium	Magnesium
		gm	gm	kcal	gm	gm	gm	mg	mg	mg	mg	mg	mg
15137	Crab, Alaska king, cooked, moist heat 1 leg	134	103.92	129.98	25.93	0	0	79.06	375.2	1.02	1436.48	351.08	84.42
15140	Crab, blue, cooked, moist heat 1 cup (not packed)	135	104.53	137.7	27.27	0	0	140.4	278.1	1.23	376.65	437.4	44.55
15226	Crab, dungeness, cooked, moist heat 1 crab	127	93.1	139.7	28.35	1.21	0	74.93	222.25	0.55	480.06	518.16	73.66
15227	Crab, queen, cooked, moist heat 3 oz	85	63.84	97.75	20.16	0	0	28.05	108.8	2.45	587.35	170	53.55
15243	Crayfish, mixed species, farmed, cooked, moist heat 3 oz	85	68.68	73.95	14.89	0	0	43.35	204.85	0.94	82.45	202.3	28.05
15148	Lobster, northern, cooked, moist heat 3 oz	85	64.63	83.3	17.43	1.09	0	51.85	157.25	0.33	323	299.2	29.75
15165	Mussel, blue, cooked, moist heat 3 oz	85	51.98	146.2	20.23	6.28	0	28.05	242.25	5.71	313.65	227.8	31.45
15167	Oyster, eastern, wild, raw 6 medium	84	71.53	57.12	5.92	3.28	0	37.8	113.4	5.59	177.24	131.04	39.48
15169	Oyster, eastern, wild, cooked, moist heat 6 medium	42	29.53	57.54	5.92	3.28	0	37.8	85.26	5.04	177.24	118.02	39.9
15244	Oyster, eastern, wild, cooked, dry heat 6 medium	59	49.15	42.48	4.87	2.83	0	26.55	80.24	2.55	143.96	99.12	27.14
15171	Oyster, Pacific, raw 3 oz	85	69.75	68.85	8.03	4.21	0	6.8	137.7	4.34	90.1	142.8	18.7
15231	Oyster, Pacific, cooked, moist heat 3 oz	85	54.5	138.55	16.07	8.42	0	13.6	206.55	7.82	180.2	256.7	37.4
15173	Scallop, mixed species, cooked, breaded & fried 2 large scallops	31	18.12	66.65	5.6	3.14	0	13.02	73.16	0.25	143.84	103.23	18.29
15151	Shrimp, mixed species, cooked, moist heat 4 large	22	17	21.78	4.6	0	0	8.58	30.14	0.68	49.28	40.04	7.48
15176	Squid, mixed species, cooked, fried 3 oz	85	54.86	148.75	15.25	6.62	0	33.15	213.35	0.86	260.1	237.15	32.3
Vegetables and vegetable juices													
11008	Artichokes (globe or French), cooked, boiled, drained, wo/salt 1 medium artichoke	120	100.76	60	4.18	13.42	6.48	54	103.2	1.55	114	424.8	72
11011	Asparagus, raw 1 small spear (5" long or less)	12	11.09	2.76	0.27	0.54	0.25	2.52	6.72	0.1	0.24	32.76	2.16
11027	Bamboo shoots, cooked, boiled, drained, wo/salt 1 cup (1/2" slices)	120	115.1	14.4	1.84	2.3	1.2	14.4	24	0.29	4.8	639.6	3.6
11053	Beans, snap, green, cooked, boiled, drained, wo/salt 1 cup	125	111.53	43.75	2.36	9.86	4	57.5	48.75	1.6	3.75	373.75	31.25
11081	Beets, cooked, boiled, drained 1/2 cup slices	85	74	37.4	1.43	8.47	1.7	13.6	32.3	0.67	65.45	259.25	19.55
11090	Broccoli, raw 1 cup, flowerets	71	64.39	19.88	2.12	3.72	2.13	34.08	46.86	0.62	19.17	230.75	17.75
11099	Brussels sprouts, cooked, boiled, drained, wo/salt 1/2 cup	78	68.11	30.42	1.99	6.76	2.03	28.08	43.68	0.94	16.38	247.26	15.6
11109	Cabbage, raw 1 cup, shredded	70	64.51	17.5	1.01	3.8	1.61	32.9	16.1	0.41	12.6	172.2	10.5

NDB #	Zinc	Copper	Vitamin A	Thiamin	Riboflavin	Niacin	Vitamin B6	Folate	Vitamin B12	Vitamin C	Fat	Fat: Saturated	Fat: Monounsaturated	Fat: Polyunsaturated	Cholesterol
	mg	mg	IU	mg	mg	mg	mg	mcg	mcg	mg	gm	gm	gm	gm	mg
15137	10.21	1.58	38.86	0.07	0.07	1.8	0.24	68.34	15.41	10.18	2.06	0.18	0.25	0.72	71.02
15140	5.7	0.87	8.1	0.14	0.07	4.46	0.24	68.58	9.86	4.46	2.39	0.31	0.38	0.92	135
15226	6.95	0.93	132.08	0.07	0.26	4.6	0.22	53.34	13.18	4.57	1.57	0.21	0.27	0.52	96.52
15227	3.05	0.53	147.05	0.08	0.21	2.45	0.15	35.7	8.82	6.12	1.28	0.16	0.28	0.46	60.35
15243	1.26	0.49	42.5	0.04	0.07	1.42	0.11	9.35	2.64	0.43	1.11	0.18	0.21	0.35	116.45
15148	2.48	1.65	73.95	0.01	0.06	0.91	0.07	9.44	2.64	0	0.5	0.09	0.14	0.08	61.2
15165	2.27	0.13	258.4	0.26	0.36	2.55	0.09	64.26	20.4	11.56	3.81	0.72	0.86	1.03	47.6
15167	76.28	3.74	84	0.08	0.08	1.16	0.05	8.4	16.35	3.11	2.07	0.65	0.26	0.81	44.52
15169	76.28	3.18	75.6	0.08	0.08	1.04	0.05	5.88	14.71	2.52	2.06	0.65	0.26	0.81	44.1
15244	43.42	2.04	0	0.05	0.05	0.99	0.06	10.62	16.4	2.42	1.12	0.32	0.14	0.48	28.91
15171	14.13	1.34	229.5	0.06	0.2	1.71	0.04	8.5	13.6	6.8	1.96	0.43	0.3	0.76	42.5
15231	28.25	2.28	413.1	0.11	0.38	3.08	0.08	12.75	24.48	10.88	3.91	0.87	0.61	1.52	85
15173	0.33	0.02	23.25	0.01	0.03	0.47	0.04	5.64	0.41	0.71	3.39	0.83	1.39	0.89	18.91
15151	0.34	0.04	48.18	0.01	0.01	0.57	0.03	0.77	0.33	0.48	0.24	0.06	0.04	0.1	42.9
15176	1.48	1.8	29.75	0.05	0.39	2.21	0.05	4.51	1.04	3.57	6.36	1.6	2.34	1.82	221

Vegetables and vegetable juices

NDB #	Zinc	Copper	Vitamin A	Thiamin	Riboflavin	Niacin	Vitamin B6	Folate	Vitamin B12	Vitamin C	Fat	Fat: Saturated	Fat: Monounsaturated	Fat: Polyunsaturated	Cholesterol
11008	0.59	0.28	212.4	0.08	0.08	1.2	0.13	61.2	0	12	0.19	0.04	0.01	0.08	0
11011	0.06	0.02	69.96	0.02	0.02	0.14	0.02	15.36	0	1.58	0.02	0.01	0	0.01	0
11027	0.56	0.1	0	0.02	0.06	0.36	0.12	2.76	0	0	0.26	0.06	0.01	0.12	0
11053	0.45	0.13	832.5	0.09	0.12	0.77	0.07	41.63	0	12.13	0.35	0.08	0.01	0.18	0
11081	0.3	0.06	29.75	0.02	0.03	0.28	0.06	68	0	3.06	0.15	0.02	0.03	0.05	0
11090	0.28	0.03	1094.82	0.05	0.08	0.45	0.11	50.41	0	66.17	0.25	0.04	0.02	0.12	0
11099	0.26	0.06	560.82	0.08	0.06	0.47	0.14	46.8	0	48.36	0.4	0.08	0.03	0.2	0
11109	0.13	0.02	93.1	0.04	0.03	0.21	0.07	30.1	0	22.54	0.19	0.02	0.01	0.09	0

NDB #	Description & Serving	Grams	Water	Calories	Protein	Carbohydrates	Fiber	Calcium	Phosphorus	Iron	Sodium	Potassium	Magnesium
		gm	gm	kcal	gm	gm	gm	mg	mg	mg	mg	mg	mg
11110	Cabbage, cooked, boiled, drained, wo/salt 1/2 cup shredded	75	70.2	16.5	0.77	3.35	1.73	23.25	11.25	0.13	6	72.75	6
11112	Cabbage, red, raw 1 cup, shredded	70	64.09	18.9	0.97	4.28	1.4	35.7	29.4	0.34	7.7	144.2	10.5
11113	Cabbage, red, cooked, boiled, drained, wo/salt 1/2 cup shredded	75	70.2	15.75	0.79	3.48	1.5	27.75	21.75	0.26	6	105	8.25
11115	Cabbage, savoy, cooked, boiled, drained, wo/salt 1 cup, shredded	145	133.4	34.8	2.61	7.84	4.06	43.5	47.85	0.55	34.8	266.8	34.8
11117	Cabbage, Chinese (pak-choi), cooked, boiled, drained, wo/salt 1 cup, shredded	170	162.44	20.4	2.65	3.03	2.72	158.1	49.3	1.77	57.8	630.7	18.7
11124	Carrots, raw 1 cup, grated	110	96.57	47.3	1.13	11.15	3.3	29.7	48.4	0.55	38.5	355.3	16.5
11960	Carrots, baby, raw 1 medium	10	8.98	3.8	0.08	0.82	0.18	2.3	3.8	0.08	3.5	27.9	1.2
11125	Carrots, cooked, boiled, drained, wo/salt 1/2 cup slices	78	68.16	35.1	0.85	8.17	2.57	24.18	23.4	0.48	51.48	177.06	10.14
11135	Cauliflower, raw 1 cup	100	91.91	25	1.98	5.2	2.5	22	44	0.44	30	303	15
11136	Cauliflower, cooked, boiled, drained, wo/salt 1/2 cup (1" pieces)	62	57.66	14.26	1.14	2.55	1.67	9.92	19.84	0.2	9.3	88.04	5.58
11965	Cauliflower, green, raw 1 cup	64	57.47	19.84	1.89	3.9	2.05	21.12	39.68	0.47	14.72	192	12.8
11967	Cauliflower, green, cooked, no salt 1/5 head	90	80.52	28.8	2.74	5.65	2.97	28.8	51.3	0.65	20.7	250.2	17.1
11143	Celery, raw 1 cup, diced	120	113.57	19.2	0.9	4.38	2.04	48	30	0.48	104.4	344.4	13.2
11148	Chard, Swiss, cooked, boiled, drained, wo/salt 1 cup, chopped	175	162.14	35	3.29	7.25	3.68	101.5	57.75	3.96	313.25	960.75	150.5
11151	Chicory, witloof, raw 1/2 cup	45	42.53	7.65	0.41	1.8	1.4	8.55	11.7	0.11	0.9	94.95	4.5
11162	Collards, cooked, boiled, drained, wo/salt 1 cup, chopped	190	174.53	51.3	2.57	11.65	5.32	43.7	15.2	0.3	30.4	248.9	13.3
11168	Corn, sweet, yellow, cooked, boiled, drained, wo/salt 1 baby ear	8	5.57	8.64	0.27	2.01	0.22	0.16	8.24	0.05	1.36	19.92	2.56
11203	Cress, garden, raw 1 cup	50	44.7	16	1.3	2.75	0.55	40.5	38	0.65	7	303	19
11205	Cucumber, with peel, raw 1/2 cup slices	52	49.93	6.76	0.36	1.44	0.42	7.28	10.4	0.14	1.04	74.88	5.72
11210	Eggplant, cooked, boiled, drained, wo/salt 1 cup (1" cubes)	99	90.85	27.72	0.82	6.57	2.48	5.94	21.78	0.35	2.97	245.52	12.87
11213	Endive, raw 1/2 cup, chopped	25	23.45	4.25	0.31	0.84	0.78	13	7	0.21	5.5	78.5	3.75
11234	Kale, cooked, boiled, drained, wo/salt 1 cup, chopped	130	118.56	41.6	2.47	7.32	2.6	93.6	36.4	1.17	29.9	296.4	23.4
11242	Kohlrabi, cooked, boiled, drained, wo/salt 1 cup, sliced	165	149	47.85	2.97	11.04	1.82	41.25	74.25	0.66	34.65	561	31.35
11247	Leeks (bulb & lower leaf-portion), cooked, boiled, drained, wo/salt 1/4 cup chopped or diced	26	23.61	8.06	0.21	1.98	0.26	7.8	4.42	0.29	2.6	22.62	3.64

NDB #	Zinc	Copper	Vitamin A	Thiamin	Riboflavin	Niacin	Vitamin B6	Folate	Vitamin B12	Vitamin C	Fat	Fat: Saturated	Fat: Monounsaturated	Fat: Polyunsaturated	Cholesterol
	mg	mg	IU	mg	mg	mg	mg	mcg	mcg	mg	gm	gm	gm	gm	mg
11110	0.07	0.01	99	0.04	0.04	0.21	0.08	15	0	15.08	0.32	0.04	0.02	0.15	0
11112	0.15	0.07	28	0.04	0.02	0.21	0.15	14.49	0	39.9	0.18	0.02	0.01	0.09	0
11113	0.11	0.05	20.25	0.03	0.02	0.15	0.11	9.45	0	25.8	0.15	0.02	0.01	0.07	0
11115	0.33	0.08	1289.05	0.07	0.03	0.03	0.22	67.14	0	24.65	0.13	0.02	0.01	0.06	0
11117	0.29	0.03	4365.6	0.05	0.11	0.73	0.28	69.02	0	44.2	0.27	0.04	0.02	0.13	0
11124	0.22	0.05	30941.9	0.11	0.06	1.02	0.16	15.4	0	10.23	0.21	0.03	0.01	0.08	0
11960	0.02	0	197.2	0	0.01	0.09	0.01	3.3	0	0.84	0.05	0.01	0	0.03	0
11125	0.23	0.1	19152.12	0.03	0.04	0.39	0.19	10.84	0	1.79	0.14	0.03	0.01	0.07	0
11135	0.28	0.04	19	0.06	0.06	0.53	0.22	57	0	46.4	0.21	0.03	0.01	0.1	0
11136	0.11	0.02	10.54	0.03	0.03	0.25	0.11	27.28	0	27.47	0.28	0.04	0.02	0.13	0
11965	0.41	0.03	97.28	0.05	0.07	0.47	0.14	36.48	0	56.38	0.19	0.03	0.02	0.09	0
11967	0.57	0.04	126.9	0.06	0.09	0.61	0.19	36.9	0	65.34	0.28	0.04	0.03	0.12	0
11143	0.16	0.04	160.8	0.06	0.05	0.39	0.1	33.6	0	8.4	0.17	0.04	0.03	0.08	0
11148	0.58	0.29	5493.25	0.06	0.15	0.63	0.15	15.05	0	31.5	0.14	0.02	0.03	0.05	0
11151	0.07	0.02	13.05	0.03	0.01	0.07	0.02	16.65	0	1.26	0.05	0.01	0	0.02	0
11102	0.21	0.06	5181.3	0.04	0.1	0.55	0.1	11.4	0	22.99	0.36	0.05	0.03	0.17	0
11168	0.04	0	17.36	0.02	0.01	0.13	0	3.71	0	0.5	0.1	0.02	0.03	0.05	0
11203	0.12	0.09	4650	0.04	0.13	0.5	0.12	40.2	0	34.5	0.35	0.01	0.12	0.11	0
11205	0.1	0.02	111.8	0.01	0.01	0.11	0.02	6.76	0	2.76	0.07	0.02	0	0.03	0
11210	0.15	0.11	63.36	0.08	0.02	0.59	0.09	14.26	0	1.29	0.23	0.04	0.02	0.09	0
11213	0.2	0.02	512.5	0.02	0.02	0.1	0.01	35.5	0	1.63	0.05	0.01	0	0.02	0
11234	0.31	0.2	9620	0.07	0.09	0.65	0.18	17.29	0	53.3	0.52	0.07	0.04	0.25	0
11242	0.51	0.22	57.75	0.07	0.03	0.64	0.25	19.97	0	89.1	0.18	0.02	0.01	0.09	0
11247	0.02	0.02	11.96	0.01	0.01	0.05	0.03	6.32	0	1.09	0.05	0.01	0	0.03	0

NDB #	Description & Serving	Grams	Water	Calories	Protein	Carbohydrates	Fiber	Calcium	Phosphorus	Iron	Sodium	Potassium	Magnesium
		gm	gm	kcal	gm	gm	gm	mg	mg	mg	mg	mg	mg
11250	Lettuce, butterhead (incl Boston & bibb types), raw 1 cup, shredded or chopped	55	52.57	7.15	0.71	1.28	0.55	17.6	12.65	0.17	2.75	141.35	7.15
11251	Lettuce, cos or romaine, raw 1/2 cup shredded	28	26.57	4.48	0.45	0.66	0.48	10.08	12.6	0.31	2.24	81.2	1.68
11252	Lettuce, iceberg (incl crisphead types), raw 1 cup, shredded or chopped	55	52.74	6.6	0.56	1.15	0.77	10.45	11	0.28	4.95	86.9	4.95
11253	Lettuce, looseleaf, raw 1/2 cup shredded	28	26.32	5.04	0.36	0.98	0.53	19.04	7	0.39	2.52	73.92	3.08
11260	Mushrooms, raw 1 cup, whole	96	88.14	24	2.01	4.46	1.15	4.8	99.84	1.19	3.84	355.2	9.6
11950	Mushrooms, enoki, raw 1 large	5	4.47	1.7	0.12	0.35	0.13	0.05	5.65	0.04	0.15	19.05	0.8
11268	Mushrooms, shiitake, dried 1 mushroom	3.6	0.34	10.66	0.34	2.71	0.41	0.4	10.58	0.06	0.47	55.22	4.75
11269	Mushrooms, shiitake, cooked, wo/salt 1 cup (pieces)	145	121.05	79.75	2.26	20.71	3.05	4.35	42.05	0.64	5.8	169.65	20.3
11279	Okra, cooked, boiled, drained, wo/salt 8 pods (3" long)	85	76.42	27.2	1.59	6.13	2.13	53.55	47.6	0.38	4.25	273.7	48.45
11282	Onions, raw 1 cup, chopped	160	143.49	60.8	1.86	13.81	2.88	32	52.8	0.35	4.8	251.2	16
11283	Onions, cooked, boiled, drained, wo/salt 1 cup	210	184.51	92.4	2.86	21.32	2.94	46.2	73.5	0.5	6.3	348.6	23.1
11291	Onions, spring (incl tops & bulb), raw 1 tablespoon, chopped	6	5.39	1.92	0.11	0.44	0.16	4.32	2.22	0.09	0.96	16.56	1.2
11297	Parsley, raw 1 cup	60	52.63	21.6	1.78	3.8	1.98	82.8	34.8	3.72	33.6	332.4	30
11299	Parsnips, cooked, boiled, drained, wo/salt 1/2 cup slices	78	60.62	63.18	1.03	15.23	3.12	28.86	53.82	0.45	7.8	286.26	22.62
11305	Peas, green, cooked, boiled, drained, wo/salt 1 cup	160	124.59	134.4	8.58	25.02	8.8	43.2	187.2	2.46	4.8	433.6	62.4
11333	Peppers, sweet, green, raw 1 cup, chopped	149	137.36	40.23	1.33	9.58	2.68	13.41	28.31	0.69	2.98	263.73	14.9
11951	Peppers, sweet, yellow, raw 10 strips	52	47.85	14.04	0.52	3.29	0.47	5.72	12.48	0.24	1.04	110.24	6.24
11363	Potatoes, baked, flesh, wo/salt 1 potato (2-1/3" x 4-3/4")	156	117.66	145.08	3.06	33.63	2.34	7.8	78	0.55	7.8	609.96	39
11364	Potatoes, baked, skin, wo/salt 1 potato skin	58	27.44	114.84	2.49	26.72	4.58	19.72	58.58	4.08	12.18	332.34	24.94
11365	Potatoes, boiled, cooked in skin, flesh, wo/salt 1 potato (2-1/2" dia, sphere)	136	104.69	118.32	2.54	27.38	2.45	6.8	59.84	0.42	5.44	515.44	29.92
11423	Pumpkin, cooked, boiled, drained, wo/salt 1 cup, mashed	245	229.54	49	1.76	11.98	2.7	36.75	73.5	1.4	2.45	563.5	22.05
11952	Radicchio, raw 1 cup, shredded	40	37.26	9.2	0.57	1.79	0.36	7.6	16	0.23	8.8	120.8	5.2
11429	Radishes, raw 1 cup, slices	116	110.01	19.72	0.7	4.16	1.86	24.36	20.88	0.34	27.84	269.12	10.44
11436	Rutabagas, cooked, boiled, drained, wo/salt 1 cup, mashed	240	213.31	93.6	3.1	20.98	4.32	115.2	134.4	1.27	48	782.4	55.2

NDB #	Zinc	Copper	Vitamin A	Thiamin	Riboflavin	Niacin	Vitamin B6	Folate	Vitamin B12	Vitamin C	Fat	Fat. Saturated	Fat. Monounsaturated	Fat. Polyunsaturated	Cholesterol
	mg	mg	IU	mg	mg	mg	mg	mcg	mcg	mg	gm	gm	gm	gm	mg
11250	0.09	0.01	533.5	0.03	0.03	0.17	0.03	40.32	0	4.4	0.12	0.02	0	0.06	0
11251	0.07	0.01	728	0.03	0.03	0.14	0.01	38	0	6.72	0.06	0.01	0	0.03	0
11252	0.12	0.02	181.5	0.03	0.02	0.1	0.02	30.8	0	2.15	0.1	0.01	0	0.06	0
11253	0.08	0.01	532	0.01	0.02	0.11	0.02	13.94	0	5.04	0.08	0.01	0	0.04	0
11260	0.7	0.47	0	0.1	0.43	3.95	0.09	20.26	0	3.36	0.4	0.05	0.01	0.16	0
11950	0.03	0	0.35	0	0.01	0.18	0	1.5	0	0.6	0.02	0	0	0.01	0
11268	0.28	0.19	0	0.01	0.05	0.51	0.03	5.88	0	0.13	0.04	0.01	0.01	0.01	0
11269	1.93	1.3	0	0.05	0.25	2.18	0.23	30.31	0	0.44	0.32	0.08	0.1	0.04	0
11279	0.47	0.07	488.75	0.11	0.05	0.74	0.16	38.85	0	13.86	0.14	0.04	0.02	0.04	0
11282	0.3	0.1	0	0.07	0.03	0.24	0.19	30.4	0	10.24	0.26	0.04	0.04	0.1	0
11283	0.44	0.14	0	0.09	0.05	0.35	0.27	31.5	0	10.92	0.4	0.07	0.06	0.15	0
11291	0.02	0	23.1	0	0	0.03	0	3.84	0	1.13	0.01	0	0	0	0
11297	0.64	0.09	3120	0.05	0.06	0.79	0.05	91.2	0	79.8	0.47	0.08	0.18	0.07	0
11299	0.2	0.11	0	0.06	0.04	0.56	0.07	45.4	0	10.14	0.23	0.04	0.09	0.04	0
11305	1.9	0.28	955.2	0.41	0.24	3.23	0.35	101.28	0	22.72	0.35	0.06	0.03	0.16	0
11333	0.18	0.1	941.68	0.1	0.04	0.76	0.37	32.78	0	133.06	0.28	0.04	0.02	0.15	0
11951	0.09	0.06	123.76	0.01	0.01	0.46	0.09	13.52	0	95.42	0.11	0	0	0	0
11363	0.45	0.34	0	0.16	0.03	2.18	0.47	14.2	0	19.97	0.16	0.04	0	0.07	0
11364	0.28	0.47	0	0.07	0.06	1.78	0.36	12.53	0	7.83	0.06	0.02	0	0.02	0
11365	0.41	0.26	0	0.14	0.03	1.96	0.41	13.6	0	17.68	0.14	0.04	0	0.06	0
11423	0.56	0.22	2650.9	0.08	0.19	1.01	0.11	20.83	0	11.52	0.17	0.09	0.02	0.01	0
11952	0.25	0.14	10.8	0.01	0.01	0.1	0.02	24	0	3.2	0.1	0.02	0	0.04	0
11429	0.35	0.05	9.28	0.01	0.05	0.35	0.08	31.32	0	26.45	0.63	0.03	0.02	0.05	0
11436	0.84	0.1	1346.4	0.2	0.1	1.72	0.24	36	0	45.12	0.53	0.07	0.06	0.23	0

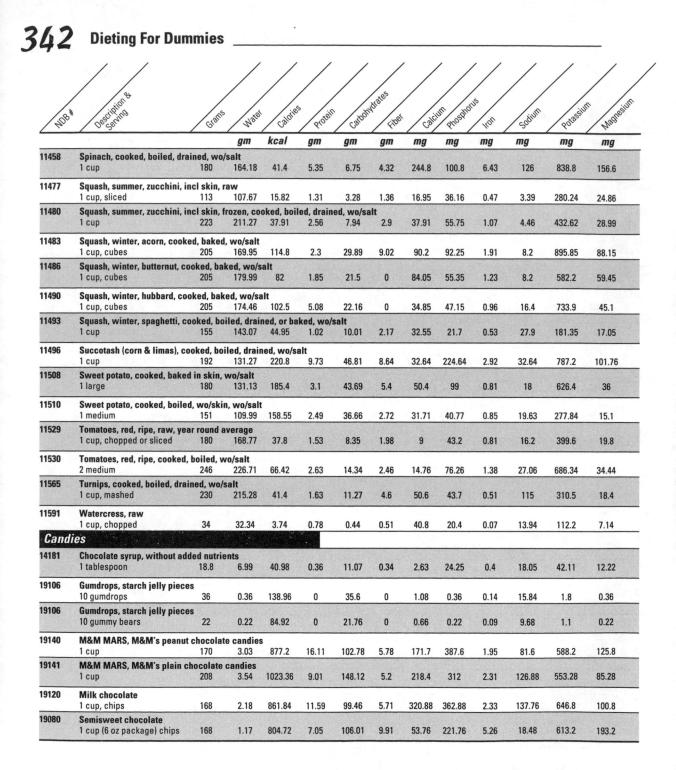

NDB #	Description & Serving	Grams	Water	Calories	Protein	Carbohydrates	Fiber	Calcium	Phosphorus	Iron	Sodium	Potassium	Magnesium
			gm	kcal	gm	gm	gm	mg	mg	mg	mg	mg	mg
11458	Spinach, cooked, boiled, drained, wo/salt 1 cup	180	164.18	41.4	5.35	6.75	4.32	244.8	100.8	6.43	126	838.8	156.6
11477	Squash, summer, zucchini, incl skin, raw 1 cup, sliced	113	107.67	15.82	1.31	3.28	1.36	16.95	36.16	0.47	3.39	280.24	24.86
11480	Squash, summer, zucchini, incl skin, frozen, cooked, boiled, drained, wo/salt 1 cup	223	211.27	37.91	2.56	7.94	2.9	37.91	55.75	1.07	4.46	432.62	28.99
11483	Squash, winter, acorn, cooked, baked, wo/salt 1 cup, cubes	205	169.95	114.8	2.3	29.89	9.02	90.2	92.25	1.91	8.2	895.85	88.15
11486	Squash, winter, butternut, cooked, baked, wo/salt 1 cup, cubes	205	179.99	82	1.85	21.5	0	84.05	55.35	1.23	8.2	582.2	59.45
11490	Squash, winter, hubbard, cooked, baked, wo/salt 1 cup, cubes	205	174.46	102.5	5.08	22.16	0	34.85	47.15	0.96	16.4	733.9	45.1
11493	Squash, winter, spaghetti, cooked, boiled, drained, or baked, wo/salt 1 cup	155	143.07	44.95	1.02	10.01	2.17	32.55	21.7	0.53	27.9	181.35	17.05
11496	Succotash (corn & limas), cooked, boiled, drained, wo/salt 1 cup	192	131.27	220.8	9.73	46.81	8.64	32.64	224.64	2.92	32.64	787.2	101.76
11508	Sweet potato, cooked, baked in skin, wo/salt 1 large	180	131.13	185.4	3.1	43.69	5.4	50.4	99	0.81	18	626.4	36
11510	Sweet potato, cooked, boiled, wo/skin, wo/salt 1 medium	151	109.99	158.55	2.49	36.66	2.72	31.71	40.77	0.85	19.63	277.84	15.1
11529	Tomatoes, red, ripe, raw, year round average 1 cup, chopped or sliced	180	168.77	37.8	1.53	8.35	1.98	9	43.2	0.81	16.2	399.6	19.8
11530	Tomatoes, red, ripe, cooked, boiled, wo/salt 2 medium	246	226.71	66.42	2.63	14.34	2.46	14.76	76.26	1.38	27.06	686.34	34.44
11565	Turnips, cooked, boiled, drained, wo/salt 1 cup, mashed	230	215.28	41.4	1.63	11.27	4.6	50.6	43.7	0.51	115	310.5	18.4
11591	Watercress, raw 1 cup, chopped	34	32.34	3.74	0.78	0.44	0.51	40.8	20.4	0.07	13.94	112.2	7.14
Candies													
14181	Chocolate syrup, without added nutrients 1 tablespoon	18.8	6.99	40.98	0.36	11.07	0.34	2.63	24.25	0.4	18.05	42.11	12.22
19106	Gumdrops, starch jelly pieces 10 gumdrops	36	0.36	138.96	0	35.6	0	1.08	0.36	0.14	15.84	1.8	0.36
19106	Gumdrops, starch jelly pieces 10 gummy bears	22	0.22	84.92	0	21.76	0	0.66	0.22	0.09	9.68	1.1	0.22
19140	M&M MARS, M&M's peanut chocolate candies 1 cup	170	3.03	877.2	16.11	102.78	5.78	171.7	387.6	1.95	81.6	588.2	125.8
19141	M&M MARS, M&M's plain chocolate candies 1 cup	208	3.54	1023.36	9.01	148.12	5.2	218.4	312	2.31	126.88	553.28	85.28
19120	Milk chocolate 1 cup, chips	168	2.18	861.84	11.59	99.46	5.71	320.88	362.88	2.33	137.76	646.8	100.8
19080	Semisweet chocolate 1 cup (6 oz package) chips	168	1.17	804.72	7.05	106.01	9.91	53.76	221.76	5.26	18.48	613.2	193.2

NDB #	Zinc	Copper	Vitamin A	Thiamin	Riboflavin	Niacin	Vitamin B6	Folate	Vitamin B12	Vitamin C	Fat	Fat: Saturated	Fat: Monounsaturated	Fat: Polyunsaturated	Cholesterol
	mg	mg	IU	mg	mg	mg	mg	mcg	mcg	mg	gm	gm	gm	gm	mg
11458	1.37	0.31	14742	0.17	0.42	0.88	0.44	262.44	0	17.64	0.47	0.08	0.01	0.19	0
11477	0.23	0.06	384.2	0.08	0.03	0.45	0.1	24.97	0	10.17	0.16	0.03	0.01	0.07	0
11480	0.45	0.1	963.36	0.09	0.09	0.86	0.1	17.39	0	8.25	0.29	0.06	0.02	0.12	0
11483	0.35	0.18	877.4	0.34	0.03	1.81	0.4	38.34	0	22.14	0.29	0.06	0.02	0.12	0
11486	0.27	0.13	14352.05	0.15	0.03	1.99	0.25	39.36	0	30.96	0.18	0.04	0.01	0.08	0
11490	0.31	0.09	12371.75	0.15	0.1	1.14	0.35	33.21	0	19.48	1.27	0.26	0.09	0.53	0
11493	0.31	0.05	170.5	0.06	0.03	1.26	0.15	12.4	0	5.43	0.4	0.1	0.03	0.2	0
11496	1.21	0.34	564.48	0.32	0.18	2.55	0.22	62.98	0	15.74	1.54	0.28	0.3	0.73	0
11508	0.52	0.37	39279.6	0.13	0.23	1.09	0.43	40.68	0	44.28	0.2	0.04	0.01	0.09	0
11510	0.41	0.24	25751.54	0.08	0.21	0.97	0.37	16.76	0	25.82	0.45	0.1	0.02	0.2	0
11529	0.16	0.13	1121.4	0.11	0.09	1.13	0.14	27	0	34.38	0.59	0.08	0.09	0.24	0
11530	0.27	0.23	1827.78	0.17	0.14	1.84	0.23	31.98	0	56.09	1.01	0.14	0.15	0.42	0
11565	0.46	0.15	0	0.06	0.05	0.69	0.15	21.16	0	26.68	0.18	0.02	0.01	0.1	0
11591	0.04	0.03	1598	0.03	0.04	0.07	0.04	3.13	0	14.62	0.03	0.01	0	0.01	0
Candies															
14181	0.14	0.1	5.64	0	0	0.06	0	0.75	0	0.04	0.17	0.1	0.05	0	0
19106	0	0	0	0	0	0	0	0	0	0	0	0	0	0	0
19106	0	0	0	0	0	0	0	0	0	0	0	0	0	0	0
19140	3.91	0.87	158.1	0.17	0.28	6.37	0.14	59.5	0.31	0.85	44.61	17.56	18.7	7.14	15.3
19141	1.99	0.58	422.24	0.11	0.44	0.46	0.06	12.48	0.56	1.04	43.95	27.21	14.32	1.31	29.12
19120	2.32	0.65	310.8	0.13	0.51	0.54	0.07	13.44	0.65	0.67	51.57	31.05	16.75	1.78	36.96
19080	2.72	1.18	35.28	0.09	0.15	0.72	0.06	5.04	0	0	50.4	29.82	16.75	1.63	0

Index

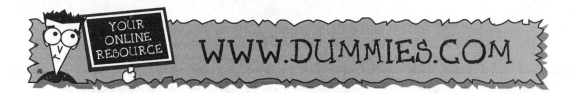

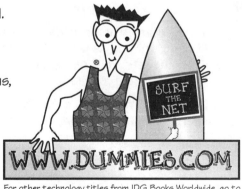

IDG BOOKS WORLDWIDE
BOOK REGISTRATION

We want to hear from you!

Register This Book and Win!

Visit **http://my2cents.dummies.com** to register this book and tell us how you liked it!

✔ Get entered in our monthly prize giveaway.

✔ Give us feedback about this book — tell us what you like best, what you like least, or maybe what you'd like to ask the author and us to change!

✔ Let us know any other *...For Dummies*® topics that interest you.

Your feedback helps us determine what books to publish, tells us what coverage to add as we revise our books, and lets us know whether we're meeting your needs as a *...For Dummies* reader. You're our most valuable resource, and what you have to say is important to us!

Not on the Web yet? It's easy to get started with *Dummies 101*®*: The Internet For Windows*® *98* or *The Internet For Dummies*,® 5th Edition, at local retailers everywhere.

Or let us know what you think by sending us a letter at the following address:

...For Dummies Book Registration
Dummies Press
7260 Shadeland Station, Suite 100
Indianapolis, IN 46256-3945
Fax 317-596-5498

BESTSELLING BOOK SERIES FROM IDG